D0204032

THE Cancer-Fighting Kitchen

Nourishing, Big-Flavor Recipes for Cancer Treatment and Recovery

Rebecca Katz *with* Mat Edelson

Celestial Arts
Berkeley

For Waz Thomas, who showed me the way

The information in this book is based on the experience and research of the authors. It is not intended as a substitute for consulting with your physician or other health-care provider. Any attempt to diagnose and treat an illness should be done under the direction of a health-care professional. The publisher and authors are not responsible for any adverse effects or consequences resulting from the use of any of the suggestions, preparations, or procedures discussed in this book.

Copyright © 2009 by Rebecca Katz
Foreword copyright © 2009 by Keith I. Block, MD
Photographs copyright © 2009 by Leo Gong

All rights reserved.
Published in the United States by Ten Speed Press, an imprint of the Crown Publishing Group, a division of Random House, Inc., New York.
www.crownpublishing.com
www.tenspeed.com

Ten Speed Press and the Ten Speed Press colophon are registered trademarks of Random House, Inc.

Library of Congress Cataloging-in-Publication Data is on file with the publisher

ISBN 978-1-58761-344-9

Printed in China

Cover and text design by Chloe Rawlins
Food styling by Jen Strauss
Prop styling by Harumi Shimizu

10 9 8 7 6 5 4 3 2

First Edition

Contents

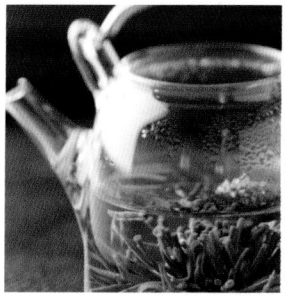

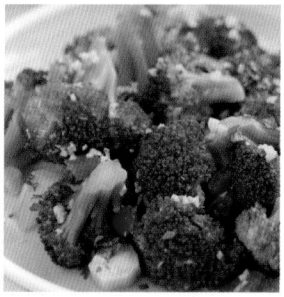

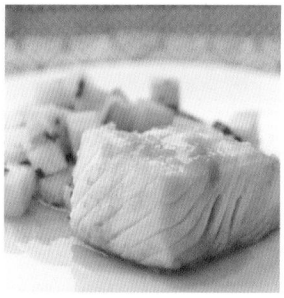

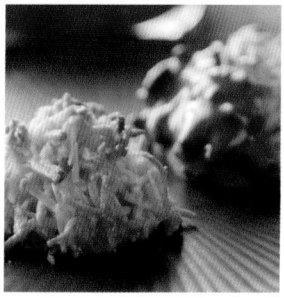

Foreword · vii

Acknowledgments · ix

Introduction · 1

Chapter 1: Cancer-Fighting Tool Kit · 8

Chapter 2: Strategies for Thriving during Treatment · 42

Chapter 3: Nourishing Soups and Broths · 52

Chapter 4: Vital Vegetables · 76

Chapter 5: Protein-Building Foods · 100

Chapter 6: Anytime Foods · 124

Chapter 7: Tonics and Elixirs · 154

Chapter 8: Dollops of Yum! · 172

Chapter 9: Sweet Bites · 190

Resources · 208

Bibliography · 213

Index · 217

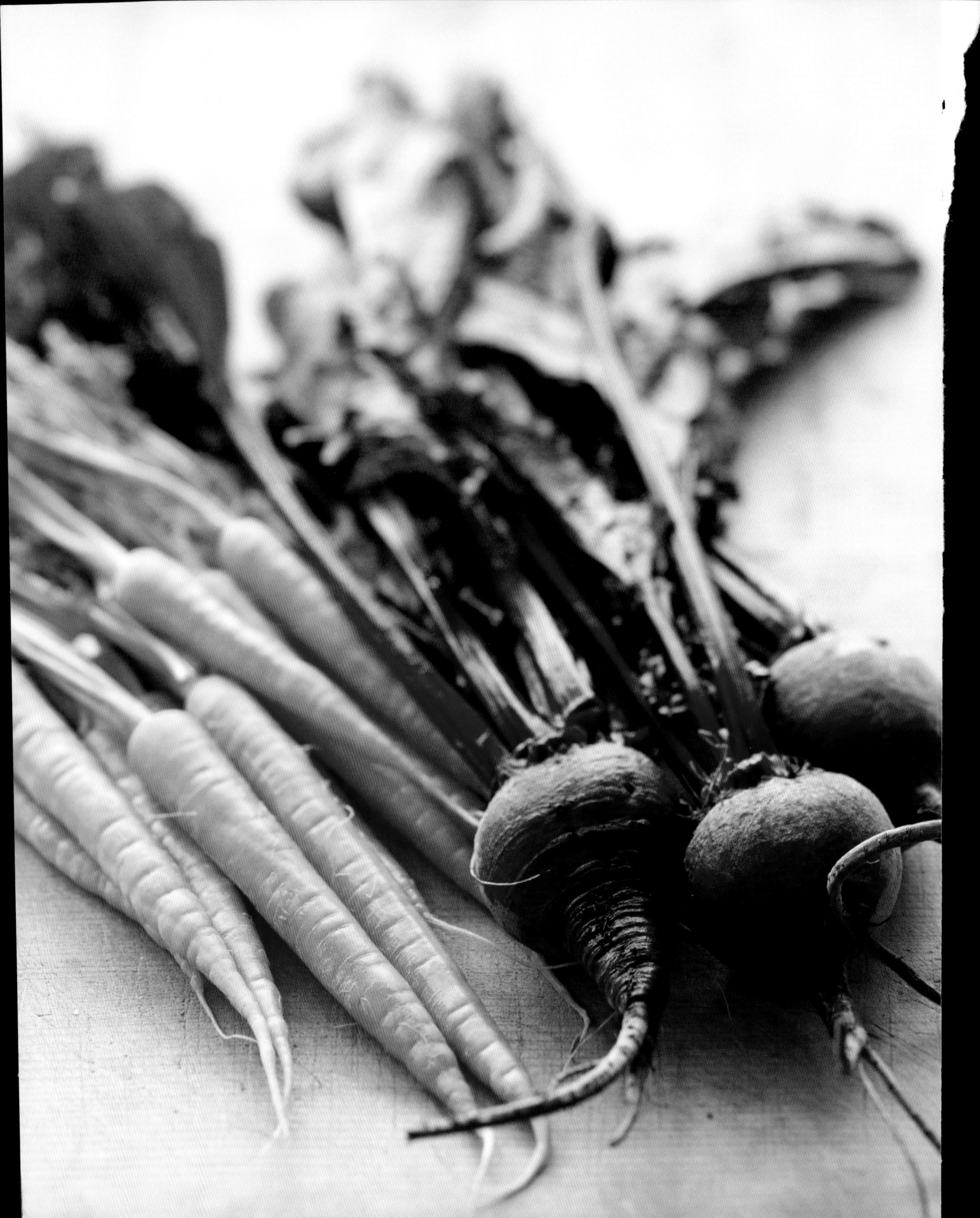

Jeremy Geffen, MD; Teressa Koetters, RN, MS; Annemarie Colbin, PhD; and Nancy Novack, PhD for their time and expertise. To my colleagues at Commonweal's Cancer Help Program, I am so honored to have been witness to your collective wisdom and incredible program participants. To Michael Lerner for his continued guidance and support; Lenore Lefer, MS, MFCC, MFT, whose sagacity and compassion helps so many people find meaning in their lives during fragile times; Waz Thomas for making the phone call that changed my life; Claire Heart for being a wonderful cook and culinary alchemist; Ethan Funk for being the quickest prep cook in the west; and Rachael Remens, MD, Kate Holcombe, Stuart Horance, Susan Braun, Jhani Chapman, Irene Gallway, Sabriga Turgon, Elizabeth Evans, Jenepher Stowell, and Mimi Mindel for making Commonweal such a special and magical place for people to find healing. Thanks to the folks at Smith Farm Center for Healing and the Arts, especially Shanti Norris, co-founder and executive director, and Laura Pole, RN, MSN, for keeping me in the know.

A special thanks to Jim Gordon, MD, founder and director of the Center for Mind Body Medicine, for his vision to improve the quality of health care, and his insights found within the pages of this book; Kathie Swift, MS, RD, LDN, co–course director of the Food As Medicine nutritional training program; the staff and faculty of Food as Medicine and Cancer Guides; and Jo Cooper, dear friend and colleague, for your passion for food and your big heart. A hug to my friends at the Pine Street Clinic, Michael Broffman, the ever supportive Louise, Jane, Johanna, and Michael McCulloh, PhD; to Phyllis Cox, Elizabeth Blickman, Rebecca Farrell, Tanya Coller, Chris Hall, and all the talented people I work with at Berkeley Heart Labs; and to my editors Celeste McCauley and Anne Simpkinson at *Guideposts*. Many bows to Paula Bartholomy, MS, co-founder of Hawthorn University and Liz Lipski PhD, who supported this project in its embryonic stages; Sarah Bearden, MS, for helping me on my nutritional journey; Montse Vallory, Ruth Fehr, and Cathryn Couch for teaching others how to cook for people with cancer; and the gracious Caroline Nation, founder of My Food My Health.

A shout-out to Gina Gallo, Gia Passalaqua, Patricia Lewis, and the charming Jean Charles Boisset. A salute to the following friends and cheerleaders: Victor Marchese for his love of the farmer's market; the gang on Rustic Way; Jennifer Omholt for always telling it like it is with a extra dash of humor; Jill Leiner for her courage and lifelong friendship; Jodie Chase for her PR savvy; Karen Omholt for her strategic marketing expertise; Paul and Vicki Remer and John, Henry, and William Silva for being willing to taste many of the recipes in this book during various stages of development; and Judy Witts Francini, Italian life coach and amazing cook who, many years ago, steered me towards the kitchen where I belonged.

My gratitude to my parents, Barbara and Jay Katz, for their love and support throughout my journey, along with their wonderful community of friends; my brother Jeff for his advise and counsel; my talented nephew and niece Harry and Amelia; Bella, my muse and kitchen dog; and my husband Gregg Kellogg, for his belief in my work, unwavering support, and patience. And, finally, thank you to all my clients and students for all you have taught me along the way.

Acknowledgments

This book would never have come to pass without the following people. I'm awed by their generosity of spirit and time, as well as their heartfelt desire to make this book all that it could be.

My heartfelt thanks to Keith I. Block, MD, and Penny B. Block, PhD, of the Block Center for Integrative Cancer Treatment, for their commitment to state-of-the-art integrative cancer care and their understanding of the critical role nutrition and nourishment play in healing; and thanks to Leni Kass for facilitating communications with professionalism and grace.

I bow to the master, Jeremy Katz, my agent and friend, for sitting me down and, in no uncertain terms, saying that *this* was the book I needed to write. A heaping amount of praise and thanks to Mat Edelson, a brilliant and gifted writer, for transforming copious amounts of dense information into easy digestible and delectable words. Thanks to Wendy Remer, dear friend and baker supreme; Christine Kaddaras, my assistant, whose hard work, good cheer, and positive attitude are essential ingredients in this book; Catherine McConkie, amazing person and recipe tester along with her intern, Drake Cameron. Katherine Wilson for her love of the Vita Mix; Emily Marciniak for her organizational charts; and Wendy Hess, for her expert nutritional analysis that accompanies each recipe. A big 16-quart hug to Julie Burford, my soup sister, and a special kiss on the head to both her husband, Stan, and Josie, pooch supreme, for their moral support.

Humble appreciation to Phil Wood, Lorena Jones, and Jo Ann Deck, who saw the possibilities for my first book, *One Bite at a Time: Nourishing Recipes for Cancer Survivors and Their Friends*. Kudos to the amazing talented team at Ten Speed Press under the leadership of Aaron Wehner for their steadfast belief in this project: my awesome editor and master juggler, Melissa Moore, for her deft skills in shaping this manuscript and her keen editorial eye; Chloe Rawlins for the absolutely beautiful design; Nancy Austin for her sensitive art direction; Jasmine Star for her excellent copyediting; proofreader Linda Bouchard; Veronica and Victoria Randall for their inspirational stories; and Patricia Kelly, Michele Crim, Debra Matsumoto, and Kara Van De Water for their sales, marketing, and publicity expertise. Blessings to photographer Leo Gong and his wife and studio manager, Harumi Shimizu, and stylists Jen Straus and Alexa Hyman for the beautiful images.

A huge debt of thanks to Donald Abrams, MD; Debu Tripathy, MD; Gerry Mullin, MD; Joel Evans, MD; Linda Bartoshuk, PhD; Jeanne Wallace, PhD; Suzanne Dixon, MPH, MS, RD;

Eating a plant-based diet is fundamental to a successful fight. The conundrum is that no one likes to feel like they're going on a *diet*, especially when they're ill. As you read this, you might be thinking, "Am I going to have to live on food resembling a pot of brown, cardboard-textured hippie chow in order to prevent or help treat cancer?"

The answer is a resounding "no, absolutely not!" And here lies the value of *The Cancer-Fighting Kitchen*. Patients need a variety of colorful, delicious, savory dishes that satisfy their palates while helping set the stage to more effectively battle cancer—and to inspire living, as well. Rebecca Katz's book does just this in a way that takes the negativity and fear out of changing one's food choices. I can attest to the pleasure of eating her nutrient-rich meals, having enjoyed her cooking many times over the years.

When it comes to chefs with the unique skill set and creative talent for preparing health-promoting foods that taste more like an indulgence then the healing therapy they are, Rebecca is a true culinary artist.

—Keith I. Block, MD, author of *Life Over Cancer*, medical director of the Block Center for Integrative Cancer Treatment, and director of integrative medical education at University of Illinois College of Medicine

Foreword

Every day in my practice, I'm asked if food can really make a difference in the fight against cancer. The quick answer is yes, but, since you've picked up Rebecca's Katz's latest book, *The Cancer-Fighting Kitchen*, I think you deserve a little more than a simple affirmative. So, here's the backstory: Until very recently, most cancer research has focused on cancer cells, rather than the environment in the human body in which these cells function and sometimes flourish. The impact of this research omission has played a significant role in our often failing efforts to beat cancer.

For nearly three decades at the Block Center for Integrative Cancer Treatment, my research staff and I have studied the biological environment these cells reside in. This "soup" is a biochemical milieu that, when optimized through things patients can do for themselves—such as diet and lifestyle changes—can help inhibit malignant growth, mitigate treatment toxicity, improve quality of life, and provide a survivor's edge.

For example, breast cancer patients who keep their insulin levels under control—a factor most often associated with diet and lifestyle—*cut* their risk of cancer recurrence in half and decrease cancer mortality by two-thirds. It's also well known that decreasing inflammation can help reduce cancer growth, boost treatment efficacy, and diminish side effects. We know that refined flours and sugars, most fast food and soda pop, increase the enzymes that promote inflammatory cascades. This is why I encourage patients to avoid these pro-inflammatory foods and increase ingredients that have anti-inflammatory properties. Rebecca understands this and her book includes countless spices, herbs, and foods that can optimize the environment necessary for battling cancer and reducing treatment toxicity. But, importantly, Rebecca presents delicious, enticing recipes that will keep you coming back for more. This is vital, as patients who are well-fed during treatment enhance their quality of life, and improve their chances for recovery.

The fact is, everything you eat and drink changes the chemistry of your blood. Our cell membranes are lined with fats that are comprised primarily of those we've eaten in the last 90 days. If you've been making unhealthy choices, which include the "typical" American diet, there's a price to pay.

Introduction

If you've picked up this book, it's probably because you or someone very close to you is going through a difficult time. A cancer diagnosis and the prospect of cancer treatment is scary, even for the most upbeat soul. There are probably a million questions and thoughts running around your head, and while I can't address them all, I can speak to one: Am I going to enjoy eating during treatment? Heck, am I going to be able to eat at all?

This book is all about enhancing your appetite during treatment, and much more. For me, the key concept is something I think of as "the power of yum," a phrase I've used throughout my career as a "culinary translator," if you will. I work with oncologists, nutritionists, and cancer wellness professionals to help their patients stay well fed during treatment by translating nutritional recommendations into delicious, nourishing meals. To me, this was always the power of yum in action: showing people that great nutrition and great taste could join together joyously on the same plate. Working with cancer patients for the past decade, I've seen heartening results. People who had truly disconnected from food could be brought back to the table and nourished, so long as the food was appealing to all the senses; was presented in a manner that fit their often shifting tastes and appetite (think small, nutrient-dense portions that are easily stored and reheated); and could easily be shopped for, prepped, and cooked by either the patient or their caregivers.

> The power of yum in action is showing people that good nutrition and great taste can join together joyously on the same plate.

If that was all there was to the power of yum, I'd be eternally grateful. It turns out that this is only half of the story. Over the past five years, the study of nutrition has expanded, exploded really, especially when it comes to understanding the many incredible properties foods have to fight cancer and limit the side effects of treatment. This isn't fly-by-night science either; it's the result of thousands of credible studies done by the country's finest academic research institutes and presented in first-rate peer-reviewed scientific journals such the *New England Journal of Medicine* and the *Journal of the American Medical Association*.

As a chef, I've been awed by this data and, truth be told, a little intimidated. I intuitively and experientially understood how taste and flavor could positively affect the people I worked with. It had long been known that as many as 80 percent of cancer patients were malnourished, in some cases leaving them too weakened to withstand ongoing treatment. By keeping them nourished with healthy foods, both the patients and I knew they stood a better chance of making the transition from patient to survivor.

Still, it seemed like a new study was coming out every week on this food or that, and all of this nutritional data was a bit confusing to me. And from the conversations I had with clients, I knew it was confounding to them at times. Yet this information held such promise that I decided I'd better learn to talk the talk. I was excited at the prospect of being able to make dishes that not only tasted great, but could make someone with a specific side effect feel better.

So I went and got a masters in nutrition, not to impress my clients, but to be able to converse with those doctors and scientists working in the trenches with these foods to get a feel for where the research and the cancer-food connection was strong and where it wasn't, and so I could translate all that information into more outrageously scrumptious dishes to lure people in treatment back to the table.

The result of this melding of science and taste is the cookbook and resource you hold in your hands. It's the culmination of conversations with what I think of as my counsel of experts: more than a dozen of the best minds in medical and cancer wellness in the country. Each of these individuals sees nutrition and food as a vital, complementary part of their healing arsenal, a tool that patients themselves can use to keep their bodies and minds in optimal shape while enduring treatment.

That last point is so crucial. A cancer diagnosis is shocking, disorienting, and capable of scrambling anybody's mental GPS. To find a stabilizing force, a grounding activity such as cooking and eating well can provide more than nourishment; it can offer a huge psychological boost.

Jeanne Wallace, PhD, a researcher and expert in cancer nutrition, articulates this idea of sustenance beautifully. Jeanne's voluminous, meticulously researched, personalized action plans for her clients in treatment include numerous food recommendations to combat their cancer. She says, "When you get a cancer diagnosis, suddenly you become a very powerless person. You're traipsing through the hospital as a name and number, people do all kinds of procedures to you, and you have a life-threatening condition, which many doctors maintain you have no control over. So when I'm handing someone their plan, saying, 'You could make some changes with your diet and it would give you some sense of empowerment,' many of my clients are so willing to do that. They embrace the sense of not being powerless, that even though they might not have total control over the cancer, they do have some influence."

A grounding activity such as cooking and eating well can provide more than nourishment; it can offer a huge psychological boost.

Defining that potential influence is fascinating. Can what you eat really affect cancer? Professor Jim Gordon, MD, founder and director of the Center for Mind-Body Medicine in Washington, DC, sponsors several annual symposia that address the issue. His Cancer Guides training and Food as Medicine programs attract hundreds of doctors from across the country, including top integrative oncologists, internists, and other cancer wellness professionals. Gordon, a pioneer in the use of nutrition to impact cancer, uses a bit of scientifically informed common sense when asked if what he teaches makes a difference. "People with cancer are told by their oncologists, 'This is the treatment: surgery, chemotherapy, radiation, maybe even immune therapy. Everything else is regarded as, at worst, unnecessary, peripheral, or, at best, complementary. . . .' I think that's a major misconception. The data in standard textbooks on nutrition and cancer is that cancer is related in some way to nutrition. It stands to reason that if nutrition is a significant factor in the development of cancer, you would want there to be to a focus on nutrition as part of the treatment and the prevention of recurrence in cancer." Gerry Mullin, MD, a contributing editor to *Nutrition in Clinical Practice*, agrees: "Cancer is a consequence of the complex interplay of genes and environment on the immune system, and diet, as part of the environment, plays a role that can influence cancer's development and treatment."

A key area of nutritional research is looking at the environment in which tumors function within the body. Part of what makes cancer such a difficult foe is its ability to send out signals that divert vital resources, such as blood and energy, for its own nefarious purposes. Researchers are now looking at how various nutrients in food—especially plant-based foods, spices, and herbs, with their abundant phytochemicals—can block cancer's communication. If we can cut off this internal dialogue, tumors may become much more vulnerable to treatment.

Integrative oncologist Donald Abrams, director of clinical programs for the Osher Center for Integrative Medicine at the University of California, San Francisco (UCSF), tells his patients by way of analogy that when it comes to cancer, it's perfectly acceptable to be a bad host. In fact, it's encouraged. "I tell them that cancer is a weed, you're the garden, and our job is take make your soil as inhospitable as possible to further growth and spread of the weed. The first approach I take is through diet and nutrition."

The wonderful aspect of this work is that so many common foods—everything from broccoli to blueberries—have multiple cancer-fighting properties, including controlling blood sugar so you avoid insulin issues and obesity, which are major secondary risk factors for cancer. Similarly, everyday herbs and spices ranging from ginger to cinnamon to turmeric can help quell side effects ranging from nausea to fatigue. If you'd like to learn more about these properties, see the Culinary Pharmacy, page 28, where we've detailed the beneficial properties of most of the foods used in the recipes in this book. We've included the science because many of my clients get interested in the particulars once they realize how much better they often feel as they become well nourished. Still, others couldn't care less about the science; they just want to be able to eat something, *anything*, because during treatment, their appetite has left the building.

First and foremost, I'm a chef and a teacher who believes everyone has the ability to nourish themselves, even in the most dire of circumstances. This book was designed to meet you wherever you are in your treatment journey. If you just want to eat without giving a second thought to nutrition, worry not; every recipe in this book was created to be a nutrient-dense, delicious powerhouse, full of what your body needs to support your immune system, which is called upon to do yeoman's work during treatment.

I believe everyone has the ability to nourish themselves, even in the most dire of circumstances. This book was designed to meet you wherever you are in your treatment journey.

The Cancer-Fighting Kitchen emphasizes what's known as a whole foods approach. As the name suggests, whole foods come straight from the farm to the table with their nutrients intact, unlike refined and processed foods, such as white flour and sugar, which are stripped of so much of their nutritional value. (I call them empty calories).

In addition to offering the broadest range of nutrients, the whole foods approach serves another purpose. People often ask me, "If science knows specific foods that fight cancer, why don't I just eat those?" Ah, if only a single food had such abilities. But that's not the way it works . . . at least not yet. Eating a wide variety of foods allows you to hedge your bets, as each of us absorbs nutrients differently. Since we haven't gotten to the point yet where we can identify which specific foods work best for each individual, a wide-ranging diet is the only way to guarantee you'll get the nourishment you need.

I realize I've just put a lot on your plate. Now let me put your mind at ease. I understand that stepping into the kitchen to cook for someone with cancer (whether that's you or someone else) takes a lot of courage. You so want them to like the food so they'll eat. I'm here to let you know I'll be holding your hand all the way. Life is serious enough for you and your loved ones right now. Although this book deals with a difficult topic, it comes at eating from a stance of joy and fun. Believe me, when you see the results—and the healing effect they have on all who partake—your motivation to get into the kitchen will take a quantum leap.

When people ask me what I enjoy most about my work, I tell them I love being what I call a culinary translator. To me, that means really listening to my clients' hopes and dreams for eating well, and then, using my culinary experience and education, helping them to develop the practical kitchen skills, nourishing recipes, and support systems (like learning how to shop a farmers' market without fear) that make their desires a reality. It's a role I relish and that I've brought to the fore in this book. Similarly, my coauthor, Mat Edelson, is a whiz at taking complex medical topics and explaining them in language that's informative, entertaining, and easy to understand.

It's not only our voices you'll hear in this book, but that of experts who have dedicated their careers to helping patients to live and eat well during treatment. You'll also see tips from the real voices of experience, those who have personally dealt with cancer and want to share what they've learned about eating and other ways to stay well during treatment. Like me, they all believe in the power of yum. I'm hoping that as you read and use this book, you'll come to believe in it too.

How to Use This Book

The most important advice I have on how to use this book is to have fun. So many things following a cancer diagnosis are chores; eating from this book shouldn't be one of them. There are probably going to be days when swallowing a few sips of broth is going to be an accomplishment. By all means, celebrate that nourishment. Don't beat yourself up for the meals you miss. When you accentuate the positive, your connection to food will remain intact during treatment and even build upon itself.

Think of this book as a toolbox, full of great ideas that can entice you to eat with a minimum of stress in the kitchen for whoever is cooking. Will you utilize every tool in the box? Perhaps—but it isn't necessary. I've tried to be all-inclusive because I want to give you ways to address issues that commonly crop up during treatment.

Think of this book as a toolbox, full of great ideas that can entice you to eat with a minimum of stress in the kitchen for whoever is cooking.

Chapter 1, Cancer-Fighting Tool Kit, is a guide to scrumptious foods, recipes, and kitchen techniques that can lessen the impact of side effects, improve appetite and immunity, and overcome changes in the sense of taste or impaired taste buds, which is a common consequence of treatment. It includes very specific suggestions on what to eat before, during, and after chemotherapy. I've also included a questionnaire that's a simple way to figure out people's food preferences—your own or, if you're a caregiver, someone else's. Treatments can throw people's tastes for such a loop that old favorites may not be appetizing. When that's the case, knowing more about the person's inherent preferences is valuable information. Chapter 1 also includes information on what I call global flavorprints—lists of herbs and spices that characterize different cuisines—and an introduction to the powerhouse foods used in the recipes, including their amazing cancer-fighting properties and other nutritional effects. I call this the culinary pharmacy, and it's an incredibly powerful prescription for both health and appetite.

Chapter 2, Strategies for Thriving during Treatment, sets out a game plan for making sure that everyone is on the same page and that as many people as possible get involved in the process. Cancer is such an emotional experience that the joy of caregiving can be jeopardized if organization and communication aren't brought to the process. I'll show you how to organize a culinary support team to cover shopping and cooking tasks, and how to clearly define roles so people don't step on each other's toes—and, most importantly, the patient's. The guidance in chapter 2 will allow everyone to contribute in a way that's desired and appreciated. On a practical level, this chapter will show you how to make sure a wide variety of healthy, yummy meals and snacks are available whenever hunger hits, even in settings outside the home, such as at work, in the hospital, or during treatment sessions. Eating small portions often is the best route for delivering nourishment to the body during treatment. And it gives detailed instructions on various food preparation techniques, and advice on storage and reheating.

For those without easy access to a farmers' market or well-stocked grocery stores, the Resources section provides online sources for many of the ingredients in the recipes. It also includes information on cancer support groups and medical information. The extensive bibliography documents sources for the information used in this book.

As for the recipes and variations that are the heart and soul of the book, they have been tried and tested more times than I can count, by a battery of tasters who refused to be satisfied until they were moaning with delight. You've paid for a cookbook with the expectation that every recipe will deliver in terms of both taste and nutrition; my team and I have done the utmost to meet, and hopefully exceed, those expectations.

Throughout the recipes, you'll find suggestions on substitutions for common food sensitivities. For those who want to avoid dairy, you can generally use soy or rice milk—just be sure to use an unsweetened variety. Folks with gluten intolerance will find substitutions for wheat, as well.

Whenever possible, I suggest eating organic for all of my clients, and that's especially important for people in treatment, particularly when it comes to meat and dairy. I realize organics can cost a bit more across the board, but consider that undergoing treatment means you're already dealing with plenty of toxins in your body. It makes sense to me that you don't want to introduce more, in the form of pesticides, hormones, antibiotics, and other drugs, in your food. Plus, organically grown produce raised outdoors without pesticides produces phytochemicals to protect itself from the environment, and one school of scientific thought holds that many of these same chemicals offer chemoprotective benefits in the body. Either way, here's one thing I can tell you for sure: organic, fresh-picked produce, pasture-raised chicken, and fish caught in the wild are absolutely delicious, offering the finest flavors that can land on your plate. Speaking as a chef and the little pixie in your ear, why would you settle for anything less?

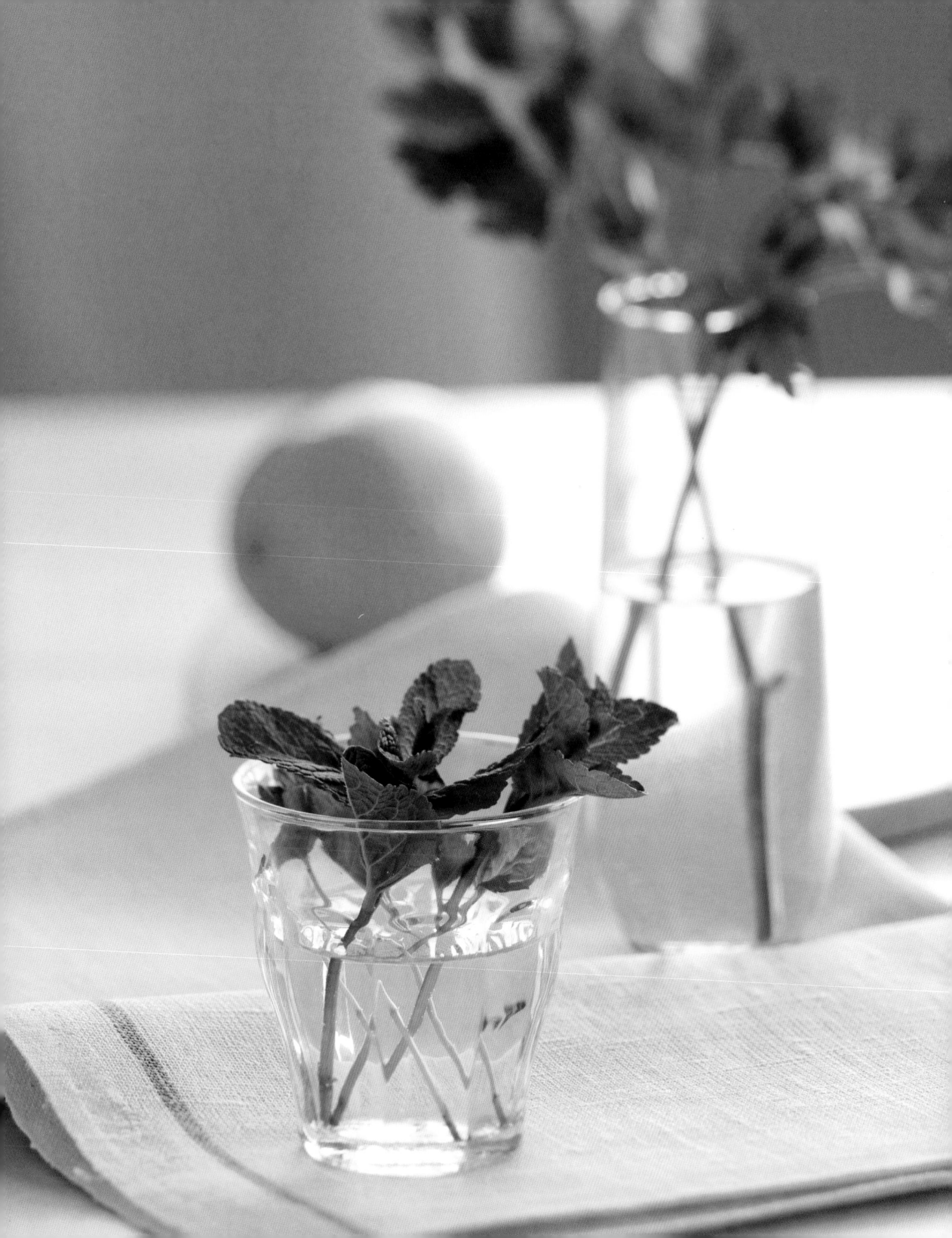

CHAPTER 1

Cancer-Fighting Tool Kit

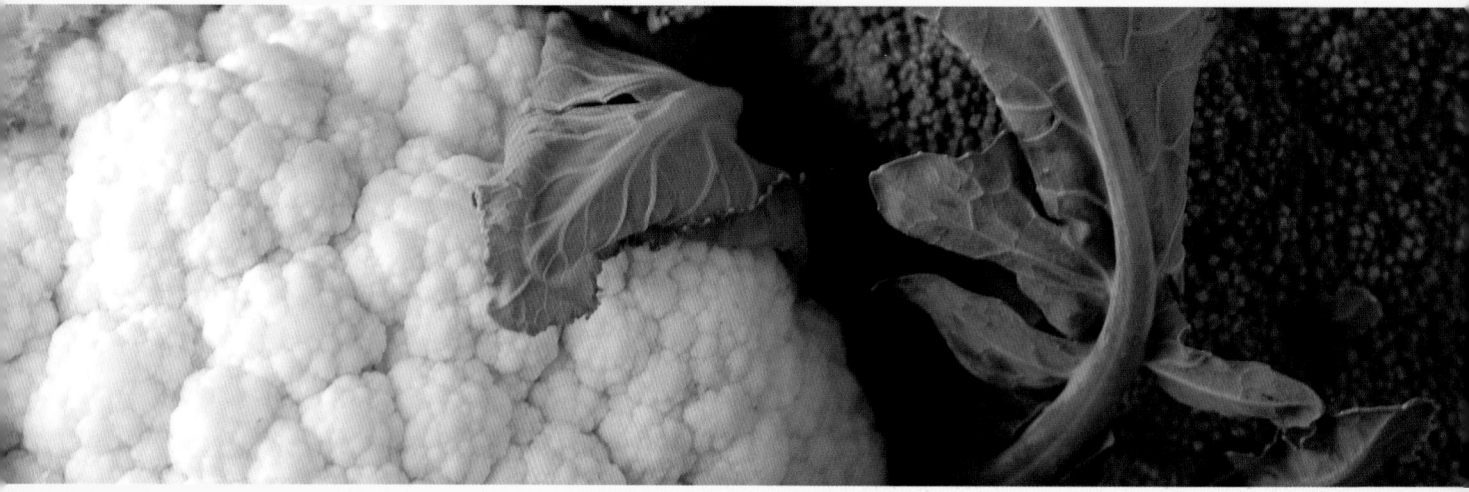

10 *Side Effects*

11 *Recipes for Specific Side Effects*

16 *Menu Planning*

20 *Enhancing Flavor and Dealing with Taste Changes*

23 *FASS Fixes for Taste Bud Troubles*

25 *Learning Your Food Preferences*

27 *The Power of Herbs and Spices*

28 *Culinary Pharmacy*

The first thing you need to remember about this chapter is there won't be a test at the end. There's no midterm or final here, no omnipotent voice of the annoyed schoolmarm standing over your shoulder in the kitchen, sighing in a way that makes her words seem to say, "This one is never going to get it." The point of all of the tools in this chapter is to use them as you like, take from them what you will, and know that they're all country roads that lead to the same joyous place: a dish, a meal, a snack, or a tea that will help you or your loved one feel a little better and live a little easier during a tough time.

Here are a few things I can tell you about these tools: They all come from firsthand experience. Folks I've worked with who have "been there, done that" have shared their culinary discoveries and recipes or foods that have made dealing with treatment less onerous. Indeed, they've often told me that eating well gives them a chance to forget what they're dealing with during the rest of the day. Many cancer wellness professionals have also generously imparted nutritional tips and explained the science behind them. I can't tell you how good it makes me feel to know that so many fantastic doctors, nurses, nutritionists, dieticians, and researchers are seriously looking into the ways that nutrition and cancer interact. But more than that, they're coming up with practical applications for their findings, in the form of suggestions on the best ways to approach eating during cancer treatment.

Then there's the trial and error of my own culinary journey in cooking for people with cancer and learning how people's tastes and taste buds literally change during treatment. Over time, working with friends, family, and clients, I've created a simple tool consisting of four pantry staples that can greatly enhance the flavor of any dish, even for those with the most impaired taste buds. I've also seen how clients felt about food as they traversed their treatment schedules and will share solutions I've come up with to cajole them into eating enjoyably—even when at first they might have wrinkled up their nose at the idea. The nice thing about this tool kit is that everything in it is easy to use. It's the culinary equivalent of handling a screwdriver, wrench, and hammer; there are no miter saws or power tools involved. (Okay, maybe a blender, but that's fun.)

Basic tools can be powerful, and the power of yum can tackle many of the difficult aspects of treatment, including the following:

- Lessening the impact of common side effects, including nausea, fatigue, and muscle loss
- Improving appetite, which will enhance the immune system and keep people stronger, allowing them to get the maximum benefit from cancer treatments
- Appealing to those with impaired taste buds by using simple ingredients to boost flavor
- Utilizing strategies to ensure that people can eat delicious nourishing foods that they like whenever they want, no matter how quickly or often their tastes and appetite changes
- Offering outstanding anticancer properties—not to mention unparalleled flavor—with generous amounts of spices

Side Effects

Ah, the things we're supposed to endure to retain or regain our health. Cancer treatments and their side effects are one nasty tag team. Most of the people I've worked with have dealt with one or more side effects due to chemotherapy, radiation, or surgery. This brings me to a few important points. The good news is that doctors should be able to medically treat most side effects. But—and this is a huge but—you have to speak up and let someone know you're not feeling well.

I know this can be a hard thing to do. Sometimes it stems from perfectionism. You want to be a good patient or the best patient, which for some translates into a "grin and bear it" attitude. And some doctors are tightly focused on the therapies they need to apply to help you beat cancer. In the usually all-too-short time of an office visit, they want to cover those therapies with you and conversations about side effects may take a backseat as a result.

The problem is, not addressing side effects can have larger consequences. Cancer treatments impact the immune system, and other side effects, especially those that make people avoid eating, can further hinder immunity. All of this can impact your treatment schedule.

Think of it this way: Thousands of researchers have spent hundreds of thousands of hours devising precise dosing schedules. The clinical goal is to take you right to that edge where you receive the maximum therapy dose to wipe out your cancer while keeping your body intact. Each treatment takes you to this precipice in an effort to get ahead of the cancer. Any side effect that isn't addressed leaves your body less than 100 percent prepared for the next treatment. At times, this may force your doctor to lessen your chemo dose or skip a treatment altogether to give your body more time to recover. Obviously, the odds suggest you don't want to be missing treatments too often.

Some therapy side effects are seemingly beyond being addressed by nutrition, at least at this point, such as neuropathy, hair loss, and loss of function due to surgery. But fortunately, in many cases what you eat can lessen the impact of side effects. A lot of my clients have heard of using ginger to soothe an upset stomach. There are dozens of other healing foods, which appear often in the recipes in this book—foods that can help you deal with fatigue, nausea, anemia, constipation, dehydration, diarrhea, mouth sores, swallowing issues, weight loss, and low immune function or low white blood cell counts.

You'll find a listing of these foods in the Culinary Pharmacy, but let me suggest that you first take a look at the listing of side effects and recommended recipes below. I'm steering you toward these sections because consulting them is quick and easy and often offers answers. A glance, a flip of the page, and you're right where you need to be. Feeling a little queasy? There you are, Ginger Peppermint Green Tea, on page 162. *Flip-flip, sip-sip,* in no time at all, you may be feeling better.

There's another reason I'm nudging you toward recipes versus individual foods. The experts I consulted generally recommend getting nutrients from multiple foods, like you'll find in most any recipe, rather than focusing on individual foods. Why? Because we're all unique, and the same DNA that determines whether you have blue eyes or brown also determines what enzymes you produce to help you break down and assimilate food. Put another way, two people eating grapes off the same bunch may get vastly different health benefits. Science doesn't yet have a way of figuring out each individual's digestive "blueprint," but they're getting there; it's a field called proteomics, which eventually will allow us to determine which proteins and enzymes each individual is capable of producing. In the meanwhile, experts suggest that you hedge your bets during treatment by eating a wide variety of healthy foods—just what a chef like me *loves* to hear.

Recipes for Specific Side Effects

Anemia

Soups: Minestrone (page 64), Pasture Beef Bone Broth (page 56), Velvety Red Lentil Dahl (page 74)

Vegetables: Kale with Carrots (page 88), Kale with Sweet Potatoes and Pecans (page 89)

Anytime Foods: Mediterranean Lentil Salad (page 142)

Constipation

General recommendations: Drink warm fluids throughout the day and eat fruit.

Soups: Chicken Magic Mineral Broth (page 55), Italian White Bean Soup (page 57), Magic Mineral Broth (page 54), Pasture Beef Bone Broth (page 56), Velvety Red Lentil Dahl (page 74)

Vegetables: Baby Bok Choy with Yam and Ginger (page 80), Basil Broccoli (page 78), Emerald Greens with Orange (page 84), Kale with Carrots (page 88), Kale with Sweet Potatoes and Pecans (page 89), Shredded Carrot and Beet Salad (page 98), Stir-Fried Baby Bok Choy with Shiitake Mushrooms (page 92)

Anytime Foods: Anytime Bars (page 126), Mediterranean Lentil Salad (page 142)

Tonics and Elixirs: Cinnamon Ginger Tea (page 163), Commonweal's Most Nourishing and Healing Tea (page 157), Ginger Peppermint Green Tea (page 162), Green Tea Ginger Lemonade (page 162)

Dollops of Yum!: Dried Fruit Compote (page 183), Seasonal Stewed Fruit (page 184)

Sweet Bites: Baked Apples Filled with Dates and Pecans (page 194), Poached Pears with Saffron Broth (page 203)

Dehydration

Soups: All of the recipes in Chapter 3

Tonics and Elixirs: All of the recipes in Chapter 7

Diarrhea

Anytime Foods: Best Oatmeal Ever (page 128), Creamiest Buckwheat (page 138), Creamy Millet (page 136), Creamy Polenta (page 134), Simple Tuscan Farro (page 148)

Tonics and Elixirs: Anee Maries Calming Kudzu Elixir (page 156)

Sweet Bites: Coconut Rice Pudding (page 198), Chocolate Tapioca Pudding (without the chocolate) (page 195)

Fatigue

Soups: Pasture Beef Bone Broth (page 56), Chicken Magic Mineral Broth (page 55), Chicken Vegetable Soup with Ginger Meatballs (page 59), Italian White Bean Soup (page 57), Lemony Greek Chicken Soup (page 60), Magic Mineral Broth (page 54), Ma's Mushroom Barley Soup (page 61), Thai It Up Chicken Soup (page 62), Velvety Red Lentil Dahl (page 74)

Vegetables: Gregg's Stuffed Acorn Squash with Quinoa, Cranberries, and Swiss Chard (page 86)

Protein-Building Foods: All of the recipes in Chapter 5

Anytime Foods: Anytime Bars (page 126), Black Bean Hummus (page 132), Cannellini Bean Dip with Kalamata Olives (page 132), Curried Hummus (page 133), Curried Hummus and

Vegetable Pinwheels (page 153), Edamame Avocado Dip with Wasabi (page 131), Navy Bean and Sun-Dried Tomato Dip (page 131), Quinoa Pilaf (page 149), Rice Paper Moo-Shu Rolls (page 150)

Tonics and Elixirs: Chocolate Banana Smoothie (page 166), Cinnamon Ginger Tea (page 163), Mango Coconut Smoothie (page 167), Commonweal's Most Nourishing and Healing Tea (page 157), Ginger Peppermint Green Tea (page 167), Green Tea Ginger Lemonade (page 162), Papaya Pineapple Smoothie (page 171), Peach Ginger Smoothie (page 169), Pineapple Ginger Smoothie (page 170), Triple Berry Smoothie (page 169)

Nausea and Vomiting

Soups: Chicken Magic Mineral Broth (page 55), Magic Mineral Broth (page 54), Pasture Beef Bone Broth (page 56)

Tonics and Elixirs: Cinnamon Ginger Tea (page 163), Ginger Ale with Frozen Grapes (page 164), Ginger Peppermint Green Tea (page 162), Ginger Tea Spritzer (page 163)

Neutropenia

Soups: Bella's Carrot, Orange, and Fennel Soup (page 65), Creamy Broccoli and Potato Soup (page 75), Curry Cauliflower Soup (page 67), Italian White Bean Soup (page 57), Magic Mineral Broth (page 54), Ma's Mushroom Barley Soup (page 61, Minestrone (page 64), Rockin' Black Bean Soup (page 71), Spiced Sweet Potato Soup (page 72), Summer's Best Zucchini Soup (page 73), Velvety Red Lentil Dahl (page 74)

Vegetables: Hungarian Roasted Root Vegetable Potpie (page 95)

Protein-Building Foods: Lemon Mustard Salmon Salad (page 109)

Anytime Foods: Best Oatmeal Ever (page 128), Beyond Just Good Cornbread (page 129), Creamiest Buckwheat (page 138), Creamy Polenta (page 134), Quinoa Pilaf (page 149), Simple Tuscan Farro (page 148)

Tonics and Elixirs: Annemarie's Calming Kudzu Elixir (page 156), Cinnamon Ginger Tea (page 163), Commonweal's Most Nourishing and Healing Tea (page 157), Ginger Peppermint Green Tea (page 162), Ginger Ale with Frozen Grapes (page 164)

Dollops of Yum!: Seasonal Stewed Fruit (page 184)

Sweet Bites: Almond Muffin Mania (page 192), Chocolate Tapioca Pudding (page 195), Coconut Rice Pudding (page 198), Great Pumpkin Custard (page 200), Triple Ginger Snap Cookies with Pecans (page 207)

Sore Mouth and Difficulty Swallowing

General recommendations: Omit spicy ingredients and ginger from all recipes.

Soups: Bella's Carrot, Orange, and Fennel Soup (page 65), Chicken Magic Mineral Broth (page 55), Cooling Cucumber Avocado Soup (page 70), Creamy Broccoli and Potato Soup (page 75), Magic Mineral Broth (page 54), Pasture Beef Bone Broth (page 56), Rockin' Black Bean Soup (page 71), Spiced Sweet Potato Soup (page 72), Summer's Best Zucchini Soup (page 73)

Anytime Foods: Best Oatmeal Ever (page128), Creamiest Buckwheat (page 138)

Tonics and Elixirs: Annemarie's Calming Kudzu Elixir (page 156), Cantaloupe Granita with Mint (page 158), Chocolate Banana Smoothie (page 166), Cinnamon Ginger Tea (page 163), Commonweal's Most Nourishing and Healing Tea (page 157), Ginger Peppermint Green Tea (page 162), Green Tea Ginger Lemonade (page 162), Mango Coconut Smoothie (page 167), Mouth-watering Watermelon Granita (page 161), Papaya Pineapple Smoothie (page 171), Peach Ginger Smoothie (page 169), Pineapple Ginger Smoothie (page 170), Triple Berry Smoothie (page 169)

Weight Loss

Soups: Bella's Carrot, Orange, and Fennel Soup (page 65), Chicken Vegetable Soup with Ginger Meatballs (page 59), Curry Cauliflower Soup (page 67), Italian White Bean Soup (page 57), Lemony Greek Chicken Soup (page 60), Ma's Mushroom Barley Soup (page 61), Minestrone (page 64), Thai It Up Chicken Soup (page 62), Velvety Red Lentil Dahl (page 74)

Vegetables: Gregg's Stuffed Acorn Squash with Quinoa, Cranberries, and Swiss Chard (page 86), Hungarian Roasted Root Vegetable Potpie (page 95), Purple Peruvian Smashed Potatoes (page 93)

Protein-Building Foods: Chicken and Broccoli Stir-Fry with Cashews (page 105), Cozy Comfy Chicken and Rice (page 106), Curried Chicken Salad (page 104), Easy Eggs in a Cup (page 102), Middle Eastern Chickpea Burgers (page 112), My Family's Favorite Chicken (page 111), Nana's Egg Salad (page 114), Orange Ginger Roasted Chicken (page 117), Poached Eggs with Basil Lemon Drizzle (page 115)

Anytime Foods: All of the recipes in Chapter 6

Tonics and Elixirs: Chocolate Banana Smoothie (page 166), Mango Coconut Smoothie (page 167), Papaya Pineapple Smoothie (page 171), Peach Ginger Smoothie (page 169), Pineapple Ginger Smoothie (page 170), Triple Berry Smoothie (page 169)

Sweet Bites: Almond Muffin Mania (page 192), Cardamom Maple Mini Macaroons (page 197), Chocolate Tapioca Pudding (page 195), Great Pumpkin Custard (page 200), Triple Ginger Snap Cookies with Pecans (page 207), Wendy's Date Nut Truffles (page 201)

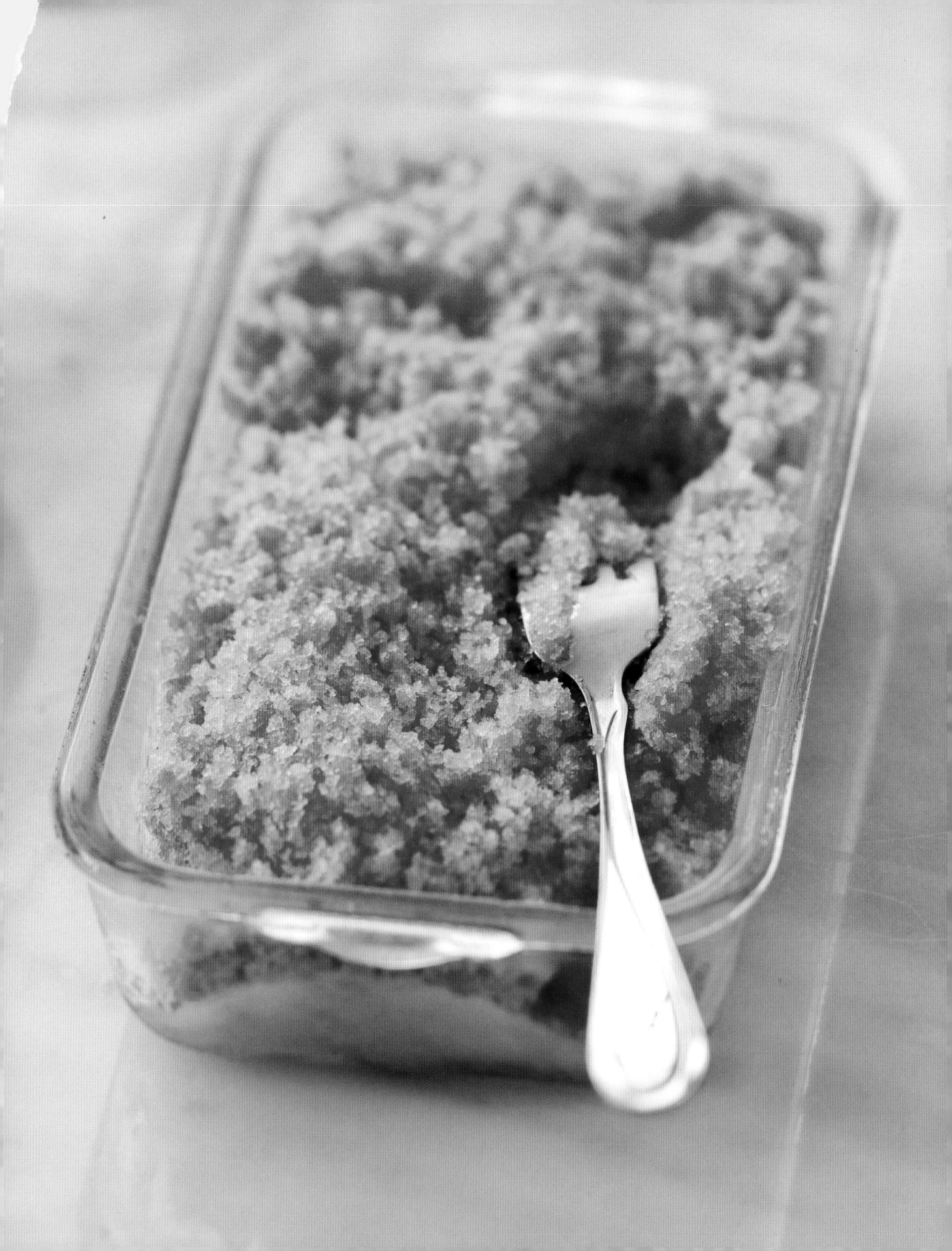

Menu Planning

If you're undergoing cancer treatment, whether it's surgery, chemotherapy, radiation, or any medical procedure, it's always worthwhile to schedule your eating in a way that maximizes the benefits of treatment and minimizes side effects. Part of this involves a conversation with your doctor or nutritionist about what you can and can't eat—and, just as importantly, when you can eat—before, during, and after treatment. There may be issues particular to your treatment that both you and she should discuss.

That said, here are some recommendations, based on what I've found effective for my clients. Good nutrition is always a key to regaining and maintaining health, but some general rules apply depending upon what treatment you're getting.

Surgery tends to dehydrate the body, partially because of stress and partially because you're often asked, because of anesthesia, to go without food and water for at least 12 hours prior to the procedure. I suggest that you concentrate on staying well hydrated for two weeks prior to a procedure, with an eye toward eating broths and smoothies with protein powder. The protein helps with wound healing, while the extra fluids help anesthesia flush from the body. I think of this extra attention to detail as "pre-hab"; research is showing that by getting your body ready for medical procedures before they take place, you often set yourself up for a quicker recovery.

Similarly, fluids play a big role with chemotherapy because they can limit nausea, which is by far the most common effect I see from that treatment. Also, fried foods, ice cream, anything with a high fat content should be avoided around treatment days. Believe me, your stomach will thank you.

As for radiation treatments, they often prompt fatigue. To help alleviate this, I suggest focusing on high-energy foods you can find in the side-effect chart section (no, they're not laced with sugar, but your body will love them nonetheless). In addition to radiation used for therapy, the many X-rays and scans that are involved in treatment expose your body to radiation. Miso, as well as nori, kombu, and other sea vegetables, pulls radiation from the body, so be sure to eat foods with sea vegetables after scans—but avoid eating them just after radiation treatment because they can reduce its effectiveness.

Now, some ideas about what to eat and when, all with the goal of making treatment as easy as possible.

Two Days before Chemotherapy

In the days leading up to your chemotherapy session, remember that eating right will give your body the extra boost it needs to stay strong and make the most of the treatments you receive—and hopefully minimize side effects as well. Here are two points to remember in the few days leading up to your chemotherapy session:

1. Avoid your favorite foods, so as to avoid developing an aversion to them in the event that you get sick from chemotherapy. (For the same reason, avoid your favorite foods for three days after chemotherapy as well.)
2. Avoid eating fat-filled, fried, and greasy foods.

Week of Chemotherapy, Including Treatment Days

During treatment, you should try to eat a small nibble every hour or so, even if you aren't especially hungry. Small meals throughout the day will keep you fueled and keep your strength up. Pay attention to the time; set an alarm, if necessary, to make sure you eat something nutritious. You're more likely to feel nauseous if your stomach is empty, so keep it supplied with good food.

If you're at a loss as to what, specifically, to eat during chemotherapy, fear not. Below you'll find recommendations for three different appetite levels: minimal, fairly normal, and hearty. If you fall into the minimal appetite category, I hope that the healing foods and delicious recipes in this book will help you work your way up to a regular appetite, and eventually a hearty appetite. It may seem inconceivable now, but I've seen this with many clients.

Bare Minimum Menu

No matter how awful you're feeling, you need nourishment. At a bare minimum, this is what you should eat each day during the week surrounding chemotherapy:

- 4 cups of Magic Mineral Broth (page 54), Chicken Magic Mineral Broth (page 55), or Pasture Beef Bone Broth (page 56)
- 2 servings of smoothies with protein powder
- 2 cups of Commonweal's Most Nourishing and Healing Tea (page 157)
- 2 cups of green tea or any variation on green tea in this book

Regular Menu

Here's a list of recipes that might work well during the week of chemotherapy treatment. All are easy to digest, comforting, nourishing, and full of the vitamins and minerals your body needs to heal. This is a perfect reference list to give to friends and family who offer to cook for you during this time.

Soups: Bella's Carrot, Orange, and Fennel Soup (page 65), Chicken Magic Mineral Broth (page 55), Chicken Vegetable Soup with Ginger Meatballs (page 59), Creamy Broccoli and Potato Soup (page 75), Magic Mineral Broth (page 54), Pasture Beef Bone Broth (page 56), Spiced Sweet Potato Soup (page 72), Summer's Best Zucchini Soup (page 73), Thai It Up Chicken Soup (page 62)

Vegetables: Hungarian Roasted Root Vegetable Potpie (page 95), Mashed Cinnamon Butternut Squash (page 90), Purple Peruvian Smashed Potatoes (page 93)

Protein-Building Foods: Cozy Comfy Chicken and Rice (page 106), Easy Eggs in a Cup (page 102), Nana's Egg Salad (page 114), Poached Eggs with Basil Lemon Drizzle (page 115)

Anytime Foods: Best Oatmeal Ever (page 128), Black Bean Hummus (page 132), Cannellini Bean Dip with Kalamata Olives (page 132), Catherine's Magic Green Tea Rice (page 135), Creamy Millet (page 136), Creamy Polenta (page 136), Creamiest Buckwheat (page 138), Curried Hummus (page 133), Curried Hummus and Vegetable Pinwheels (page 153), Edamame Avocado Dip with Wasabi (page 131), Maple-Glazed Walnuts (page 141), Navy Bean and Sun-Dried Tomato Dip (page 131), Quinoa Pilaf (page 149), Rice Paper Moo-Shu Rolls (page 150), Spiced Toasted Almonds (page 139)

Tonics and Elixirs: Annemarie's Calming Kudzu Elixir (page 156), Cantaloupe Granita with Mint (page 158), Chocolate Banana Smoothie (page 166), Cinnamon Ginger Tea (page 163), Commonweal's Most Nourishing and Healing Tea (page 157), Ginger Peppermint Green Tea (page 162), Green Tea Ginger Lemonade (page 162), Mango Coconut Smoothie (page 167), Mouthwatering Watermelon Granita (page 161), Papaya Pineapple Smoothie (page 171), Peach Ginger Smoothie (page 169), Pineapple Ginger Smoothie (page 170), Triple Berry Smoothie (page 169)

Sweet Bites: Chocolate Tapioca Pudding (page 195) Coconut Rice Pudding (page 198), Great Pumpkin Custard (page 200), Strawberries with Mango Coconut "Sabayon" (page 204)

Hearty Appetite Menu

If you're lucky to have a voracious appetite, eat up! Here's a list of additional foods that are beneficial during treatment.

Soups: Italian White Bean Soup (page 57), Minestrone (page 64), Velvety Red Lentil Dahl (page 74)

Vegetables: Basil Broccoli (page 78), Warm and Toasty Cumin Carrots (page 93)

Protein-Building Foods: Chicken and Broccoli Stir-Fry with Cashews (page 105), Middle Eastern Chickpea Burgers (with Tomato Mint Chutney or Sweet and Savory Yogurt) (page 112), My Family's Favorite Chicken (page 111), Orange Ginger Roasted Chicken (page 117)

Anytime Foods: Orange Pistachio Couscous (page 145)

Dollops of Yum!: Sweet and Savory Yogurt (page 189), Tomato Mint Chutney (page 176)

Sweet Bites: Almond Muffin Mania (page 192), Triple Ginger Snap Cookies with Pecans (page 207)

One Week after Chemotherapy

At some point during the week after chemo, your mouth is going to wake up and want to taste food again. Pay attention to this list of recipes that can jump-start your taste buds and get your appetite up and running again.

Soups: Bella's Carrot, Orange, and Fennel Soup (page 65), Curry Cauliflower Soup (page 67), Lemony Greek Chicken Soup (page 60), Rockin' Black Bean Soup (page 71), Spiced Sweet Potato Soup (page 72), Thai It Up Chicken Soup (page 62), Velvety Red Lentil Dahl (page 74)

Vegetables: Baby Bok Choy with Yam and Ginger (page 80), Cucumber, Jicama, and Mango Salad (page 83), Emerald Greens with Orange (page 84), Gregg's Stuffed Acorn Squash with Quinoa, Cranberries, and Swiss Chard (page 86), Kale with Carrots (page 88), Kale with Sweet Potatoes and Pecans (page 89), Mashed Cinnamon Butternut Squash (page 90), Mixed Greens with Edamame, Radish, and Avocado (page 91), Shredded Carrot and Beet Salad (page 98), Stir-Fried Baby Bok Choy with Shiitake Mushrooms (page 97), Warm Napa Cabbage Slaw (page 92)

Protein-Building Foods: Baked Citrus Halibut with Tomato Sauce (page 123), Middle Eastern Chickpea Burgers (page 112), Poached Salmon with Moroccan Pesto (page 121), Triple-Citrus Ginger Black Cod (page 118)

Anytime Foods: Black Bean Hummus (page 132), Cannellini Bean Dip with Kalamata Olives (page 132), Curried Hummus (page 133), Edamame Avocado Dip with Wasabi (page 131), Mediterranean Lentil Salad (page 142), Navy Bean and Sun-Dried Tomato Dip (page 131)

Tonics and Elixirs: Cantaloupe Granita with Mint (page 158), Commonweal's Most Nourishing and Healing Tea (page 157), Green Tea Ginger Lemonade (page 162), Mango Coconut Smoothie (page 167), Mouthwatering Watermelon Granita (page 161), Pineapple Ginger Smoothie (page 170)

Dollops of Yum!: Apricot Pear Chutney (page 175), Avocado Dressing (page 178), Basil Lemon Drizzle (page 177), Cashew Cream (page 180), Cilantro Lime Vinaigrette (page 181), Parsley Basil Drizzle (page 187), Pistachio Cream (page 181), Seasonal Stewed Fruit (page 184), Signora's Tomato Sauce (page 188), Sweet and Savory Yogurt (page 189), Tomato Mint Chutney (page 176), Zesty Lemon Fennel Vinaigrette (page 182)

Sweet Bites: Baked Apples Filled with Dates and Pecans (page 194), Cardamom Maple Mini Macaroons (page 197), Poached Pears with Saffron Broth (page 209)

Between Treatments

Once your appetite returns to what feels like normal, continue to eat in a healthy and nourishing manner. One colorful way to stay well nourished is to eat a rainbow of deeply hued fruits and vegetables, as they generally contain the highest level of cancer-fighting nutrients. All of the recipes in this cookbook are appropriate then—or anytime. In addition, I recommend the following immune boosters on a daily basis:

- Smoothie or protein shake
- Commonweal's Most Nourishing and Healing Tea (page 157)
- Chicken Magic Mineral Broth (page 55), Magic Mineral Broth (page 54), or Pasture Beef Bone Broth (page 56)
- Cinnamon Ginger Tea (page 163), Ginger Peppermint Green Tea (page 162), Green Tea Ginger Lemonade (page 162), or any other green tea

Enhancing Flavor and Dealing with Taste Changes

There's one side effect I didn't discuss above because in the context of a cookbook, it really deserves a whole section unto itself. The technical term is "transient taste change," but I just say it's what happens when your taste buds go kaflooey during treatment. A good number of the people I've worked with complain of a metallic taste in their mouth as they go through their cancer therapies, most notably chemotherapy. They're not imagining things. Cancer therapies can not only damage taste buds or throw off their balance but also cause sudden sensitivities to hot and cold. That's the bad news. The good news is that many of these changes wax and wane even between treatments, and they often disappear after treatment. The reason, according to Dr. Linda Bartoshuk of the University of Florida Dental School, is that taste buds and taste nerves regenerate rapidly, often within weeks.

The great news is that, even if your taste buds have been drained of vitality, I have a tool that can help revitalize them. It's called FASS, which stands for Fat, Acid, Salt, and Sweet. In my kitchen, olive oil represents the fat, lemons are the acid, sea salt is the only salt I'll touch, and Grade B organic maple syrup is my preferred sweet. You'll find this Fantastic Four of seasonings right next to my stove, as ever-present and important to me as a spreadsheet is to an accountant.

FASS started off as a culinary tool to help any dish whose flavor strayed off course during the cooking process, and to bring food to the table bursting with flavor. Think of cooking as a game of darts, with the bull's-eye being that absolute moment of yum. Each element of FASS represents a culinary quadrant of the dartboard. When they're balanced and work in harmony, you'll hit the bull's-eye. Acid and salt add high notes to taste, each in their own way; fat and sweet tend to bring roundness and fullness to a dish. FASS is really just an acronym to remind you of these fundamentals, which chefs and many cooks do by intuition much of the time.

The great news is that even if your taste buds have been drained of vitality, I have a tool that can help revitalize them.

When I make a soup, I taste it throughout the cooking process. When I teach, I always suggest that people develop this habit. It's a fun way to fix into your memory what each new player brings to the table, and constant tasting is the only way to ensure a dish has optimum flavor without running the risk of having to resort to drastic measures after it's completed. If you've ever tried to put wiring into a house after the walls are up, you know what I'm talking about. By adding a spritz of lemon here or a pinch of salt there, you can alchemize the ingredients so that what hits the tongue in the end is pure bliss.

That's FASS as a culinary tool, and it's a mighty powerful use of yum. But it only scratches the surface of what FASS can do to address taste changes in people undergoing treatment. It's a strange thing about chefs and taste—we all depend on it to make a living, yet very few chefs, or even physicians and scientists, know how the taste buds work. But to most effectively compensate for malfunction of the taste buds, you need to know how they work when things are normal.

For nearly a century, the conventional wisdom said that individual taste buds resided in different regions of the tongue: Sweet up front, bitter in back, and sour and salt on different sides. Fat wasn't even seen as a taste but more as a sense. As it turns out, this conventional wisdom wasn't so wise. Researchers now think there are small islands of different types of taste buds spread around the tongue and—get this—even on the soft palate, upper esophagus, and epiglottis.

Our taste guru, Linda Bartoshuk, says, "If you want to prove this to yourself, put a little salt on your finger and touch it to the area about halfway back in your mouth where the hard palate meets the soft palate." We did, and she's right; you can taste salt there. When you think about it, this built-in redundancy makes sense. The ability to taste sweet versus bitter—which allowed our ancient ancestors to differentiate what was edible from what was poisonous—was crucial for allowing our species to get where it is today.

So what's going on when suddenly your mouth feels like it's full of aluminum, or when everything starts tasting like cardboard? And, more importantly, what can we do to bring the sense of taste back to life?

Normally, the brain combines sensory input from the taste buds and the sense of smell, and the resulting neuronal input is taste. It's kind of like a color wheel; mix blue and yellow in equal portions and you get green, without fail. Now imagine the painter who one day starts mixing paints only to find that blue and yellow are yielding a very pale shade of green, certainly not the tone she wants and expects. Frustrated and annoyed, she throws down her palette in disgust and stalks off to watch *Judge Judy.* So it is with taste buds damaged by cancer therapy: Their sensory output becomes distorted or impaired, so the brain can only pick up a whisper of the flavor and therefore produces a taste in conflict with what the eater expects. As a result, your all-time favorite treat, say warm banana bread fresh from the oven, may *look* delicious, and it may even *smell* delicious, but when you taste it, it's anything but. So you push back from the table, disappointed and disengaging from one of the most important things you must do during treatment: eat.

And as for those phantom metallic tastes? Well, that would be like our painter looking down at her palette and realizing that no matter what colors she wants to mix, there's always a splotch of orange to contend with. Again, who wants to deal with that?

I recently conducted a cooking class for a bunch of second-year medical students at UCSF who were in a program entitled "Caring for the Seriously Ill." I wanted to give them a feel of what it's like to live with transient taste change during cancer therapy. They watched hungrily as I cooked up a batch of carrot-ginger soup, which unbeknownst to them I had watered down just enough to throw off the taste. Still the bright orange color looked just about right, and a hint of the smell was also there. They lined up to taste the soup, anticipation in their eyes, but upon taking a sip they looked disappointed, to say the least.

What can we do to bring the sense of taste back to life when suddenly your mouth feels like it's full of aluminum, or when everything starts tasting like cardboard?

Now that I had their attention, I explained the role that FASS plays for the taste impaired. Salt is where I often start. Not regular table salt, mind you, as it's bitter and devoid of trace minerals. Sea salt, on the other hand, has more than eighty minerals and a much fuller flavor as a result. For people experiencing deadened taste buds, a tiny amount of sea salt can make a huge difference as it stimulates nerve endings and ignites taste. It's kind of like cranking up the volume on your stereo. By contrast, lemons, citrus in general, and other acidic ingredients are like turning up the treble and can brighten up whatever tastes you've brought out with the salt.

Sweet—in this case Grade B organic maple syrup—adds a depth or roundness to flavor that's the equivalent of hearing an orchestra in a concert hall, rather than on your stereo. Just a bit of sweetness can transform a two-dimensional taste encounter into a memorable 3-D culinary experience.

As for fat, think of it as the taxi that provides transportation to the concert hall for all of the tastes sweet, salt, and acidity generate; without a ride, they can't get there. Fat serves as a chauffeur supreme, carrying tastes to the different islands of taste buds throughout the mouth, guaranteeing that all the buds—impaired *and* healthy—have an opportunity to at least listen to the concert.

FASS isn't foolproof. In some cases there's damage to the nerve roots, the highways that take the information from taste buds to the brain. But fortunately there's some built-in redundancy here, too, and I've yet to meet anyone in treatment who wasn't helped by an application of the FASS principle. For those with little or no change in the sense of taste, FASS makes a good meal great. For those with more challenging taste issues, it can spell the difference between finding meals palatable, which keeps the appetite engaged, and losing interest in eating. A case in point is Susan, a woman in treatment for breast cancer who was in the audience at a cooking demonstration I gave at a hospital. I was making butternut squash soup and had used FASS to get it to yum for everyone—everyone that is, except Susan. When the little cups of soup were passed out to the audience, the crowd responded with "yummms" and "ahhhs." But Susan wasn't smiling. "Okay," I told the audience, "nobody's leaving until Susan is happy!"

Susan explained that even before treatment she'd had especially sensitive taste buds (making her fall into that category of people known as "supertasters"), and that treatment had left her with a bitter taste in her mouth. I asked Susan to rate the soup on a scale of 1 to 10, and she gave the soup a 7. To me, that's the culinary equivalent of dressing up in a beautiful gown only to hear someone say, "Gee, she's a nice gal"—not exactly a raving endorsement. I knew I could do better, so I called Susan up to make sure she really did have sensitivity to bitterness. It wasn't that I doubted her; sometimes people aren't sure exactly what their taste deficit is, so they take their best guess. In Susan's case, she was spot on, but I wanted to give her taste buds a little workout. First I added just two little pinches of sea salt to the pot, which contained about four cups of soup.

For those with more challenging taste issues, FASS can spell the difference between finding meals palatable, which keeps the appetite engaged, and losing interest in eating.

"Better," she said.

Then I added just five drops of lemon juice. Yes, this was bitter, but would this tiny amount affect Susan? Again, a taste—and a face.

"I liked it better before," she said.

The audience was astounded that such small amounts could affect the taste of that volume of soup. Then came the clincher: an eighth of a teaspoon (no, that's not a misprint) of maple syrup. Taste. Nod. Grin. "Now that's more like it!" said Susan.

FASS Fixes for Taste Bud Troubles

If your taste buds are saying _____, use this FASS fix.

Things have a metallic taste. Add a little sweetener, like maple syrup or agave nectar, and a squeeze of lemon. You could also try adding fat, such as a nut cream or butter.

Things taste too sweet. Start by adding 6 drops of lemon or lime juice. Keep adding it in small increments until the sweet taste becomes muted.

Things taste too salty. Add 1/4 teaspoon of lemon juice. It erases the taste of salt.

Things taste too bitter. Add a little sweetener, like maple syrup or agave nectar.

Everything tastes like cardboard. Add more sea salt until the flavor of the dish moves toward the front of the mouth. A spritz of fresh lemon juice also helps.

If you are having trouble swallowing or dealing with mouth sores, add fat, such as a nut cream, to your food. Eat blended or pureed foods, such as blended soups, smoothies, and granitas. Stay away from ginger, curry, red pepper flakes, and other strong spices.

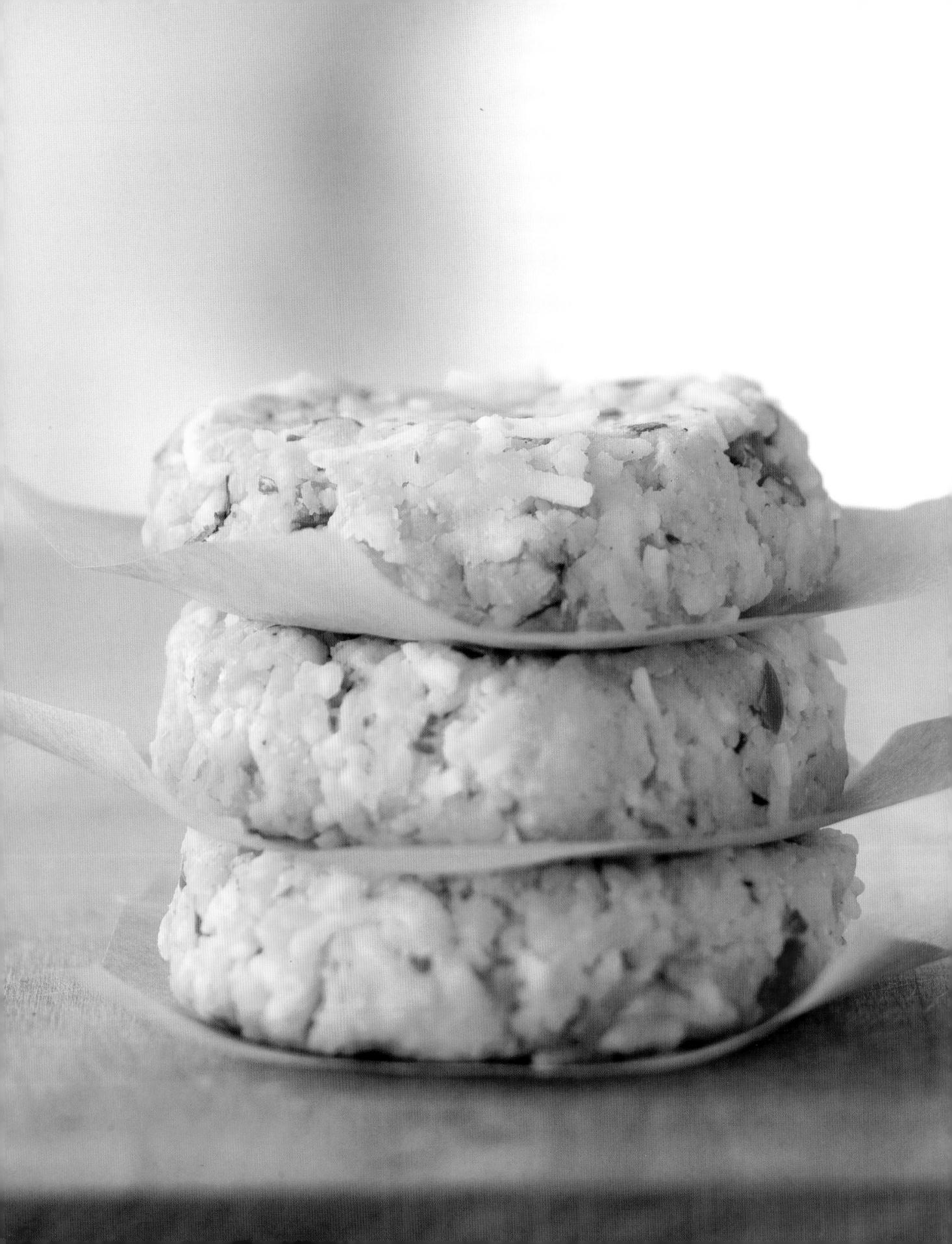

Learning Your Food Preferences

Okay, we've covered some fundamentals about taste, but that's only half the game. An often-ignored part of appetite allure is texture. Let's use mushrooms as an example. People tend to love 'em or hate 'em (in my experience there's rarely a middle ground). And the reason usually has nothing to do with taste; it's the slippery texture they often have once they're cooked.

So how do you figure out taste and texture preferences—whether yours or someone else's? For those in treatment, this isn't an idle question; it's absolutely vital. Sometimes the question "What do you like to eat?" can be so hard to answer. Yet a detailed answer is necessary if people with cancer are to find healthier, more nutritious, and appealing substitutes for the foods they prefer. I've learned that sustainable change only occurs if you meet people where they are, rather than insisting that they start where you'd like them to be. Especially at first, changes to a more healthful diet might have to take place gradually, with lots of hand-holding and understanding. I wouldn't take someone who is basically a meat-and-potatoes guy and expect to perform a culinary coup d'état that lands him in a strict vegan diet. That's counterproductive. It will never last, and he'll resent the change every step of the way. It doesn't matter how nutritious and healthful the new regime is; in the long run, as Chinese medicine and nutrition expert Michael Broffman notes, "If it doesn't taste good and you won't eat it, by definition it can't be good food."

I've come up with a tool that gets to the heart of people's connection or disconnection with food. It's a questionnaire I use during what I call my "culinary intake," an hour-or-so process where I sit down with a new client and their caregivers (usually family members) to get to know the person and his or her situation. It's a fun process—and often funny. I'll ask people what their favorite food is and because they think of me as the "healthy" chef in the room, they'll say something like "Oh, I really like broccoli."

And I'll say, "Really? Broccoli? That's funny, because I love cinnamon jelly beans. Used to eat 'em by the handful."

The only way to get an honest answer is to drop any judgments. The point is to find the person's comfort level and work within those parameters. If someone's straight with me and admits to being a Ding Dong addict, that's fine—great, in fact. Why? Because it tells me they have a sweet tooth. How can I make that work in the person's favor? By remembering to add something a little sweet—a *healthy* sweet—into each meal. For example, I'd be sure to top Velvety Red Lentil Dahl (page 74) with Apricot Pear Chutney (page 175). Similarly, if my interview turns up the fact that a person really likes crunchy foods like pretzel sticks, I'd make darn sure to include croutons or another crunchy topping on every healthy soup.

Doing this accomplishes two nutritional goals, both of which serve people in treatment. First, by including their favorite textures and tastes as often as possible, I'm creating allure to bring them to a dish they might not otherwise try. By giving them that hit of a taste or texture they like, I help them experience the delicious, nutritious nature of the other outstanding foods in the meal. So a woman who wouldn't go near a broccoli stalk suddenly finds herself enjoying creamy broccoli potato soup. Why? Because potatoes, which she likes, are in the foreground, and the broccoli, instead of being presented in chunks—a texture she eschews—is creamy and colorful, a background canvas for the rest of the meal. Put a small shaving of Cheddar on top—another food she craves—and there's no way she'll turn her nose up at this soup. Secondly, by getting that satisfying hit of a taste they like, they won't feel so deprived, making it far less likely that they'll go on a binge.

Many of the questions below are pretty straightforward, but I recommend that you really give them some thought, and even write down your answers. I also recommend paying special attention to one question that may seem a bit unusual: If your taste buds could travel around the world, where would they go? After the questionnaire you'll find a tool I call global flavorprints, which can help you make the most of the insight you gain from this questionnaire.

Discovering Your Culinary Preferences

- Do you have any food allergies, for example, to nuts?
- What are your favorite foods? (Don't hold back; chocolate and jelly beans count!)
- Why do you like them? What, specifically, about them do you like?
- What are your comfort foods, or what foods make you happy?
- If you were banished to a desert island, what's the one food you would take with you and why?
- What kinds of food do you crave and why?
- What are your favorite tastes? If your taste buds could travel around the world, where would they go? Multiple landings are allowed!
- What are your favorite or least favorite textures? Do you enjoy crispy, crunchy, or smooth textures? For example, do you like chunky, hearty soups, or smooth and creamy soups, or both?
- What foods do you not like or not want included in your meals? For example, do you love or hate cilantro?
- What kind of relationship do you have with food? Did you grow up with family members who cooked? Was gathering at the dinner table a happy or upsetting experience?
- Where are your ancestors from?
- Do you have any specific comforting food memories?
- How many meals do you eat a day—small meals more often, or one big meal?

- How do you feel when you're eating? Do you feel nourished and satiated?
- Do you eat to live or live to eat?
- Do you cook or does someone else in your family cook?
- Do you want to cook or be a part of the cooking process?
- If you cook, how often do you cook?
- What are your goals pertaining to food; for example, do you want to become re-inspired or make a transition to new dietary guidelines?

The Power of Herbs and Spices

When it comes to increasing the yum factor of food, nothing does the trick better than herbs and spices. (And as you'll learn below, these flavorful ingredients also have powerful healing properties.) Here's a little tip about how to use herbs and spices to release maximum flavor and phytochemicals. When using dried herbs and spices, don't sprinkle them on at the end. Instead, add them near the beginning of the process, especially if the dish is cooked. The reason? Heat, especially in combination with a bit of fat, like olive oil, breaks down the oils in the spices and releases them into the food. These oils carry much of the taste, and with it the healing benefits of the spice. As far as fresh herbs like cilantro, mint, and parsley are concerned, it's best to add them at the end, to retain maximum flavor and color.

A lot of people I teach are afraid of adding herbs and spices, fearful of overdoing it. Use the recipes in the book as a guide for how much of each herb or spice to add and when. After a while, you'll get a feel for the amounts that work for you. You'll also find that certain groups of spices like to hang out together, as indicated in the following chart of global flavorprints. It lists many of the herbs and spices associated with a variety of popular cuisines. To capture the essence of a cuisine, I generally recommend using three spices from its list. This will allow you to bring the flavors of your favorite restaurants home in far healthier versions to create in your own kitchen.

Global Flavorprints

Italian: Garlic, basil, oregano, parsley, rosemary, bay leaves, nutmeg, fennel seeds, red pepper flakes, marjoram, sage (and mint in Sicilian cooking)

French: Tarragon, chervil, parsley, thyme, rosemary, nutmeg, saffron, bay leaves, garlic, green and pink peppercorns

Spanish: Saffron, paprika, garlic, parsley, cumin seeds

Greek: Oregano, mint, garlic, cinnamon, dill weed, nutmeg

Middle Eastern: Allspice, oregano, marjoram, mint, sesame seeds, garlic, dill weed, cinnamon, cumin seeds, coriander seeds, cilantro, anise seeds

North African (Moroccan): Red pepper flakes, cumin seeds, coriander seeds, cilantro, mint, saffron, garlic, cinnamon, ginger, turmeric

German: Caraway seeds, dill seeds and weed, cinnamon, ginger, nutmeg, white pepper, juniper berries, allspice, mustard seeds

Hungarian: Paprika, poppy seeds, caraway seeds, garlic, white pepper

Russian: Dill weed, cilantro, parsley, mint

Chinese: Ginger, anise seeds, garlic, red pepper flakes, sesame seeds, star anise, five-spice powder (a blend of star anise, Szechuan pepper, cinnamon, fennel, and clove)

Thai: Lemongrass, galangal root, ginger, Thai basil, mint, kaffir lime leaves, lime, curry powder, turmeric, coriander seeds, chiles, garlic, cilantro, five-spice powder, red pepper flakes, bay leaves

Indian: Red pepper flakes, chiles, saffron, mint, cumin seeds, coriander seeds, cilantro, garlic, turmeric, nutmeg, cinnamon, ginger, anise seeds, dill weed, cloves, mace, cardamom seeds, mustard seeds, sesame seeds, fenugreek, curry powder

Mexican: Chiles, oregano, cumin seeds, sesame seeds, cinnamon, cilantro

(This list was adapted from the Information Bureau of the American Spice Trade Association.)

Culinary Pharmacy

Clearly, herbs and spices play an important role in the appeal of food and can help bring reluctant eaters back to the table. But they have other benefits too: an unparalleled concentration of cancer-fighting compounds. Hundreds if not thousands of studies have looked at the effects of various spices or the compounds within them on tumors, cell regeneration, and numerous other biological processes that play a role in determining the effectiveness of cancer treatments. (For a list of some of these studies, consult the Bibliography.)

The following Cancer-Fighting Ingredients section outlines some of these healing properties, everything from cinnamon's ability to keep blood sugar levels stable (which is important because people on chemo can be more prone to insulin swings and diabetes) to curcumin's role in helping regulate nuclear factor kappa B (NF-kB), a protein complex involved in immune and inflammatory processes. Incorrect regulation of NF-kB and inflammation is thought to play a role in many diseases, including cancer. A fantastic study by Dr. Bharat B. Aggarwal at the University of Texas M. D. Anderson Cancer Center shows that many other herbs and spices, including basil, rosemary, cloves, ginger, and fennel contain compounds with similar effects on NF-kB, and that these compounds may actually stop the "master switch" that turns on cancer genes from being activated. Similarly, cancer treatments often tax the immune system, making people more vulnerable to infection and illness from viruses, bacteria, and the like. I've noted the foods that have antiviral and antimicrobial properties, such as rosemary, cloves, and mustard seed, which may offer protective benefits.

One final point about my benchmark for all these citations, namely peer-reviewed scientific studies. You'll see a lot of qualifiers in how I describe the medicinal activity of foods—lots of 'may's and 'could's, as in 'this may help reduce the risk of colon cancer.' There's a reason for this. While the number of studies looking at the food/cancer-fighting connection has exploded over the past ten years, much of the work has been done in the lab or on animals. Promising? Yes. But it's too early in many cases to definitively say that something that works in a mouse will work in humans. Similarly, when studies of human diet show a particular population to be less prone to a certain cancer, it often takes a long time to tease what particular food—and what compound in that food—is responsible. Generally, the greatest amount of study in humans has come with research that looks at antioxidants and beta-carotene and how they affect cancer rates. The newer research, more limited to the lab and animals at this point, looks at phytochemicals—the properties that make up everything in a plant from its pigment to its enzymes—and how they interact when consumed. All this research is, in my opinion, great news. But the fact that the jury is still out in many areas argues—and my medical experts concur—for playing the odds when it comes to eating by consuming a wide-ranging diet. That way, you'll consume more potentially beneficial nutrients, which is really the name of the game.

I like to think of the culinary pharmacy as a shop that's open 24/7, with something in every aisle that can help people thrive during treatment. It's one of my favorite tools in the tool kit. To find recipes that include each ingredient, consult the index.

Cancer-Fighting Ingredients

Agave Nectar: **Anti-inflammatory.** For all its sweetness, agave nectar actually has a lower glycemic index (in other words, sugar content) than many other sweeteners. This makes it an excellent substitute for folks worried about their blood sugar levels during chemotherapy, especially if they're also receiving steroids that affect blood sugar.

Allspice/Allspice Berries: **Digestion aid, antimicrobial.** Allspice is great if you're feeling bloated or gassy, as it relieves indigestion and soothes discomfort, especially in the upper intestines. Its volatile oil component is also a weak antimicrobial agent.

Almonds: **Anti-inflammatory.** Almonds are a fantastic source of fiber, which may help prevent colon cancer. They have twice the antioxidant power with their skins on. They're also good blood sugar regulators, important if you're on chemo or steroids that can elevate blood sugar.

Anise/Aniseed: **Digestion aid, anti-inflammatory, NF-kB regulator.** As a phytoestrogen, that is, a plant (from the Greek *phyto*)-based estrogen, anise can mildly boost production of female sex hormones. Since these hormones are sometimes used to treat prostate cancer in men (to counter the effects of testosterone), there's some medical thought that anise could assist such treatments, though this has yet to be proven conclusively.

Apples: **Anti-inflammatory.** Apples, scientists say, have been shown in the lab to keep liver, breast, and colon cancer cells at bay.

Apricots: **Anti-inflammatory.** Dehydration from treatments can wreak havoc on electrolyte balance. Apricots, wonderful sources of potassium, can help rebalance your system, including regulating your blood pressure. Apricots' iron content, which benefits oxygen transport, keeps hemoglobin and energy levels steady as well.

Asparagus: **Anti-inflammatory.** Inflammation in the body is now thought to contribute to cancer proliferation. Many foods, such as asparagus, have anti-inflammatory properties. In fact, the phytochemicals in asparagus mimic a type of anti-inflammatory called a COX-2 inhibitor. Asparagus is also rich in potential cancer-fighting nutrients such as vitamin A (in lab and animal models it takes on skin, breast, liver, colon, and prostate cancers), vitamin K (prostate and lung cancers), and folic acid (many cancers including colorectal, esophageal, stomach, and breast).

Avocados: **Anti-inflammatory.** The oleic acid that's part of avocado's monounsaturated fats may protect against breast cancer, while other phytochemicals and vitamin E are believed to combat prostate cancer growth. Glutathione, a combination of amino acids abundant in avocados, works as an internal vacuum cleaner, taking carcinogens (outside substances known to promote cancer, such as cigarette smoke) away from healthy cells they can damage. California's Hass avocados have shown promising effects in taking on oral and prostate cancers.

Bananas: The high potassium levels in bananas replace electrolytes that can be lost during treatments. As with apples, they're full of pectin, which soothes the stomach, and their natural fiber sweeps toxins from the intestinal tract, improves bowel function, and lowers the risk of colon cancer.

Barley: **Anti-inflammatory.** A certain percentage of breast cancers and other hormone-dependent cancers is linked to too much estrogen; lignan, a phytochemical in barley, binds with estrogen receptors in the body, which may interfere with estrogen production. As with bananas, barley is a high fiber food, benefiting digestion, and bowel function, and lowering the risk of colon cancer.

Basil: **Digestion aid, anti-inflammatory, antimicrobial, antibacterial, NF-kB regulator.** Radiation destroys cancer cells but can also be harmful to healthy cells. Two flavonoids (chemicals that are part of a plant's metabolism) in basil, orientin and vicenin, protect human cells from radiation damage, as well as oxygen damage (too much oxygen in the cells, also known as free radicals, can be harmful). Basil's oils also have anti-inflammatory effects similar to those found in asparagus. If your taste buds are off, or a sore throat or irritated mouth is affecting taste, basil can have a corrective effect.

Bay Leaf: If you need relief from abdominal cramps and gas, seek out bay leaves. They have a soothing and relaxing effect on the digestive tract, which can be thrown off-kilter by treatment.

Beans and Lentils: **Anti-inflammatory.** Having cancer once can put you at greater risk for recurrence, but beans and lentils can lower the odds. Studies show that diets high in beans or lentils lowered breast cancer recurrence in women. As with many high fiber foods, both lower colon cancer risk. They're also linked to controlling blood sugar and carrying toxins from the body, both of which are important when undergoing treatment. They are fantastic sources of protein and numerous minerals including phosphorus, iron, protein, and the impossible to pronounce molybdenum, which, when deficient in the body, has been linked to stomach and esophageal cancers.

Beets: **Anti-inflammatory.** The rich red color of beets comes from the phytochemical betacyanin; studies show that it combines with the fiber in beets to fight colon cancer. Beet fiber is also unusual in that it helps increase levels of glutathione, which cleanses toxins from cells and the bloodstream.

Bell Peppers: **Anti-inflammatory.** Lycopene—also found in tomatoes—along with vitamin C and lots of fiber in bell peppers may offer protection against colon, cervical, bladder, prostate, and pancreatic cancers. The vitamin A–promoting carotenoid beta-cryptoxanthin works its wonders against lung cancer, lowering the risk of development. A host of antioxidants, including vitamins A, C, K, folic acid, and B_6, also absorbs cancer-causing free radicals.

Black Pepper: **Digestion aid, antibacterial, NF-kB regulator.** Black pepper stimulates the taste buds to signal the stomach to produce hydrochloric acid, which aids digestion. The outer layer of peppercorns also contains piperine, an alkaloid that increases the body's ability to assimilate cancer-fighting nutrients including beta-carotene, curcumin, and selenium. The National Cancer Institute says piperine also may have anti-inflammatory and antitumor properties.

Blueberries: **Anti-inflammatory.** Blueberries rule when it comes to anticancer properties. Their phytochemicals include ellagic acid, which interferes with the metabolic pathways that feed certain cancers. Another ingredient, kaempferol, can help reduce risk of pancreatic cancer. Another set of acids, called phenols, causes colon cells to self-destruct. Blueberries are also high in pectin (see Bananas).

Brazil Nuts: **Anti-inflammatory.** Brazil nuts contain high amounts of selenium, which helps fight colon and prostate cancers. The American Cancer Society notes that another Brazil nut antioxidant, quercetin, may trigger cell death in certain cancer cells.

Broccoli: **Anti-inflammatory, antibacterial.** Sulforaphane, a well-studied phytochemical in broccoli, appears to slow the growth of leukemia and melanoma. Another metabolite, glucosinolate, can inhibit breast and cancer growth. When broccoli and tomatoes are eaten together, their cancer-fighting capabilities are more powerful because their active compounds work on different anti-cancer pathways.

Buckwheat: **Anti-inflammatory.** Another grain that eases digestion, buckwheat has a high fiber content that regulates bowel function and carries toxins quickly and efficiently out of the body, which may help decrease the risk of colon cancer.

Cabbage: **Anti-inflammatory, antibacterial.** Cabbage, along with cruciferous kin such as cauliflower, kale, Brussels sprouts, broccoli, bok choy, and turnips, is extremely high in anticancer phytochemicals. One such property, indole-3-carbinol (called I3C for short), nearly doubles how quickly the liver can break down estrogen so it doesn't remain in the body. Cooking cabbage for the right amount of time (in other words, not too long) is important to retain a compound called sinigrin, which reacts with an enzyme to release molecules that detoxify carinogens and inhibit the division and growth of tumor cells.

Cantaloupe: **Anti-inflammatory.** Studies at Kansas State showed that a carcinogen in cigarette smoke depletes vitamin A, which may lead to emphysema and lung inflammation. Cantaloupes, a rich source of vitamin A, can help make up for this deficiency in those exposed to second hand smoke. The American Cancer Society also suggests eating melons to protect against colorectal cancer.

Caraway: **Appetite stimulant, digestion aid, NF-kB regulator.** Like the peel of an orange, caraway contains the volatile oil limonene, which has been shown to protect against breast, skin, liver, and lung cancers in animals. It also has long been used to promote appetite and soothe digestion.

Cardamom: **Digestion aid, anti-inflammatory, NF-kB regulator.** A favorite of practitioners of Chinese medicine, cardamom is used to treat a whole host of digestive issues common to people on chemotherapy, including constipation, gas, and stomachaches. Just chewing on cardamom seeds can ease indigestion and brighten the breath. Indian animal studies offered preliminary evidence that cardamom may reduce inflammation and protect against growth of colon cancer cells.

Carrots: **Anti-inflammatory.** Studies show that just a carrot a day could cut lung cancer risk in half. That's probably due to their extremely high vitamin A content, which is vital to promoting lung health. They're also rich in beta-carotene (that's what accounts in part for their beautiful orange color), which is associated with preventing lung, mouth, throat, stomach, intestinal, bladder, prostate, and breast cancers.

Cashews: Cashews provide a rich source of copper, which is important because copper deficiency is associated with increased risk of colon cancer. Like avocados (see page 30), they're also high in oleic acid, an anticancer component of monounsaturated fat.

Cauliflower: **Anti-inflammatory.** See Cabbage.

Cayenne and Chili Flakes: **Appetite stimulant, digestion aid, anti-inflammatory, antibacterial.** Capsaicin protects chili peppers from disease, and may also extend its protective properties to humans. Studies show that it decreases PSA levels—that's the antigen whose level normally rises as prostate cancer develops. Capsaicin may also prevent stomach cancer and perhaps affect the spread of brain and spinal cord tumors known as gliomas.

Celery: **Anti-inflammatory.** Coumarin are radar-like phytochemicals that help white blood cells seek out potentially harmful cells, in this case cancer cells and the free radicals that cause normal cells to mutate into a cancerous state. Celery's coumarins help to prevent free radicals from damaging cells, thereby decreasing the mutations that can cause cells to become cancerous. In addition, acetylinic compounds in celery can stop the growth of tumor cells.

Cherries: **Anti-inflammatory.** The tartness in cherries comes from perillyl alcohol, which, studies suggest, deprives cancer of the proteins it needs to flourish. It's done well in lab studies against advanced breast, prostate, and ovarian cancers. Two other cherry phytochemicals, isoquercitrin and quercetin, inhibit colon cancer cells.

Chicken: Organic, free-range fowl such as chickens are nice sources of niacin and selenium, both of which have cancer-preventive qualities. Selenium is like a DNA repair kit that induces cancer cells to stop functioning and replicating, especially colon and prostate cancer cells.

Chickpeas: **Anti-inflammatory.** Aside from being a fantastic source of protein, chickpeas are good regulators of blood sugar and cholesterol, which can be affected by treatments. As with other high fiber veggies, chickpeas help flush toxins from the body and may reduce colon cancer risk.

Chives: **Anti-inflammatory, antibacterial.** Eat a lot of chives and studies say you'll help decrease your risk of stomach and colon cancers. The magic ingredient appears to be sulfur; it's abundant in chives and helps carry carcinogens out of the body.

Chocolate: **Anti-inflammatory.** We know about the incredible psychological benefits of chocolate, but it's a physiological powerhouse as well. Chemically, the body literally sucks in chocolate's nutrients, especially flavonoids (that's the proanthcyanidins), which have chemoprotective effects. If you want to get the most bang for your chocolate buck, eat dark chocolate: It has four times the antioxidants found in tea.

Cilantro and Coriander: **Digestion aid, anti-inflammatory, antimicrobial, antibacterial, NF-kB regulator.** Cilantro packs a punch in the lab; its antimicrobial and antibacterial properties have taken out salmonella under the microscope. With regard to chemo treatments, cilantro is good if you have an upset stomach or nausea, as it relieves both. It's been shown to help with general anxiety.

Cinnamon: **Appetite stimulant, digestion aid, anti-inflammatory, antimicrobial, antibacterial, NF-kB regulator.** One of my favorite spices for soothing the stomach, cinnamon—or more precisely one of its compounds, cinnamaldehyde—lessens inflammation associated with certain cancers. For those on steroids during chemotherapy, cinnamon also helps to keep blood sugar levels balanced, while its antioxidant and calcium/fiber combination lowers cholesterol and reduces the risk of colon cancer.

Cloves: **Digestion aid, anti-inflammatory, antibacterial, NF-kB regulator.** The kaempferol in cloves (and also in almonds, Brazil nuts, and broccoli) may especially benefit women: Human studies show that a higher kaempferol intake lowered ovarian cancer risk. As with cinnamon, cloves aid digestion. Cloves also contain a wonderful oil, eugenol, that seems to throw up a shield against digestive cancers, offering anti-inflammatory benefits while attacking toxicities from environmental pollutants. Another phytochemical, rhamnetin, kicks up clove's antioxidant factor.

Coconut Milk and Coconut Oil: **Anti-inflammatory, antimicrobial, antibacterial.** Coconut is a great antibiotic. Half of its saturated fat content comes from lauric acid, which the body converts into monolaurin, a powerful antibacterial and antiviral compound. Monolaurin is the absolute enemy of many disease-causing germs, and may play a role in attacking cancer as well.

Corn: Cornell researchers found that the longer they cooked sweet corn on high heat, the more antioxidants were released from the kernels' fibers and walls. This included ferulic acid, which appears to have cancer-fighting properties. Beta-cryptoxanthin, a corn carotenoid partly responsible for its lovely color, also may lower the risk for lung cancer.

Cranberries: **Anti-inflammatory.** No fruit is better at inhibiting the growth of liver cancer cells in humans. Many of cranberry's compounds appear to be toxic to other cancer cells, while leaving healthy cells alone. This includes lung, cervical, prostate, and breast cancers, as well as leukemia. New studies say that whole cranberries may also target skin, lung, and brain cancers.

Cumin: **Appetite stimulant, digestion aid, antimicrobial, NF-kB regulator.** Like many spices used in Indian and Asian cooking, cumin has received increased laboratory attention for its potential cancer-fighting activities. Studies looking into cumin seeds showed a potential ability to slow down the growth of stomach and cervical tumors. Other studies suggest that it's good for an upset stomach and relieving cramping, especially when the seeds are toasted.

Dates: Some of the sugars found in Libyan dates were shown to have potent antitumor properties. Another sugar, beta-D-glucan, regulates cholesterol and blood sugar levels by slowing down gut absorption of glucose.

Edamame: **Anti-inflammatory.** Edamame (or soybeans) jumpstart the immune system, and in one study soybeans kept cancer from developing in animals exposed to carcinogens. Their isoflavones act like roadblocks, starving cancer cells by preventing the formation of new blood vessels in the body.

Eggs: **Anti-inflammatory.** A huge study of 121,000 women suggested that eating three eggs a week during adolescence dropped the risk of breast cancer by 18 percent. Other components of eggs, such as choline and lecithin, improve brain and gallbladder function.

Fennel: **Digestion aid, anti-inflammatory, NF-kB regulator.** Fennel is good for the stomach because it's very soothing, while anethole—a compound that largely accounts for fennel's licorice aroma—lowers inflammation that may affect the development of cancer cells.

Flaxseeds: **Anti-inflammatory.** Flaxseeds are perhaps the best source in nature for lignans, a phytoestrogen that may help women who are dealing with estrogen-sensitive breast cancer by blocking estrogen receptor sites in the body.

Garlic: **Anti-inflammatory, antimicrobial, antibacterial.** Allicin, a compound in garlic that's also found in onions, accounts for garlic's pungeant smell and cancer-protective punch, especially with regard to colon cancer. A strong antibacterial and antiviral compound, allicin appears to keep carcinogens from affecting healthy colon cells.

Ginger: **Nausea reducer, anti-inflammatory, antibacterial, NF-kB regulator.** Even your grandmother knew that ginger was good for nausea and an upset stomach; that effect is increased when it's consumed with some protein, which can be especially helpful for chemotherapy-induced nausea. Ginger's active component, spicy gingerol, controlled the growth of human bowel cancer cells in animal models.

Green Tea: **Anti-inflammatory.** Green tea's polyphenols appear to help keep carcinogens inactive in the body; they seem to have the greatest effect blocking cancers of the gastrointestinal tract, though they may also help prevent breast, prostate, and lung cancers. One potentially negative note: In a 2009 study, USC researchers found that some compounds in green tea, notably EGCG, appeared to block the anticancer action of the drug Velcade (also known as Bortezomib), used for multiple myeloma treatment. They suggested that patients taking this drug might want to avoid green tea.

Halibut: **Anti-inflammatory.** The omega-3 fatty acids found in fish such as halibut have great health-promoting properties. A few servings a week of fish rich in omega-3 fatty acids could reduce the risk of cancers including non-Hodgkin's lymphoma, multiple myeloma, and childhood leukemia. This protection may extend to common forms of kidney cancer, as well as colon, breast, prostate, and lung cancers.

Honey: **Antimicrobial.** Most of the health buzz around honey comes from propolis, a resin-like substance that bees use to seal off unused combs in the hive. Animal studies have found that propolis has antimicrobial and anticancer factors. It also aids liver function.

Kale: **Anti-inflammatory.** Brassicas, the family of crucerifous vegetables that includes kale, contain loads of a compound called indole-3-carbinol. Animal studies in particular are looking at the compound's ability to change the way estrogen metabolizes. That could affect estrogen-sensitive tissues, perhaps preventing lesions from turning cancerous or keeping cancer cells from proliferating.

Kombu: The presence of chlorophyllins in sea vegetables such as kombu may offer benefits to those dealing with breast cancer. Kombu also contains lignans (as do edamame and barley), which may prevent cancer from spreading beyond its original site.

Kudzu: Kudzu, a vine, and its vegetable offshoot may have many medicinal properties. Among its phytochemicals are daidzin and genistin, which in animal studies slowed the development of prostate cancer.

Leeks: **Anti-inflammatory, antibacterial.** Leeks, like their kin onions and garlic, are linked to a reduced risk of colon and prostate cancers. Kaempferol (which is also present in almonds, Brazil nuts, and cloves) may offer some protection with regard to development of ovarian cancer.

Lemongrass: Native to India, lemongrass is known for its powerful citrus taste. This comes in part from citral, an oil also found in lemon peel, that's an infection fighter and muscle relaxant. It's great if you're dealing with cramps or muscle-related headaches.

Lemons: **Anti-inflammatory, antimicrobial.** The high vitamin C content in citrus fruits helps the immune system stay strong. Additionally, citrus provides the body with several anti-inflammatory and anticancer compounds, including limonene (in the zest), which promotes cell death in cancer cells. Liminoids are helpful if you're dealing with cancers of the skin, lung, breast, colon, stomach, or mouth.

Limes: **Anti-inflammatory, antimicrobial.** Limes not only brighten up your taste buds, but they may boost white blood cell activity as well. Studies show that lime juice may help fight infections related to cancer, while lime sugars known as glycosides have demonstrated the ability to stop division of some cancer cells.

Mangoes: This fruit has many helpful properties, but it's especially important for the gallbladder; regular mango eaters reduce their risk for gallbladder cancer by up to 60 percent. Mango extract may also keep healthy cells from turning cancerous.

Maple Syrup, Grade B: Maple syrup contains lots of zinc, which is good because the prostate concentrates more zinc than any other organ in the body, but if you're low on zinc, your risk for prostate cancer goes up.

Millet: **Anti-inflammatory.** Millet contains laetrile (another name for amygdalin), which in the 1980s was touted by some as being a miracle cure for cancer; science quickly disproved that, and laetrile was discredited. But at least one recent study suggests that amygdalin may have some beneficial properties after all, especially the ability to induce cell death in prostate cancer cells. Millet's high fiber also cleans out the bowel, which may decrease colon cancer risk.

Mint: **Digestion aid, antimicrobial, NF-kB regulator.** Mint is more than a great-tasting ingredient; it can actually make foods that don't taste quite right more palatable to the taste buds. It's also quite effective in relieving indigestion. As with cherries, mint contains perillyl alcohol, which in the lab stalls growth of liver, mammary, and pancreatic tumors. Mint is also loaded with vitamin C and beta-carotene, which lower colorectal cancer risk.

Mushrooms: **Anti-inflammatory.** Shiitake, maitake, and reishi mushrooms all appear to pump up the body's immune system, potentially making it more resistant to cancer. The secrets may lay in their sugars—polysaccharides, to be precise—especially lentinan. Gastric cancer cells that were exposed to lentinan literally disintegrated. Another compound, lectin, stopped cancer cell division in its tracks. Some mushrooms also trigger the body's ability to create interferon, which can help chemotherapy do its job more effectively.

Mustard Seed: **Appetite stimulant, digestion aid.** Mustard seed contains sulfur and nitrogen compounds known as glucosinolates, which break down into isothiocynates that slow down cancer growth in the GI tract and colon. Mustard seed also has a nice hit of selenium, which may offer protection against prostate cancer. On the tongue, mustard prompts salivation, which in turn promotes appetite. And it can help prevent indigestion.

Nutmeg: **Appetite stimulant, digestion aid, nausea reducer, anti-inflammatory, antibacterial, NF-kB regulator.** Preliminary studies suggest that one of nutmeg's compounds, myristicin (also found in parsley), might prompt tumor-fighting ability in the body.

Olives/Olive Oil: **Anti-inflammatory, antibacterial.** The abundance of vitamin E and monounsaturated fats in olive oil translates into lowered colon cancer rates, while the oleic acid in olive oil cuts gene expression of a particular breast-cancer gene by 46 percent.

Onions: **Anti-inflammatory, antibacterial.** Onions—shallots, in particular—were effective in taking on leukemia in animal studies. Onion extract also showed antitumor properties, possibly because it helps carcinogens leave the body quickly.

Oranges: **Anti-inflammatory, antimicrobial.** Citrus helps against many cancers, notably mouth, throat, and stomach cancers. Indiana University researchers found that some of the oils in citrus, called monoterpenes, help eat up carcinogens in animals, slowing tumor growth. Vitamin C, which is abundant in oranges, has been associated with cutting colon cancer risk.

Oregano: **Digestion aid, anti-inflammatory, antimicrobial, antibacterial, NF-kB regulator.** Two antioxidants in oregano, thymol and rosmarinic acid (found in rosemary as well), scavenge for oxygen molecules that, left to their own devices, could damage healthy cells and lead to cancerous changes. Oregano is also a good source of antibacterial and antimicrobial agents, which are helpful when your immune system is being taxed by treatment.

Papayas: Nitrosamines, which are often found in the soil and in processed foods, can cause cancer, but vitamin C may negate this effect. Other papaya vitamins, such as folic acid and vitamin E, have cancer-fighting properties, and the fruit's high fiber content can reduce colon cancer risk. Papayas are also a good source of lycopene, more commonly associated with tomatoes (see page 40).

Parsley: **Appetite stimulant, digestion aid, anti-inflammatory, NF-kB regulator.** As with oregano, parsley's oils, such as myristicin, have strong antitumor properties, especially with regard to lung tumors. Parsley also appears to neutralize particular types of carcinogens, like the benzopyrenes that are present in cigarette smoke, charcoal grill smoke, and fried foods.

Parsnips: An active ingredient in parsnips called psoralen shows promise for cancer treatment. Because light appears to trigger its activity, it has been used in drug form, in combination with UV light, to treat skin nodules of a type of lymphoma. Parsnips also have a high fiber content, which is good for staying regular.

Peppermint: **Digestion aid, nausea reducer, anti-inflammatory, antibacterial.** Mint makes our entire GI tract happy, from the tip of the tongue to the bottom of the stomach. It's an extremely useful herb, which relaxes abdominal and stomach muscles, making it great for relieving cramps, decreasing gas, and aiding overall digestion.

Pineapple: **Anti-inflammatory.** It turns out there's more to pineapple than a sweet taste and a load of vitamin C. Australian scientists looking at one of pineapple's enzymes, bromelain, found two molecules that block cancer-related proteins and turn on immune cells that then attack cancer cells in animals. The researchers found this combination most effective in taking on lung, ovarian, bowel, and breast cancers.

Potatoes: Vitamin B_6 in potatoes appears to control activation of a tumor-suppression gene, which is like turning on a power switch with the potential to zap cancer. And potatoes may have an overall detoxifying effect, as other compounds present seek out cancer-causing free-radicals.

Quinoa: **Anti-inflammatory.** Quinoa contains lignans; in the body, the gut converts lignans into enterolactone, which some scientists believe mimics estrogen, but in a way that might protect against hormone-dependent breast cancer.

Radishes: **Anti-inflammatory.** Eating a radish gives your liver some love. The sulfur compounds in radishes go right to the liver and gallbladder, increasing the flow of bile to maintain organ health and, as a nice by-product, improving digestion.

Raisins: The phenolic activity in raisins is simply phenomenal when it comes to controlling some cancers in animals. Cornell researchers found that mice that were fed a phenol-rich diet had a 70 percent reduction in intestinal tumors. These same phenols have excellent antioxidant action.

Raspberries: **Anti-inflammatory.** Certain pigments in raspberries, called anthocyanidins, kick-start a process that blocks the ability of tumors to grow. Ohio State researchers also found that black raspberries in particular prevented the beginning of esophageal cancer in animals and interfered with precancerous growths that already existed.

Rice: **Anti-inflammatory.** Rice derived from whole grains, such as brown rice, is a fantastic source of fiber and may also protect premenopausal women against breast cancer, particularly those who are overweight. Whole grain rice fiber can also reduce colon cancer risk.

Rosemary: **Digestion aid, anti-inflammatory, NF-kB regulator.** One of rosemary's antioxidants, carnosol, inhibited skin and breast tumor development in animals. Rosemary has salutary effects on people as well, improving digestion, circulation, and immune function. It even gets the blood flowing to the brain.

Saffron: **Digestion aid, anti-inflammatory, NF-kB regulator.** A pigment in saffron, crocin, seems to convince human cancer cells to induce their own death—including leukemia and liver cancer cells. Saffron is also great if you're having trouble digesting.

Sage: Another member of the mint family, sage is similar to rosemary in many of its medicinal properties. An extract of its essential oils is being highly investigated by cancer researchers who believe it may have therapeutic benefits.

Salmon: **Anti-inflammatory.** Researchers think that fatty fish like salmon have compounds that trip a series of cellular reactions leading to the release of ceramide, which could be a key factor in cell metabolism—it may tell cells, especially cancer cells, when it's time to stop functioning. Salmon's selenium may also offer protection against colon and pancreatic cancers.

Sea Salt: **Appetite stimulant.** Unlike table salt, which is generally stripped of minerals and to which iodine is added, sea salt contains numerous essential minerals, including calcium, magnesium, and potassium. Aside from its cooking benefits, sea salt is a wonderful source of elements that you don't always get in your diet.

Sesame Seeds: **Anti-inflammatory.** As with flaxseeds, sesame seeds are rich in lignans, which may offer protection against hormone-related cancers. Similarly, sesame seeds are rich in gamma-tocopherols (a form of vitamin E), which studies say may help men dealing with prostate cancer.

Spelt: **Anti-inflammatory.** Unique among grains, spelt contains the tongue-twisting sugars known as mucopolysaccharides, which play a role in connective tissues such as cartilage. These same sugars invigorate the immune system and assist in blood clotting.

Spinach: Spinach carotenoids may offer help in taking on human prostate cancer, while another by-product, kaempferol, is being looked at with regard to lowering ovarian cancer risk. Spinach extracts are also being researched for their ability to inhibit stomach cancer cells from dividing.

Squash: Research on squash is not extensive, but preliminary reports suggest that the juice from squash may limit the ability of healthy cells to mutate into a cancerous state. Generally speaking, the fiber in squash, particularly winter squash, is thought to offer colon-cleansing benefits.

Star Anise: **Antimicrobial.** A popular food in Asia, Chinese star anise's (*Illicium verum*) oils contain anethole, which has antimicrobial properties. It's traditionally been used as a stimulant, as an expectorant, and to aid digestion.

Strawberries: **Anti-inflammatory.** As with raspberries, strawberries are loaded with anthocyanidins that inhibit tumor growth, as well as ellagitannins, which appear to have similar health benefits. (In one study, ellagitannins taken from pomegranates limited the growth of prostate cancer in the lab.) Strawberries also slow the growth of liver cancer cells.

Sweet Potatoes and Yams: Those beautiful orange-yellows of yams and sweet potatoes are the tip-off that these vegetables are loaded with cancer-fighting beta-carotene and vitamin C. One note: Wild yams created concern for a time among medical professionals because of their alleged ability to affect estrogen levels (they were thought for a time to be an alternative to hormone replacement therapy). More recent studies show no such link between yams and estrogen levels.

Swiss Chard: **Anti-inflammatory.** Perhaps one of the most powerful cancer-fighting foods, Swiss chard is loaded with beta-carotene, fiber, and vitamins A and C. Betalain, a pigment in Swiss chard, is also being studied for potential anticancer properties.

Thyme: **Antimicrobial, antibacterial.** Think of thyme as nature's version of a throat lozenge. Soothing to the mouth and oral cavity in general, it's also helpful with nagging coughs and congestion. It also has antiseptic and antibacterial properties.

Tomatoes: Tomatoes contain the powerful antioxidant lycopene. Put that antioxidant together with a healthy oil (such as olive oil) and the combination reduces risk for cancers of the pancreas, prostate, breast, and colon. Speaking of prostate cancer, it appears that eating tomatoes and broccoli together has a synergistic protective effect.

Turmeric: **Appetite stimulant, digestion aid, anti-inflammatory, NF-kB regulator.** When turmeric is consumed with a crucerifous vegetable, the curcumin in turmeric lowered the growth of prostate tumors as well as the tumors' ability to spread to other parts of the body. Curcumin is also an anti-inflammatory. Traditional eastern Indian medicine, also known as Ayurveda, has long used turmeric for digestive disorders.

Walnuts: **Anti-inflammatory.** Walnuts contain ellagic acid (as do many berries), which caused cancer cells to self-destruct in the lab. It also appears to limit estrogen's growth potential regarding breast cancer cells and it may help the liver to remove cancer-causing elements in the blood.

Yogurt: Plain yogurt, especially when fortified with probiotics such as lactobacillus, can moderate diarrhea and fight GI tract infections. It can also help keep the immune system strong.

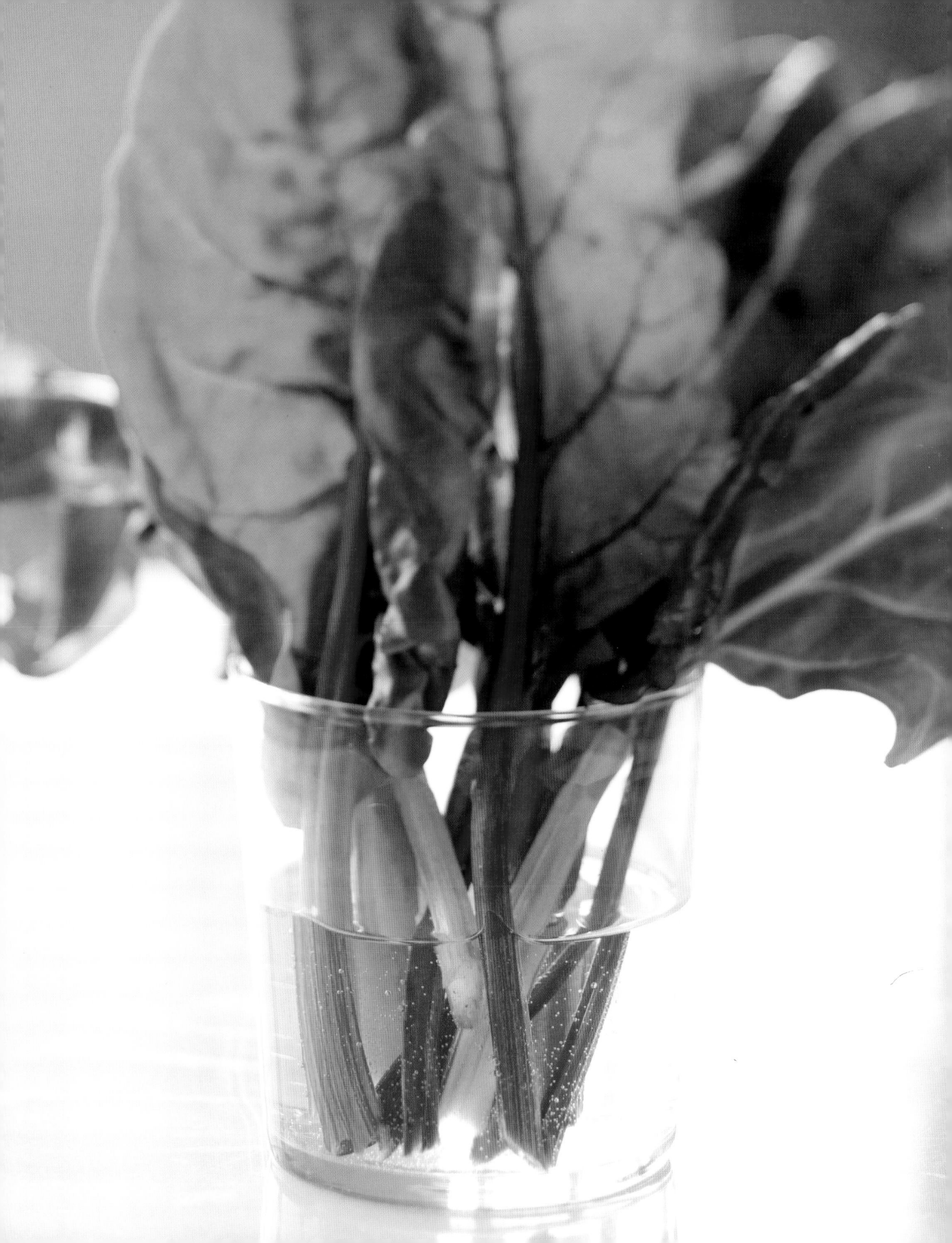

CHAPTER 2

Strategies for Thriving during Treatment

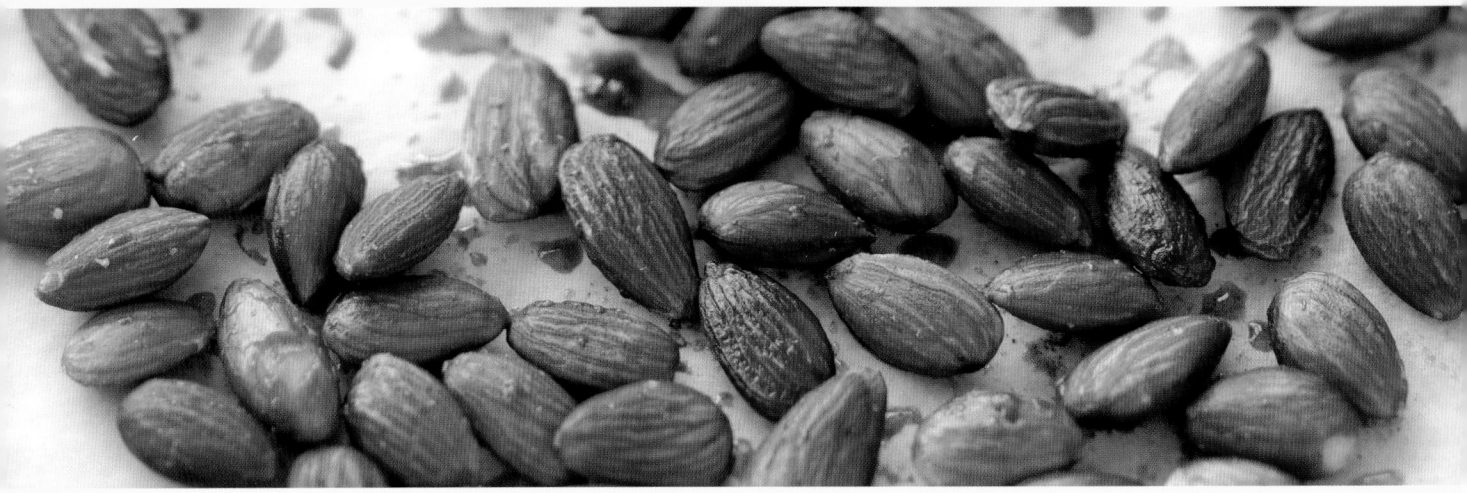

43 *Being Open to Receiving Support*

45 *Optimizing Nutrition*

47 *The Benefits of Exercise and a Healthy Attitude*

50 *Kitchen Smarts*

Cancer treatment can be a daunting process. Remember, the goal is to come through it with body and soul intact. To that end, there's one piece of advice I want to offer above all others: Please don't try to go it alone. I know how hard this is for many people. A cancer diagnosis is so frightening and can threaten the foundation of your self-image. In the days following a diagnosis, you may feel you're drowning in confusing torrents of information and emotion. A bewildering array of treatment options and potential consequences may tie you in knots as you try to make some sense of this thunderbolt striking deep in your life and reverberating off everyone and everything you hold dear.

That is a whole lot of shaking going on. Like most people caught in an emotional earthquake, you may feel one of two instinctive desires: to pull a blanket over your head and duck for cover, or to run out of the house and flee the situation as quickly as possible. Unfortunately, neither reaction will work as well as it might in a real earthquake.

But don't despair! I'm going to show you how to put together a support team no matter what your circumstances. Don't think that asking for support is a sign of weakness; you think Neil Armstrong walked on the moon by himself? Your support team can help you accomplish the all-important goal of staying well nourished during treatment. Equally as important, the team approach will keep your family, your friends, and, most importantly, *you* from feeling overwhelmed or fatigued. It's important to avoid burnout, because treatment and caregiving can go on for quite some time.

Being Open to Receiving Support

Think of creating a support team as a business investment, with team members being your capital. I'm sure you've seen businesses fail not because the idea wasn't great, but because the owners hadn't raised enough capital to get the company up and running properly. By raising your human capital first—the right number of people doing jobs they like and organized to make the best use of their time and energy—you can make sure someone always has your back, at least in terms of meals. And good organization will be a great relief to you because you'll know that those who are helping you aren't being drained or burned-out in the process.

This may sound funny coming from a nice Jewish girl, but it's all about letting go of the guilt—and maybe some pride as well. A lot of people who get a cancer diagnosis feel guilty, or believe that they brought the disease on themselves in some way. Not only is that kind of thinking self-defeating, it can interfere with your recovery. According to Lenore Lefer, a psychotherapist who works with cancer patients and their families, "The best thing for a healing experience is a very positive, loving inner experience." This isn't some sort of new age philosophy; stress actually increases levels of corticosteroids, hormones that can impair immune function. While cancer by its very nature can be an emotional roller-coaster ride, Lefer says it's important to try to manage the stress. "When you're in a healthier frame of mind, your cancer has a harder time being present."

Hopefully I've sold you on the idea of creating a support team. Now you're probably wondering how best to go about it. The place to start is a serious discussion with your significant other or whoever is likely to be your point person for the endeavor. This is usually a spouse or partner, but it can be a child, parent, friend, or neighbor. If you're used to taking care of yourself or if you live alone, this is the time to reach out to support groups or other organizations that can help, be they spiritual, fraternal, or community resources or social service providers in your area.

Regardless of who the point person for your culinary team will be, the conversation will be much the same and should focus on clearly defining roles, as it's almost impossible to drive when two or more people have their hands on the steering wheel.

Cancer nutrition specialist and registered dietician Suzanne Dixon provides a good perspective on this issue: "I used to see people in my clinic practically coming to blows over whether the caregiver was doing what they thought they should be doing and whether the patient was doing what they thought they were supposed to be doing. I'd see a patient and he'd say, 'She's always trying to cram food down my throat. I don't feel like eating, and she's shoving food under my nose and I feel sick!' And then the caregiver would say, 'I fixed him this wonderful milkshake and I put in everything that he asked for, and then he wouldn't touch it. He wouldn't even look at it. And he knows he's doing it just to be an ass!'"

The truth is, just as patients need to let go of guilt and pride to prosper, caregivers need to temper their neuroses. It's so easy, and incredibly unproductive, for caregivers, especially spouses, to look at a cancer diagnosis as the ultimate judgment of their caregiving skills. They project all of their fears of possible loss onto the patient, thinking "If I don't do this perfectly, I'm going to lose this person. Then what will become of me?" The hypervigilance that results can be suffocating, and loved ones can turn into combatants firing repeated first strikes, rather than cooperative collaborators. Where's the joy in that?

As strange as it sounds, there can be great healing of not just the body but the heart and spirit during treatment. An outpouring of support—even something as seemingly everyday as dropping by with food—can provide an uplifting counterbalance when you're feeling down. "Patients see how many people love them, how many people are willing to come and visit and bring meals," says Lenore Lefer. "It encourages them to open up to love, hope, and nourishment in ways they might not have before." Lefer has watched as patients embrace the help they're receiving, and in the process become more interested in their health and looking toward the future. "People begin a meditation or yoga practice; they start things that enhance the quality of their life even though they're sick," she says.

Reconciliations, recognition of roads you might rather have taken, and even movement in that direction aren't the first things that pop into mind when you think of a cancer diagnosis, yet they are real. Perhaps they confirm the Chinese concept of crisis—written in their language as two characters. One signifies peril or danger. But it's the other character that I choose to pay attention to. It signifies opportunity—opportunity for change, for nourishment, for happiness, for community. For a chance—not a guarantee, mind you, but a chance—to embrace life even while in the throes of serious illness.

Optimizing Nutrition

Okay, enough philosophy. If the name of the game is eating well during treatment, what exactly does that mean and how are you going to get there? Succinctly, these are the goals:

- Switching from fewer, large meals to smaller, more frequent nourishment
- Having a wide variety of prepared food always available, 24/7, so you can eat whenever the mood strikes, including during treatment sessions or hospital stays (for the best way to store and transport food, take a peek at Kitchen Smarts on page 50).
- Creating a stimulating environment that engages you in enjoyable mental and physical activities, which will lead to improved appetite
- Organizing the team so that everyone benefits from the effort, instead of exhausting themselves or ending up at each other's throats

Now let's look at the details. Many experts say that instead of looking at three large meals a day, the goal should be less food more often. How much more? UCSF oncology nurse Theresa Koetters says, "I try to preach six small meals a day, using a small plate so it's not overwhelming. Take just three bites." If Koetters's suggestion sounds impossible, just think of all the times in a day you reach for food—we're talking anything from a pretzel to a potato. That makes it pretty easy to come up with six.

For someone whose appetite is lagging, the best advice I received in researching this book was that sheep have it right. You never see ewes sitting down to a three-course meal. They graze, and that's the best approach for anyone whose appetite is on the wane. Instead of chowing down, just try nibbling throughout the day, especially those days when the thought of food doesn't exactly appeal. It's not the amount that matters, it's the attempt.

Suzanne Dixon says, "I tell my patients, 'Just set your watch alarm to go off every fifteen or twenty minutes, and then take literally one bite of food. Then go about your business. Twenty minutes later, take another bite of food and again go about your business. Because no matter what's going on—taste changes, nausea, or just plain lack of appetite—you can probably tolerate a bite here and there. You have to let go of what constitutes normal eating for you. You have to be flexible.'"

Some of my clients, those who like to make lists and check off items as they go through their day, really enjoy the challenge of getting in their six "good bites" a day. A friend who was helping her father when he was sick says he carried around a little clipboard and faithfully marked off what he had eaten and when. Another woman I know takes a thermos to work with her so she has something nutritious to sip on all day: Some days it contains mineral broth or soup, other days tea, and sometimes a protein-rich smoothie.

That brings up an important point: Lots of people work during treatment. With a little planning, it's easy to get lots of nourishment on the job (and I don't mean out of a vending machine). If you have a refrigerator and microwave at work, you can easily bring a reheatable meal from home. Take a look at chapter 6, Anytime Foods. It includes a section on foods that are especially portable, like wraps and spiced toasted nuts. The only problem you might run into is moochy office mates who try to hone in on your goodies.

Of course, work isn't the only situation that might take you away from home for an extended period of time. Sometimes treatment takes a long time, and sometimes a stay in the hospital is unavoidable. Talk about disconnecting from delicious, nourishing food! "You love your patients," says Gerry Mullin, MD, "and when you see what they're fed in the hospital, the junk, it's just heartbreaking, especially because their appetites are gone to begin with." Typical hospital food is so devastatingly unappetizing that it directly contradicts the crucial message "Eat! Eat!!" touted by more progressive doctors. In the hospital setting the food is undesirable at best.

But it doesn't have to be that way. In terms of food, even the hospital setting can allow for an affirmation of health as opposed to a constant reminder of illness. Few hospitals have regulations against bringing food in (and if they do, switch hospitals the first chance you get). If you plan on having food brought in during a hospital stay, I suggest using a large thermal carafe or airpot, which can keep large amounts of liquids hot or cold for hours. Then all you'll need is a good supply of paper cups and napkins, and you can reach for nourishment whenever the mood hits. If you have meals brought in, my suggestion is to do so in a way that will make the nurses love you: using disposable paper plates and cups and plastic utensils, and having your support people take the garbage away. Depending on what you're eating and your relationship with the nursing staff, you might want to have a little extra food on hand for whoever is on duty. If you need access to a microwave, you can often find one in the cafeteria, or there may be one you can use that's closer to your room. Ask the nursing staff about that possibility.

When psychotherapist Lenore Lefer's thirty-year-old son, Matt, was undergoing treatment for sarcoma, she often brought him his favorite meals. "Eating was a very big thing for Matt," says Lenore, whose son found an interesting relationship between eating and alleviating nausea early on. Matt reflects, "When I was eating, I was stimulating a physiological response. I discovered that nausea and appetite didn't coexist well. Eating reduced the nausea. Also, when I was eating, I visualized all the nutrients going to all the cells in my body and boosting my immune system." Matt's mom took advantage of her son's desire to eat. "I would bring anything he wanted to the hospital," says Lenore. "If he wanted a steak sandwich, he got a steak sandwich. If he wanted tofu, he got tofu. As his mother, I was thrilled that there was some way I could be useful to him: to make him chicken soup on a Friday night, and to make sure he had those things that were meaningful to him."

That sense of being able to contribute is so important, not just for frontline caregivers, but for friends, neighbors, coworkers, or anyone who is watching you go through this illness and wants to help but doesn't know how.

The Benefits of Exercise and a Healthy Attitude

I used to think about building a culinary support team in terms of food; finding people who wanted to shop, transport, prep, and cook. But people in treatment need additional support: friends willing to stop by for a chat, some fun, maybe a movie, and many of the other activities you did together before your diagnosis. This is especially true of exercise, which when combined with the power of yum can really crank up the appetite. The irony is that doctors used to restrict activity for cancer patients . . . until numerous studies convinced them otherwise. "Years ago physicians told cancer patients not to exercise because it was too strenuous during treatment," says Jeanne Wallace, a nutritional researcher with a clinical cancer practice. "Then they ran clinical trials in the U.K. and found that those put on exercise programs thrived. Their energy levels were better, and they tolerated treatment better. They found it was beneficial to initiate an exercise program during chemotherapy."

I've seen firsthand the effect exercise has on appetite and how friends can help patients stay active. One of my clients had a ritual where she and a friend would go off on a long walk or bike ride before I came by to give her a cooking lesson. Even though she was in the middle of breast cancer treatment, the exercise always left her hungry, and it wasn't too often that she left any food on her plate.

This particular client embodied the idea that a cancer diagnosis doesn't mean you have to act like you're sick. This is a concept I've seen embraced even by people who were in a terminal stage. Did it improve their outcomes? A statistician strictly measuring quantity of time might say no. But having seen these people bound and determined to wring every pleasurable moment out of whatever time they have, I'd have to vote in the affirmative. Many was the day when I'd walk up the driveway of this client's house and see her and her friends in the kitchen bopping to big band music blaring from the speakers. (She said the music reminder her of her favorite cook, her grandmother.) If there was anyone in that kitchen who identified with being sick, I sure couldn't tell.

That's what having a culinary support team is all about. No, I'm not Pollyannaish about treatment; sometimes it just plain stinks. No dancing. No smiling. Just long days. At those times, a culinary support team is a lifeline that provides a bit of respite, and you'll appreciate knowing that there's one less burden to bear. Just knowing that a healthy meal for you or your family is waiting on the doorstep in a cooler can be a great relief. A cooler, by the way, is a great way to deliver food. Some patients refuse help because they don't want people to see them in their house while they're sick. Having food dropped off on the porch in a cooler solves that problem.

There are many ways to put together a support team. Though there are many good websites devoted to the topic (see Resources), I'd suggest starting with a book. I recommend *Share the Care*, by Cappy Capossela and Sheila Warnock. These women wrote the book after their own experience caring for a sick friend, and it speaks from the heart.

Here are a few suggestions that apply to any support team, whether it's a team of three or thirty:

- Give people tasks they enjoy.
- Have only one captain to delegate assignments.
- Rotate the captain weekly, if possible.
- Take everyone's emotional temperature every few weeks to make sure no one is getting crunched.
- Recognize that caregivers have other responsibilities they need to attend to.
- Always keep feelers out for other people who want to join the team, as it's normal for some volunteers to drop out over time. (Remember, treatment can last a year or more.)

WHO KNEW? Exercise Is Beneficial during Treatment While I don't suggest that you train for a marathon in the midst of treatment, a little exercise does improve outcomes, and Dr. Keith Block says you don't even have to get out of bed or off the couch. He recalled asking a patient bedridden with hip cancer if she'd be willing to work out. "She said, 'Are you nuts?'" Block explained to her that it's possible to get a decent workout from even a simple set of isometrics; for example taking your foot and pointing your toes first up toward your eyes and holding for five seconds and then down toward the floor for a count to five. Repeating these sorts of exercises for various muscle groups in sets of twenty over the course of a day can provide an effective workout.

- Google Calendar is a great resource that can allow the captain and all team members to see online what tasks need to be accomplished. To use it, you'll need to have a Google account. For more information, search the Internet for the term "Google Calendar."

Here are a few final thoughts, things you might want to address as soon as possible after diagnosis.

Talk to your oncologist or family physician about treating depression. Depression and cancer are a common pair, yet depression is often ignored during treatment. This has many downsides, including putting your appetite at risk. As psychiatrist Jim Gordon explains, "Chemotherapy can be depressing. I've observed it. It so saps the energy. It's very hard to be upbeat on some of the powerful regimes that are available. You have to address it; chemotherapy depresses appetite and depression depresses appetite. Many of the same nutrients that are depleted in any chronic illness are also depleted in depression, so you need to have a healthier diet. By choosing food wisely, preparing it well, and enjoying eating it, you are actively engaged in your own healing, overcoming the feelings of hopelessness and helplessness that are the hallmarks of depression."

Set up a consultation with a dietician or nutritionist who has experience with cancer patients. Here's a well-earned plug for fitting a nutritional consultation into your cancer care. According to registered dietician and nutritionist Suzanne Dixon, more than a dozen studies show that patients who do so are far more likely to complete treatment. "The people who see dieticians do much better," says Dixon. "They also have fewer side effects. There's a study looking at radiation therapy treatment, and the people who saw dieticians had 90 percent completion of therapy and the people who didn't had 50 percent completion of therapy. When giving lectures, I used to tell this to doctors all the time. When they'd say, 'You can't prove that food will prolong survival.' I'd say, 'Well, let's look at it this way: raise your hand if you're really excited when you can give your patient only half of the intended treatment.'"

Make sure you're eating what you want to eat, not what someone else wants you to eat. Here's a a situation I've encountered all too often: I'll do an interview with a person in treatment who makes it blazingly clear he or she can't stand a certain food—say sweet potatoes. When I relay that information to a caregiver or a caregiver shares that information with others, someone invariably says, "Oh, but he hasn't tried my sweet potato recipe."

Sigh. This is not about who won the blue ribbon at last month's county fair. This is about eating foods you'll enjoy. Your culinary support team shouldn't assume they know what you want to eat or should be eating. Treatment and cancer can change food preferences, sometimes drastically. If necessary, use the questionnaire from chapter 1 (see page 26) to initiate a conversation about the foods you'd like to have available. If you aren't sure on any given day, browse through the recipes in this book. Sometimes just seeing the pictures is enough to get your appetite stimulated and say, "Yeah, I'd really like that." To a caregiver, those can be the most beautiful words in the world.

Kitchen Smarts

Food Storage Tips

It's worth a moment of your time to think of how you're going to store these wonderful meals once you've made them. The first time I made soup for an ill friend, I delivered it a monstrously huge 8-quart container. It quickly dawned on me—and my friend—that unless she drowned her family in soup for dinner that night, there was no way to fit the container in her freezer, and she didn't have any smaller containers to store it. I learned a lot from that experience, and want to save you from similar pitfalls. These tips for making, storing, and delivering food in the safest and most practical manner insure everything's good to the last drop, even weeks or months later.

- Build a freezer inventory so that you have broths and cooked dishes on hand in easy-to-use portion sizes. Be sure to think about the size of your freezer so that you don't end up with more food than storage space.
- Freeze food in sizes you will use at one time. One, two, four, and eight-cup sizes are convenient and freeze well.
- Label all of your containers with the date, contents, and quantity. A permanent marker and blue painter's tape (looks like blue masking tape) work great.
- Do not use plastic with hot liquids. To speed the cooling, put the container in some ice water in the kitchen sink or a large dish and stir the soup occasionally.
- When freezing liquid, leave 1/2 to 1 inch of space at the top of the container to allow for expansion.
- As a general rule, fruit and vegetables will stay freezer fresh for about eight months, meat and poultry for three, and fish and shellfish for up to six.

Cooking and Reheating Tips

- Use cast-iron or stainless steel pots and pans for cooking instead of aluminum and nonstick surfaces.
- To prevent bacterial growth, thaw frozen food in the refrigerator or in cold water, not on the counter. If thawing in cold water, change the water every 30 minutes. Frozen meat should always be thawed in the refrigerator, which can take up to 48 hours.
- Avoid using the microwave to reheat food. If you decide to reheat food in the microwave, avoid reheating in plastic containers and use glass or ceramic containers instead.

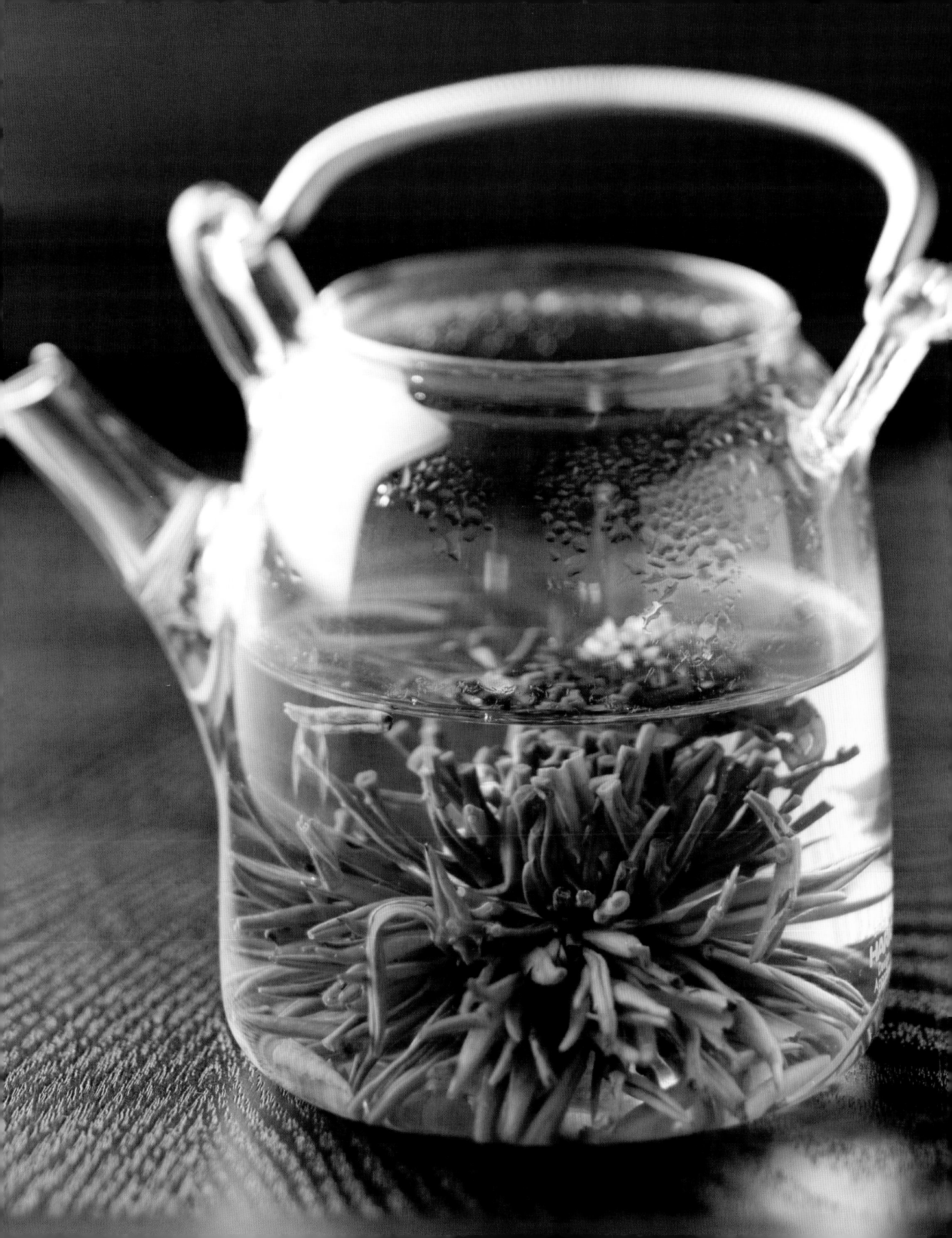

CHAPTER 3

Nourishing Soups and Broths

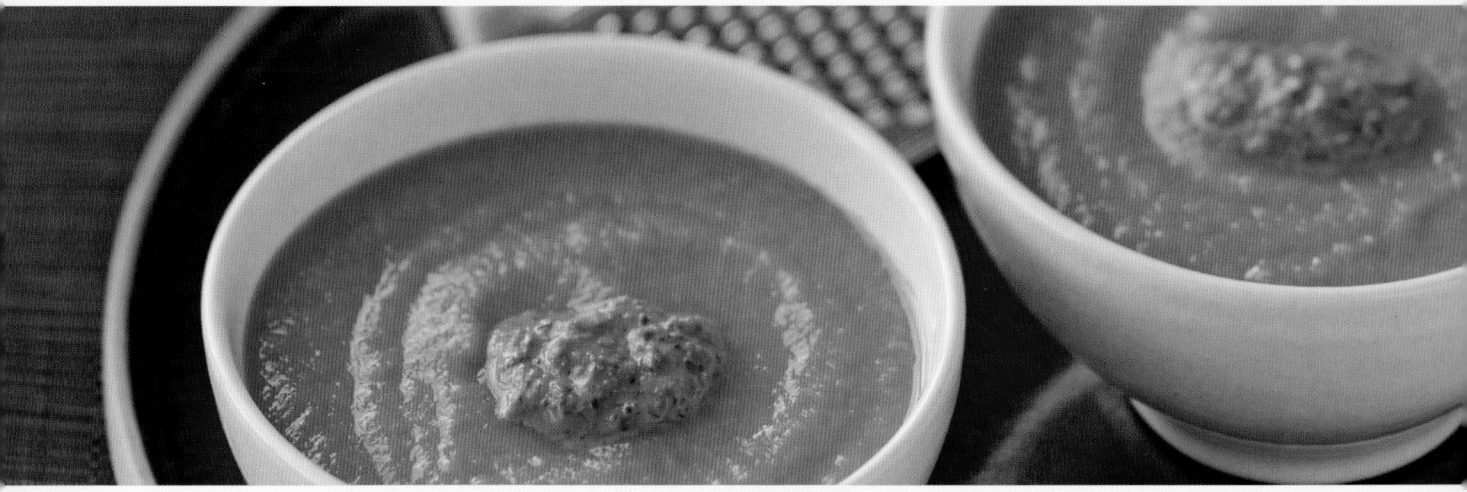

HEALING BROTHS

54 *Magic Mineral Broth*

55 *Chicken Magic Mineral Broth*

56 *Pasture Beef Bone Broth*

BROTH SOUPS

57 *Italian White Bean Soup*

59 *Chicken Vegetable Soup with Ginger Meatballs*

60 *Lemony Greek Chicken Soup*

61 *Ma's Mushroom Barley Soup*

62 *Thai It Up Chicken Soup*

64 *Minestrone*

THE CASHMERE SWEATER SOUP COLLECTION

65 *Bella's Carrot, Orange, and Fennel Soup*

67 *Curry Cauliflower Soup*

69 *Roasted Red Roma Tomato Soup*

70 *Cooling Cucumber Avocado Soup*

71 *Rockin' Black Bean Soup*

72 *Spiced Sweet Potato Soup*

73 *Summer's Best Zucchini Soup*

74 *Velvety Red Lentil Dahl*

75 *Creamy Broccoli and Potato Soup*

Just as every artist has a favorite medium, every chef has a favorite outlet. For me, that's soup, hands down. I love giving people what I call a culinary hug: a warm, comforting dish I can wrap around them like a cashmere sweater. (In fact, that's what I call some of my favorite soup recipes: my cashmere sweater collection.)

Soups allow me to throw my entire heart, soul, and cooking abilities into one incredibly nourishing pot. Soup completely captures the mind and body and engages all of the senses. It's practically aromatherapy in a bowl, with the heady smells, the enveloping heat, and the stimulating scaffolding of tastes.

Best of all, especially for people in treatment, is that soup is the perfect vehicle for delivering both enticing taste and sumptuous nourishment, especially those all-important phytochemicals and other nutrients that boost immunity and challenge cancer head-on. The combination of broth and heat alchemizes the vegetables, breaking them down and releasing more nourishment.

As you make your way through the soup recipes, you'll develop a sense of my formula for optimizing flavor. I've made sure to put in variations and combinations guaranteed to appeal to people who like everything from hearty stews to light broths, but regardless of the particulars, it all comes down to what I think of as layering the flavors. Each ingredient is added in a way that brings out its maximum taste and nutrition.

The best part is that these nutrient-dense soups will appeal to everyone around the table. Sip for sip and spoon for spoon, soup will always be my go-to dish when I want to show people I really care then. Because for me, soup is where the love is.

Magic Mineral Broth

This is my Rosetta stone of soup, a broth that can be transformed to meet a myriad nutritional needs, serving as everything from a delicious sipping tea to the powerful base for more hearty soups and stews. So no matter what a person's appetite, it can provide a tremendous nutritional boost. Chemotherapy often saps your strength due to dehydration, which pulls vital nutrients out of your system. This rejuvenating liquid, chock-full of magnesium, potassium, and sodium, allows the body to refresh and restore itself. I think of it as a tonic, designed to keep you in tip-top shape. MAKES 6 QUARTS

- 6 unpeeled carrots, cut into thirds
- 2 unpeeled yellow onions, cut into chunks
- 1 leek, white and green parts, cut into thirds
- 1 bunch celery, including the heart, cut into thirds
- 4 unpeeled red potatoes, quartered
- 2 unpeeled Japanese or regular sweet potatoes, quartered
- 1 unpeeled garnet yam, quartered
- 5 unpeeled cloves garlic, halved
- 1/2 bunch fresh flat-leaf parsley
- 1 8-inch strip of kombu
- 12 black peppercorns
- 4 whole allspice or juniper berries
- 2 bay leaves
- 8 quarts cold, unfiltered water
- 1 teaspoon sea salt

REBECCA'S NOTES Like fine wine, this broth gets better with age. The longer the simmer time, the better tasting and more nutrient dense the broth will be. You can also cut the recipe in half and make it in a slow cooker.

Rinse all of the vegetables well, including the kombu. In a 12-quart or larger stockpot, combine the carrots, onions, leek, celery, potatoes, sweet potatoes, yam, garlic, parsley, kombu, peppercorns, allspice berries, and bay leaves. Fill the pot with the water to 2 inches below the rim, cover, and bring to a boil.

Remove the lid, decrease the heat to low, and simmer, uncovered, for at least 2 hours. As the broth simmers, some of the water will evaporate; add more if the vegetables begin to peek out. Simmer until the full richness of the vegetables can be tasted.

Strain the broth through a large, coarse-mesh sieve (remember to use a heat-resistant container underneath), then add salt to taste. Let cool to room temperature before refrigerating or freezing.

PREP TIME: 10 minutes · COOK TIME: 2 to 4 hours

STORAGE: Store in an airtight container in the refrigerator for 5 to 7 days or in the freezer for 4 months.

PER SERVING: Calories: 45; Total Fat: 0 g (0 g saturated, 0 g monounsaturated); Carbohydrates: 11 g; Protein: 1 g; Fiber: 2 g; Sodium: 140 mg

CULINARY RX Kombu might sound like an exotic name for a jazz ensemble, but it's really a long, dark brown to black seaweed that is dried and folded into sheets. It keeps indefinitely if stored in a cool, dry place. Kombu contains a full range of trace minerals, which are often deficient in people with compromised immune systems, and is high in potassium, iodine, calcium, and vitamins A and C. It's also rich in a type of polysaccharide known as fucoidans, which may inhibit cancer cells. Kombu is available in the Asian section of many grocery stores, or you can order it online (see Resources, page 208).

Chicken Magic Mineral Broth Broth

Some people have soul sisters. I have a soup sister. Julie and I have one of those friendships where I can barge into her house uninvited and nine times out of ten I'll find Julie in the kitchen making soup. She's so good at it that when I return home from a long out-of-town job, the first place I call to make dinner reservations is her house. Last winter we were trying to come up with a hearty chicken broth recipe when we realized everything we needed for a foundation was already in the Magic Mineral Broth recipe (opposite page), with its rich color, aroma, and flavor and impressive nutritional profile. Here, we've enhanced Magic Mineral Broth by adding chicken bones, which infuse the soup with even more minerals, especially calcium and phosphorus, which, not surprisingly, are vital for bone health. MAKES 6 TO 7 QUARTS

- 6 unpeeled carrots, cut into thirds
- 2 unpeeled yellow onions, cut into chunks
- 2 leeks, white and green parts, cut into thirds
- 1 bunch celery, including the heart, cut into thirds
- 4 unpeeled red potatoes, quartered
- 2 unpeeled Japanese or regular sweet potatoes, quartered
- 1 unpeeled garnet yam, quartered
- 8 unpeeled cloves garlic, halved
- 1 bunch fresh flat-leaf parsley
- 1 6-inch strip of kombu
- 12 black peppercorns
- 4 whole allspice or juniper berries
- 2 bay leaves
- 1 tablespoon vinegar or freshly squeezed lemon juice
- 1 organic chicken carcass, or 2 pounds of chicken bones
- 8 quarts cold, unfiltered water
- 1 teaspoon sea salt

Rinse all of the vegetables well, including the kombu. In a 12- to 16-quart stockpot, combine the carrots, onions, leeks, celery, potatoes, sweet potatoes, yam, garlic, parsley, kombu, peppercorns, allspice berries, bay leaves, vinegar, and chicken carcass. Fill the pot with the water to 2 inches below the rim, cover, and bring to a boil.

Remove the lid, decrease the heat to low, and skim off the scum that has risen to the top. Simmer, uncovered, for at least 2 hours. As the broth simmers, some of the water will evaporate; add more if the vegetables begin to peek out. Simmer until the bones begin to soften and fall apart, about 4 hours, or as long as you're willing to let it simmer away.

Strain the broth through a large, coarse-mesh sieve, then stir in salt to taste. Let cool to room temperature, then refrigerate overnight. Skim off as much fat as you can from the top of the broth, then portion into airtight containers and refrigerate or freeze.

PREP TIME: 20 minutes · COOK TIME: 4 hours

STORAGE: Store in an airtight container in the refrigerator for 3 to 4 days or in the freezer for 3 months.

PER SERVING: Calories: 50; Total Fat: 0 g (0 g saturated, 0 g monounsaturated); Carbohydrates: 11 g; Protein: 1 g; Fiber: 2 g; Sodium: 145 mg

REBECCA'S NOTES Here's a trick of the trade: Once you've skimmed the fat from the surface of the broth, you can remove even more by dabbing the surface of the broth with paper towels to sop it up.

Pasture Beef Bone Broth

Beef broth has long been used as a healing beverage. Beef bones are filled with collagen and minerals the body uses to build connective tissues, such as calcium, magnesium, and phosphorus. It's a perfect sipping medium for people who are trying to figure out how to get five or six hits of nutrition a day. I've had clients with eating difficulties who have literally lived on this broth for days or weeks at a time.

MAKES 6 QUARTS

- 3 pounds marrow bones from grass-fed organic beef
- 6 unpeeled carrots, cut into thirds
- 2 unpeeled yellow onions, cut into chunks
- 1 leek, white and green parts, cut into thirds
- 1 bunch celery, including the heart, cut into thirds
- 4 unpeeled red potatoes, quartered
- 2 unpeeled Japanese or regular sweet potatoes, quartered
- 1 unpeeled garnet yam, quartered
- 5 unpeeled cloves garlic, halved
- 1/2 bunch fresh flat-leaf parsley
- 1 8-inch strip of kombu
- 12 black peppercorns
- 4 whole allspice or juniper berries
- 2 bay leaves
- 1 tablespoon apple cider vinegar
- 8 quarts cold, filtered water
- 1 teaspoon sea salt

Preheat the oven to 350°F.

Place the bones on a baking sheet or roasting pan and roast until the bones are well browned, about 30 minutes.

Rinse all of the vegetables well, including the kombu. In a 12-quart or larger stockpot, combine the bones, carrots, onions, leek, celery, potatoes, sweet potatoes, yam, garlic, parsley, kombu, peppercorns, allspice berries, bay leaves, and vinegar. Pour in the water, cover, and bring to a boil.

Remove the lid, decrease the heat to low, and skim off the scum that has risen to the top. Simmer gently, uncovered, for 8 to 24 hours. As the broth simmers, some of the water will evaporate; add more if the vegetables begin to peek out.

Remove and discard the bones, then strain the broth through a large, coarse-mesh sieve. Stir in salt to taste. Let cool to room temperature, and then refrigerate overnight. Skim off as much fat as you can from the top of the broth, then portion into airtight containers and refrigerate or freeze.

PREP TIME: 25 minutes · COOK TIME: 8 to 24 hours

STORAGE: Store in an airtight container in the refrigerator for up to 4 days or in the freezer for up to 4 months.

PER SERVING: Calories: 50; Total Fat: 0 g (0 g saturated, 0 g monounsaturated); Carbohydrates: 11 g; Protein: 1 g; Fiber: 2 g; Sodium: 140 mg

REBECCA'S NOTES To make a short-cut version, roast the marrow bones as directed and place in a 6 1/2-quart slow cooker. Cover with Magic Mineral Broth (page 54) and add the vinegar. Set the slow cooker on low for 8 to 24 hours, and allow the broth to simmer away. Strain the broth and refrigerate it overnight, then skim the fat, and add 2 more quarts of Magic Mineral Broth.

CULINARY RX While Western medicine hasn't reached definitive conclusions about many aspects of how nutrition may affect cancer and treatment side effects, Chinese medicine has a longer and more extensive body of scientific literature. Acupuncturist Michael Broffman notes the foods he suggests to patients facing certain challenges. For loss of taste, Broffman says, "We like Chinese pears and papaya. They're high in enzymes. Also pineapple, because it nicely enhances taste and the sense of smell." For dehydration, Broffman likes vegetables and fruits with high water content, such as chestnuts and cucumbers. For fatigue and anemia, he suggests figs, grapes, herring, barley, and a little fresh honey. And for those dealing with blood cancers, he recommends "foods that speak to bone marrow production: soups and stocks that use bones from beef, chicken, lamb, or fish."

Italian White Bean Soup

When it comes to cooking, Italians believe in region first, country second. That's why this recipe is my version of culinary heresy. By taking white beans—a notoriously Tuscan legume—and mixing them with saffron, which is more common to northern Italy's Lombardi region, I've committed what might be considered a food felony. My defense for breaking with tradition is justified in this case: saffron is a powerful cancer-fighting spice. It's best to soak the beans overnight before cooking them, so plan ahead. SERVES 6

BEANS

- 1 1/2 cups cannellini beans, or 1 15-ounce can drained, rinsed, and mixed with a spritz of fresh lemon juice and a pinch of sea salt
- 1 teaspoon extra-virgin olive oil
- 2 sprigs fresh rosemary, or 1/4 teaspoon dried
- 2 sprigs fresh thyme, or 1/4 teaspoon dried
- 3 leaves fresh sage
- 4 cloves garlic, peeled and smashed

SOUP

- 2 tablespoons extra-virgin olive oil
- 1 3/4 cups finely diced yellow onion
- 3 cups finely diced fennel
- Sea salt
- 1 1/2 cups peeled and finely diced carrots
- 1 1/2 cups finely diced celery
- 1 cup peeled and diced Yukon gold potato
- 2 cloves garlic, minced
- 1/4 teaspoon dried sage, or 1 tablespoon chopped fresh sage
- 1/4 teaspoon dried thyme, or 1 tablespoon fresh thyme
- 1/8 teaspoon saffron
- 8 cups Magic Mineral Broth (page 54), Chicken Magic Mineral Broth (page 55), or store-bought organic stock
- 1 tablespoon freshly squeezed lemon juice
- 1/4 cup fresh parsley, coarsely chopped
- 1/4 cup fresh basil, coarsely chopped

To cook the beans, follow the method on page 110, adding the olive oil and a sachet made with the rosemary, thyme, sage, and garlic to the cooking liquid. (If using canned beans, skip this step.)

To make the soup, heat the olive oil in a soup pot over medium heat, then add the onions, fennel, and a pinch of salt, and sauté until golden, about 4 minutes. Stir in the carrots, celery, potato, garlic, and 1/4 teaspoon of salt, then add the sage, thyme, and saffron and sauté until the vegetables are soft, about 15 minutes.

Pour in 1/2 cup of the broth to deglaze the pot and cook until the liquid is reduced by half. Add the remaining 7 1/2 cups broth and the beans, then lower the heat and simmer until the vegetables are tender and the beans are heated through, about 10 minutes. Stir in the lemon juice, parsley, basil, and another 1/4 teaspoon of salt and serve right away.

Variation: For a more southern Italian flair and some added lycopene, add 1 cup of canned diced tomatoes (drained) after you add the garlic. Since tomatoes are naturally acidic, skip the lemon juice.

PREP TIME: 20 minutes (after soaking the beans overnight)

COOK TIME: 1 hour 30 minutes (25 minutes with canned beans)

STORAGE: Store in a covered container in the refrigerator for 5 to 7 days or in the freezer for up to 2 months.

PER SERVING: Calories: 275; Total Fat: 4.5 g (0.7 g saturated, 3 g monounsaturated); Carbohydrates: 48 g; Protein: 12 g; Fiber: 11 g; Sodium: 680 mg

REBECCA'S NOTES This is a soup that swings well both ways, as a hearty soup or as a blended soup. If you serve it blended, top it with a generous amount of Parsley Basil Drizzle (page 187) for extra yum.

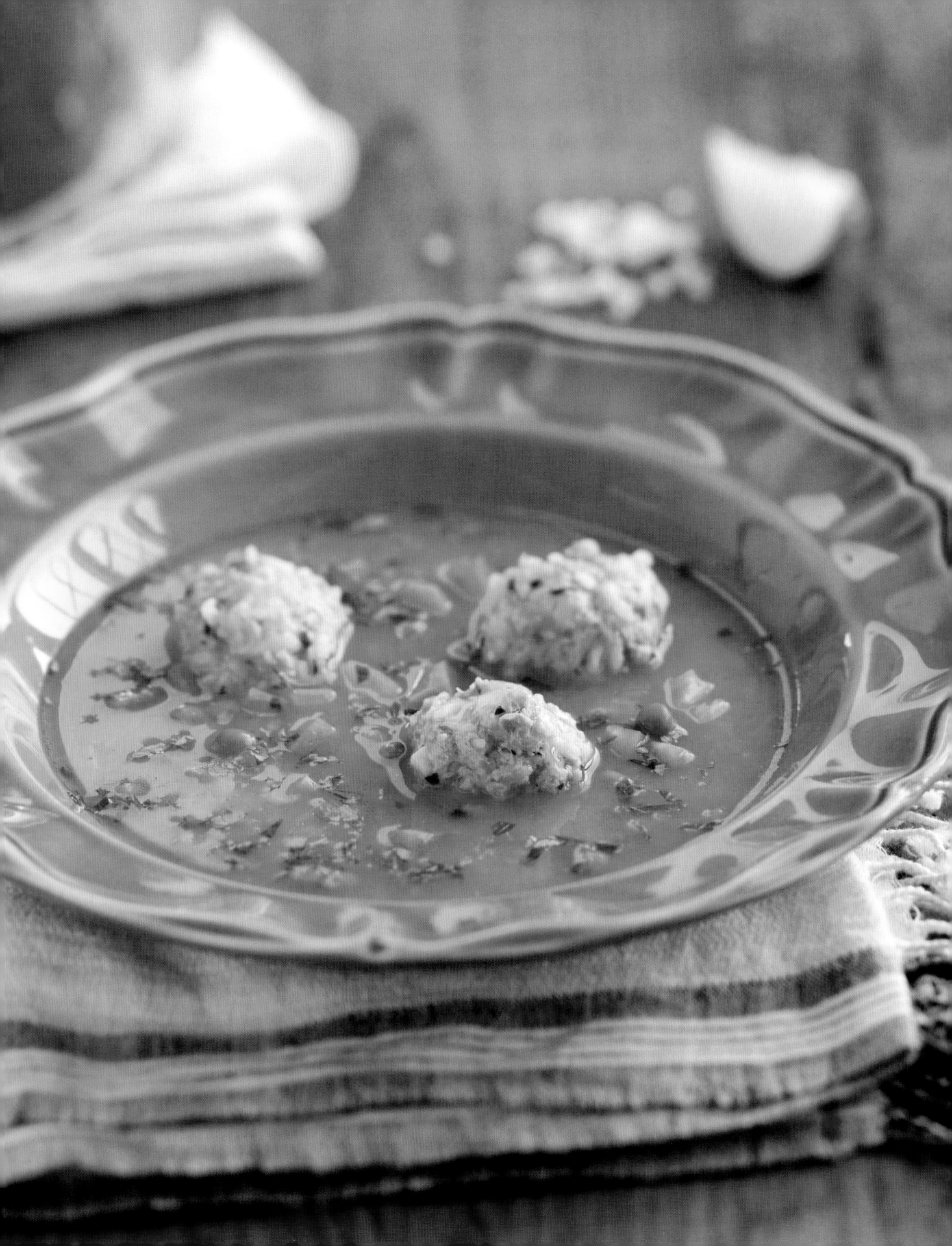

Chicken Vegetable Soup with Ginger Meatballs

If ever there was a dish that proved I wasn't Italian, it's meatballs. And that's kind of embarrassing, because not only do I love to make Italian food, I even studied (okay, suffered, but it amounted to the same thing) under an Italian signora *on the Isle of Elba. But no matter how hard I tried, I could never figure out how to keep my meatballs from falling apart, until I tried basmati rice. Now my meatballs not only taste great, they also don't disintegrate on the fork. These are actually mini meatballs, closer to the Latin-American version known as* albondiguitas, *with the ginger providing a little zing. If timing is an issue, the meatballs can be prepared ahead of time and refrigerated until you're ready to cook them. Also, this recipe makes twice as many meatballs as you'll need for the soup. To save the remainder for later, place them in the freezer for 1 hour to firm up, then transfer to an airtight container and refrigerate for up to 5 days or freeze for up to 3 months.* SERVES 4

MEATBALLS

1 pound ground organic dark-meat turkey or chicken

2 teaspoons grated fresh ginger

1 teaspoon minced garlic

1/4 cup fresh parsley, finely chopped

1/2 teaspoon sea salt

Pinch of cayenne

1 egg, beaten

1/3 cup uncooked white basmati or jasmine rice

SOUP

2 tablespoons extra-virgin olive oil

1 yellow onion, diced small

Sea salt

1 large carrot, peeled and diced small

1 large celery stalk, diced small

2 cloves garlic, minced

1 teaspoon grated fresh ginger

8 cups Chicken Magic Mineral Broth (page 55) or store-bought organic chicken broth

1/2 cup fresh or frozen sweet peas

1/4 cup fresh parsley, finely chopped

1/4 cup fresh basil, finely chopped

1 lime, cut into quarters, for garnish

To make the meatballs, line a sheet pan with wax paper. Combine the turkey, ginger, garlic, parsley, salt, cayenne, egg, and rice in a bowl and mix with your hands or a spatula until well combined. Don't overwork the mixture or the meatballs will be tough.

Wet the palms of your hands so the mixture doesn't stick, roll it into 1-inch balls, and place them on the prepared pan.

To make the soup, heat the olive oil in a soup pot over medium heat, then add the onion and a pinch of salt and sauté until translucent, about 4 minutes. Add the carrot, celery, garlic, ginger, and 1/4 teaspoon of salt and continue sautéing for about 3 minutes.

Pour in 1/2 cup of the broth to deglaze the pot and cook until the liquid is reduced by half. Add the remaining 7 1/2 cups broth and another 1/4 teaspoon of salt and bring to a boil. Lower the heat to maintain a vigorous simmer, then gently transfer half of the meatballs into the simmering broth. (Refrigerate or freeze the remainder to use later.) Cover and allow the meatballs to simmer for 15 minutes.

Add the peas and cook for 3 minutes more, then stir in the parsley and basil. Serve each bowl garnished with a wedge of lime.

Variation: If you aren't a pea person, use this recipe as an opportunity to get some dark leafy greens into your life. Simply replace the peas with 1 cup of baby spinach leaves.

PREP TIME: 20 minutes · COOK TIME: 35 minutes

STORAGE: Store in an airtight container in the refrigerator for up to 5 days or in the freezer for up to 2 months.

PER SERVING: Calories: 210; Total Fat: 7 g (1.6 g saturated, 3.4 g monounsaturated); Carbohydrates: 23 g; Protein: 15 g; Fiber: 3 g; Sodium: 380 mg

Lemony Greek Chicken Soup

A little cultural pride is a good thing, and I have to tell you I always thought my people had the market cornered when it came to making chicken soup. I mean, there's a reason they call it Jewish penicillin, right? Well, in the interest of complete fairness, let me say that the Greeks know a thing or three about chicken soup, as well. Their Mediterranean take is to fold a little lemon and egg into the mixture. And unlike the yiddishe *version, which I love but which can be a little fatty, this version is light and bright. Because of the egg, which provides protein, and the Chicken Magic Mineral Broth, this a nutrient-dense bowl of yum. You'll need to cook the farro in advance, so plan ahead.* SERVES 6

- 2 tablespoons extra-virgin olive oil
- 1 cup finely diced onion
- Sea salt
- 1/2 cup peeled and finely diced carrot
- 1/2 cup finely diced celery or fennel
- 1/4 teaspoon dried oregano
- 6 cups Chicken Magic Mineral Broth (page 55) or store-bought organic chicken stock
- 1/2 cup Simple Tuscan Farro, (page 148)
- 1/4 cup freshly squeezed lemon juice
- 2 teaspoons lemon zest
- 3 egg yolks
- 1/4 cup fresh mint, finely chopped
- 1/4 cup fresh parsley, finely chopped
- Pinch of freshly ground pepper
- 1 cup thinly sliced cooked organic chicken breast meat

Heat the olive oil in a soup pot over medium heat, then add the onion and a pinch of salt and sauté until translucent, about 4 minutes. Stir in the carrot, celery, oregano, and 1/4 teaspoon of salt, and sauté for about 30 seconds. Pour in 1/2 cup of the broth to deglaze the pot and cook until the liquid is reduced by half. Add the remaining 5 1/2 cups broth and the farro and bring to a boil, then lower the heat to maintain a simmer.

Whisk the lemon juice, lemon zest, and egg yolks together, then stir the mixture into the simmering soup and cook until it clouds and thickens a bit, about 3 minutes. Stir in the mint, parsley, pepper, and 1/2 teaspoon of salt, then add the chicken and do a FASS check. If the soup tastes too sour, add a pinch of salt.

PREP TIME: 10 minutes (after cooking the farro) · COOK TIME: 15 minutes

STORAGE: Store in an airtight container in the refrigerator for up to 5 days or in the freezer for up to 2 months.

PER SERVING: Calories: 170; Total Fat: 7.4 g (1.6 g saturated, 4.45 g mono-unsaturated); Carbohydrates: 22 g; Protein: 5 g; Fiber: 4 g; Sodium: 255 mg

REBECCA'S NOTES You can substitute 1/2 cup of cooked orzo or cooked brown rice for the farro. To make a vegetarian version, omit the chicken and use Magic Mineral Broth (page 54).

Ma's Mushroom Barley Soup

This soup is for mushroom maniacs, although if you're on the fence about them, I guarantee this soup will sway you! There's simply no taste in the culinary world that mimics mushrooms, and that flavor is backed up by a host of health-supportive properties. Between the shiitakes, the barley, and the rich broth, this is a warming meal in a bowl. Since the barley must soak overnight, you'll need to plan ahead. SERVES 6

- 1/2 cup pearl barley
- Juice of 1 lemon
- 2 tablespoons extra-virgin olive oil
- 1 small onion, diced
- 1/2 teaspoon sea salt
- 1 1/2 cups peeled and finely diced carrots
- 1 1/2 cups finely diced celery
- 1 parsnip, peeled and diced small
- 1/4 pound white mushrooms, thinly sliced
- 1/4 pound shiitake mushrooms, thinly sliced
- 2 cloves garlic, minced
- 1/4 teaspoon dried oregano
- 1/4 teaspoon dried thyme
- 1/4 teaspoon ground caraway
- Pinch of freshly ground pepper
- 9 cups Pasture Beef Bone Broth (page 56) or Magic Mineral Broth (page 54)
- 1/4 cup loosely packed chopped fresh parsley

CULINARY RX Science has discovered that many edible mushrooms have potent anticancer properties. Take shiitakes, which have anti-tumor, cholesterol-lowering, and virus-inhibiting effects. And one of those active ingredient, lentinan, is part of a larger family of complex sugar molecules known as beta-glucans, which may also kick-start the immune system.

Place the barley in a pan or bowl with the lemon juice and water to cover and soak overnight, or for at least 8 hours.

Drain and rinse the barley.

Heat the olive oil in a soup pot over medium-high heat, then add the onion and 1/4 teaspoon of the salt and sauté until golden, about 3 minutes. Add the carrots, celery, and parsnip and sauté for 3 minutes more. Add the white mushrooms, shiitake mushrooms, garlic, oregano, thyme, caraway, pepper, and barley and sauté for 3 to 4 minutes, until the mushrooms release their juices. Pour in 1 cup of the broth to deglaze the pot and cook until the liquid is reduced by three-quarters.

Add the remaining 8 cups broth and bring to a boil, then lower the heat and simmer for 20 minutes.

Stir in the the remaining 1/4 teaspoon salt and the parsley, then do a FASS check. You may want to add just a spritz of fresh lemon juice.

Variation: If you choose the vegetarian option for this soup, using Magic Mineral Broth, you may want to include some roasted portobello mushrooms to add some heft. Preheat the oven to 425°F. Cut 2 portobello mushrooms into 1/4-inch slices and toss with 1 tablespoon of olive oil, 1 teaspoon of balsamic vinegar, 1/4 teaspoon of salt, and a few grinds of black pepper. Arrange them in a single layer on a baking sheet and roast for 15 minutes. Once they're cool enough to handle, chop the portobellos into bite-size pieces. Stir them into the soup when you add the parsley.

PREP TIME: 20 minutes (after soaking the barley overnight)

COOK TIME: 45 minutes

STORAGE: Store in an airtight container in the refrigerator for up to 4 days or in the freezer for up to 2 months.

PER SERVING: Calories: 230; Total Fat: 5.4 g (0.8 g saturated, 3.4 g monounsaturated); Carbohydrates: 42 g; Protein: 6 g; Fiber: 9 g; Sodium: 460 mg

REBECCA'S NOTES If you have leftover soup, you'll find that it has much less broth, as barley loves to expand in liquid. Keep an extra cup or two of broth on hand to add when you reheat the leftovers.

Thai It Up Chicken Soup

What's the first thing you think of when somebody says, "Let's get Thai food"? Most of my friends have an involuntary response: they start to sweat. Many people think that Thai food is hot, hot, hot. Well, maybe not, not, not. True, some Thai food can set off smoke detectors. But real Thai cooking emphasizes distinctive flavor combinations regardless of the heat. This soup, a takeoff on traditional Thai tom kha gai *(a chicken soup), uses coconut milk, which is very soothing to the nerves. The ginger aids digestion, while the lime brightens up the overall flavor. The result is a soup guaranteed to jump-start even the most jaded taste buds.* SERVES 6

- 8 cups Chicken Magic Mineral Broth (page 55), Magic Mineral Broth (page 54), or store-bought organic stock
- 2 shallots, or 1 small red onion, peeled and halved
- 6 1-inch pieces of unpeeled fresh ginger
- 1 stalk lemongrass, bruised and cut into chunks
- 2 kaffir lime leaves, or 1 teaspoon lime zest
- 1/2 teaspoon sea salt
- 1 15-ounce can coconut milk
- 3 1/2 ounces rice noodles, broken into 2-inch pieces
- 1 cup peeled and finely diced carrot
- Pinch of cayenne (optional)
- 1 organic chicken breast half, cut into 1/8-inch-thick diagonal slices
- 2 tablespoons freshly squeezed lime juice
- 1/4 cup chopped fresh cilantro, for garnish
- 2 tablespoons sliced scallion, cut thinly on the diagonal, for garnish

Combine the broth, shallots, ginger, lemongrass, lime leaves, and 1/4 teaspoon of the salt in a soup pot over high heat and bring to a boil. Lower the heat to medium-low and simmer for 20 minutes.

Using a slotted spoon, scoop out all of the solids and discard. Stir in the coconut milk and continue to simmer, being careful not to boil, for another 10 minutes.

Meanwhile, put the rice noodles into a bowl of hot water and soak until tender, about 10 minutes. Drain and set aside.

Stir the carrot and cayenne into the soup, simmer for 3 minutes, then add the chicken and simmer for an additional 7 minutes, until the chicken is tender and thoroughly cooked. Stir in the noodles, lime juice, and the remaining 1/4 teaspoon salt, then do a FASS check. You my want to add a bit more salt and 1/8 teaspoon of maple syrup. Serve garnished with the cilantro and scallion.

Variation: For an extra immune booster, add 1 cup of stemmed and sliced shiitake mushrooms when you add the chicken. Want to Thai it up vegetarian style? Use Magic Mineral Broth and add thin strips of tofu in place of the chicken.

PREP TIME: 15 minutes · COOK TIME: 45 to 55 minutes

STORAGE: Store in a covered container in the refrigerator for 3 to 5 days or in the freezer for up to 2 months.

PER SERVING: Calories: 290; Total Fat: 15.5 g (13.5 g saturated, 0.7 g mono-unsaturated); Carbohydrates: 35 g; Protein: 6 g; Fiber: 4 g; Sodium: 420 mg

REBECCA'S NOTES For an easy way to slice raw chicken, place it in your freezer for 20 to 30 minutes to firm up. Slicing it straight out of the freezer will be a breeze!

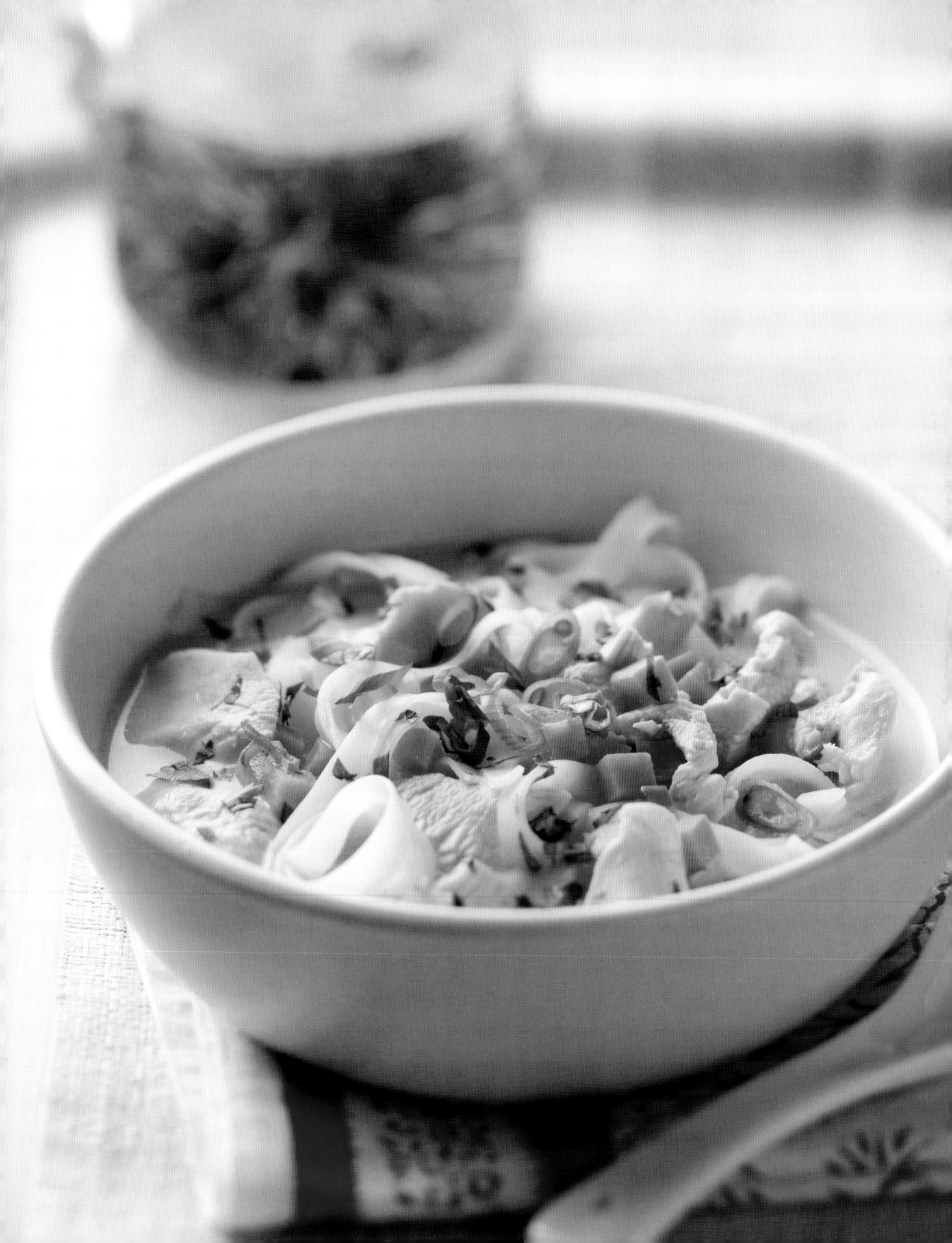

Minestrone

The Italians are beautiful because they've turned what is essentially peasant fare into an internationally renowned cuisine. Take pappa al pomodoro. *Fancy, huh? Can you say, "Day-old knot of stale bread in tomatoes and water?" A staple there, a delicacy here. The same goes for minestrone, which I've always claimed is Italian for "Whatever is in the pantry goes in the pot!" Actually, minestrone comes from the array of dishes known as* cucina povera *or "poor kitchen." It's a bit of a misnomer, though, as minestrone is rich in vital nutrients, most notably lycopene, a phytochemical in tomatoes that has anticancer properties, especially with prostate cancer.* SERVES 6

- 2 tablespoons extra-virgin olive oil
- 1 cup finely diced yellow onion
- Sea salt
- 1 cup peeled and finely diced carrot
- 1 cup finely diced celery
- 1 cup finely diced zucchini
- 1/2 teaspoon finely chopped garlic
- 1/4 teaspoon dried oregano
- 1/4 teaspoon dried thyme
- 1/4 teaspoon fennel seeds, crushed
- Pinch of red pepper flakes
- 8 cups Magic Mineral Broth (page 54), Chicken Magic Mineral Broth (page 55), or store-bought organic stock
- 1 14-ounce can crushed tomatoes
- 2 cups cooked red kidney beans, or 1 15-ounce can, rinsed, drained, and mixed with a spritz of fresh lemon juice and a pinch of salt
- 2 cups stemmed and finely chopped Swiss chard
- 4 ounces whole grain pasta, cooked
- 1/4 cup finely chopped fresh parsley
- Basil Lemon Drizzle (page 177), for garnish (optional)
- Grated organic Parmesan cheese, for garnish

Heat the olive oil in a soup pot over medium heat, then add the onion and a pinch of salt and sauté until golden, about 5 minutes. Add the carrot, celery, zucchini, garlic, oregano, thyme, fennel, red pepper flakes, and 1/4 teaspoon of salt and sauté for about 4 minutes. Pour in 1/2 cup of the broth to deglaze the pot and cook until the liquid is reduced by half.

Add the remaining 7 1/2 cups broth, the tomatoes, and the beans and bring to a boil, then lower the heat and simmer for 20 minutes.

Stir in the chard and another 1/4 teaspoon salt and cook for 3 minutes more. Stir in the pasta and the parsley. Serve topped with Basil Lemon Drizzle (if using) and a sprinkling of Parmesan.

Variations: This soup is the ultimate "clean out the refrigerator" dish. All of those slightly aged vegetables you thought you were going to eat will find a nice home in this pot of yum. During the winter, substitute diced delicata or butternut squash for the zucchini. You can bump up the nutritional value and anticancer properties even more by adding that leftover cabbage I know you have in the back of your fridge.

PREP TIME: 20 minutes · COOK TIME: 35 minutes

STORAGE: Store in an airtight container in the refrigerator for up to 5 days or in the freezer for up to 2 months.

PER SERVING: Calories: 300; Total Fat: 6 g (0.5 g saturated, 3 g monounsaturated); Carbohydrates: 55 g; Protein: 12 g; Fiber: 13 g; Sodium: 600 mg

CULINARY RX You don't have to lift weights to pump iron. Try eating kidney beans instead. Chemotherapy zaps iron, and low iron counts can lead to the blahs (that's our technical term for a lack of energy). Kidney beans are full of iron, and their complex carbohydrates guarantee a nice slow, efficient infusion of energy. For people who avoid eating red meat, being sure to consume other foods high in iron, such as kidney beans and lentils, is a must.

Bella's Carrot, Orange, and Fennel Soup

Here's a recipe where a little culinary ad-libbing met the needs of a caregiver. My husband, Gregg, was feeling a little sick but wanted to eat, but there really wasn't anything in the house. I saw some fennel and thought, "That's good for the belly." Then I found some carrots. But what to do with these limited ingredients? For years I'd made a carrot ginger soup recipe for many of my patients. Would carrot fennel soup work? I went to the fruit compartment for my trusty lemons, but only found an orange. It all went into the pot, and a little while later I put it in front of Gregg. He took one taste and started raving. A few weeks and tweaks later, I found that adding cumin, cinnamon, and allspice really brought this soup home. I named this recipe after Bella because she's quite possibly the only dog on the planet who prefers carrots to bacon; for every four carrots that go into making this soup, one goes into Bella's mouth. Otherwise she howls. (Sigh.) SERVES 6

- 2 tablespoons extra-virgin olive oil
- 1 cup chopped yellow onion
- 1 cup chopped fennel
- Sea salt
- 3 pounds carrots, cut into 1-inch pieces
- 1 1/2 teaspoons orange zest
- 1/4 teaspoon ground cumin
- 1/8 teaspoon ground cinnamon
- 1/8 teaspoon ground allspice
- Pinch of red pepper flakes
- 8 cups Magic Mineral Broth (page 54)
- 1 tablespoon freshly squeezed orange juice
- 2 teaspoons freshly squeezed lemon juice
- 1/4 teaspoon maple syrup
- Cashew Cream (page 180), for garnish

REBECCA'S NOTES Put liquid ingredients in the blender first, and then add the solids to blend more efficiently. The pressure builds up when blending hot liquids and can blow the lid right off the blender chamber, so always place a dishtowel over the blender lid before you hit the power button to prevent spin art on your kitchen wall (and possibly burns).

Heat the olive oil in a soup pot over medium heat, then add the onion, fennel, and a pinch of salt and sauté until golden, about 4 minutes. Stir in the carrots, orange zest, cumin, cinnamon, allspice, red pepper flakes, and 1/4 teaspoon of salt and sauté until well combined. Pour in 1/2 cup of the broth and cook until the liquid is reduced by half.

Add the remaining 7 1/2 cups broth and another 1/4 teaspoon salt and cook until the carrots are tender, about 20 minutes.

In a blender, puree the soup in batches until very smooth, each time adding the cooking liquid first and then the carrot mixture. If need be, add additional liquid to reach the desired thickness.

Return the soup to the pot over low heat, stir in the orange juice, lemon juice, maple syrup, and a pinch of salt, and gently reheat slowly. Do a FASS check. Does it need a squeeze of lemon, a pinch or two of salt, or a drizzle of maple syrup?

Serve garnished with a drizzle of the Cashew Cream.

Variation: With a little rearranging, you can create a carrot, coconut, and curry soup. Omit the chopped fennel, red pepper flakes, and allspice and add 1 teaspoon of curry powder with the cinnamon and cumin. At the end of the cooking process, stir in 1 cup of coconut milk before blending, then do a FASS check; you'll probably want to add an extra pinch of salt and a squeeze of lime.

PREP TIME: 30 minutes · COOK TIME: 35 minutes

STORAGE: Store in an airtight container in the refrigerator for up to 4 days or in the freezer for up to 2 months.

PER SERVING: Calories: 215; Total Fat: 5.5 g (0.8 g saturated, 3.4 g monounsaturated); Carbohydrates: 40 g; Protein: 4 g; Fiber: 10 g; Sodium: 405 mg

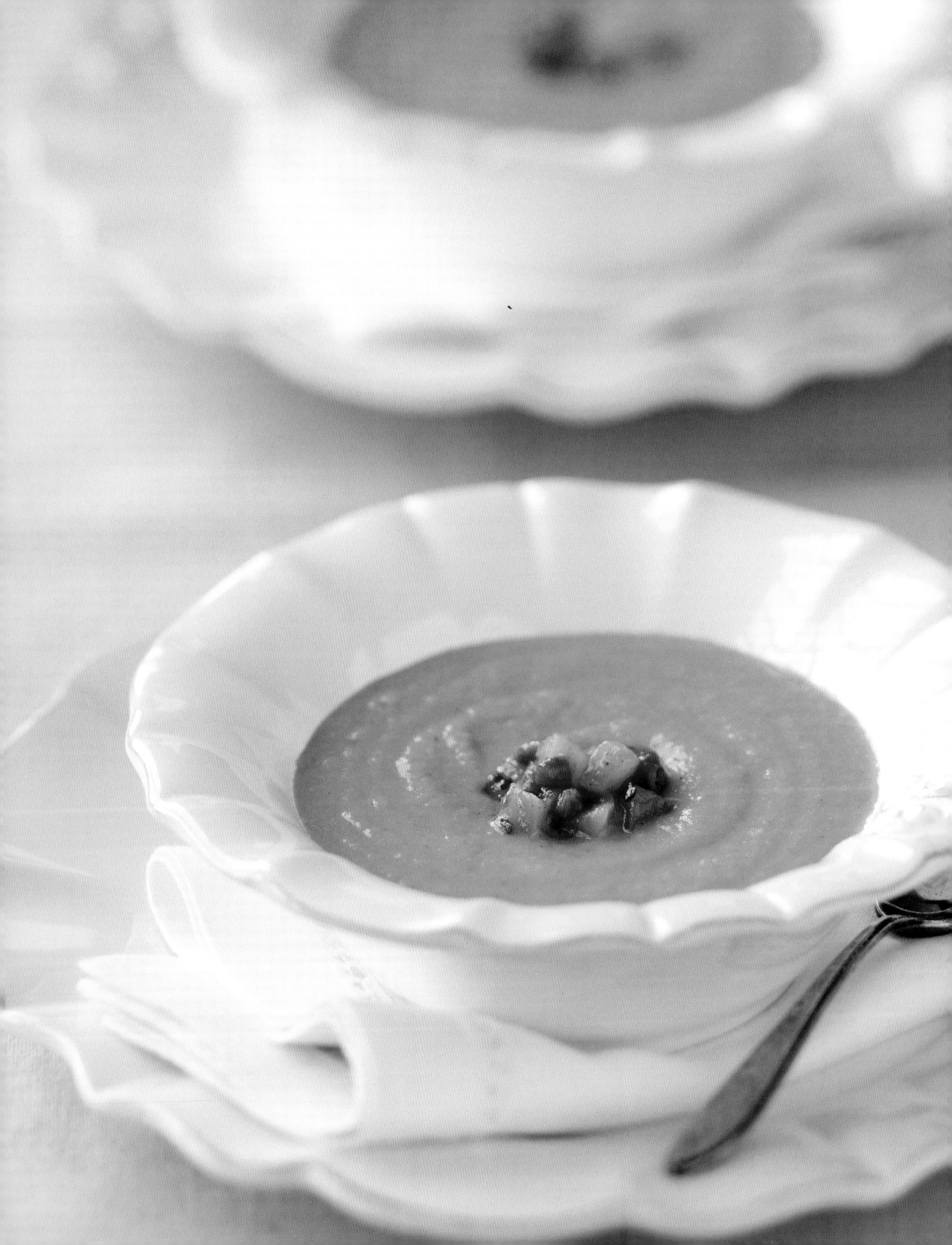

Curry Cauliflower Soup

Cauliflower is a wonderful vegetable that's full of excellent cancer-fighting enzymes, yet it's sorely in need of a PR campaign. That's because most people steam cauliflower, which makes the kitchen smell like a stink bomb detonated. Either that or, like my dad, they eat cauliflower raw and tasteless as crudités (in his case, dipped in Russian dressing). The secret is to roast cauliflower. Not only does this avoid the sulfur smell, it also produces an unbelievably sweet flavor. SERVES 6

- 1 head cauliflower, cut into florets
- 3 tablespoons extra-virgin olive oil
- Sea salt
- 1 cup finely diced yellow onion
- 2 carrots, peeled and diced small
- 1 cup finely diced celery
- 1 teaspoon curry powder
- 1/4 teaspoon ground cumin
- 1/4 teaspoon ground coriander
- 1/8 teaspoon ground cinnamon
- 6 cups Magic Mineral Broth (page 54)
- Apricot Pear Chutney (page 175), for garnish

Preheat the oven to 400°F and line a baking sheet with parchment paper.

Toss the cauliflower with 1 tablespoon of the olive oil and 1/4 teaspoon of salt, then spread it in an even layer on the prepared pan. Bake until the cauliflower is tender, about 25 minutes.

While the cauliflower is roasting, heat the remaining 2 tablespoons olive oil in a sauté pan over medium heat, then add the onion and a pinch of salt and sauté until translucent, about 3 minutes. Add the carrots, celery, and 1/4 teaspoon salt and sauté until the vegetables begin to brown, about 12 minutes.

Add the curry powder, cumin, coriander, cinnamon, and another 1/2 teaspoon of salt and stir until the spices have coated the vegetables. Pour in 1/2 cup of the broth to deglaze the pan and cook until the liquid is reduced by half. Remove from the heat.

Pour 3 cups of the remaining broth into a blender, then add half of the sautéed vegetables and roasted cauliflower. Blend until smooth, then pour the mixture into a soup pot and repeat the process with the remaining 2 1/2 cups broth and the remaining vegetables and cauliflower. For a thinner consistency, add another cup of broth.

Gently reheat the soup over low heat, then do a FASS check. You may want to add a spritz of fresh lemon juice and another 1/4 teaspoon salt.

Serve garnished with a dollop of Apricot Pear Chutney, which undoubtedly will take you to the land of yum!

PREP TIME: 10 minutes · COOK TIME: 35 minutes

STORAGE: Store in an airtight container in the refrigerator for up to 4 days or in the freezer for up to 2 months.

PER SERVING: Calories: 165; Total Fat: 7.5 g (1.1 g saturated, 5.1 g monounsaturated); Carbohydrates: 23 g; Protein: 5 g; Fiber: 7 g; Sodium: 260 mg

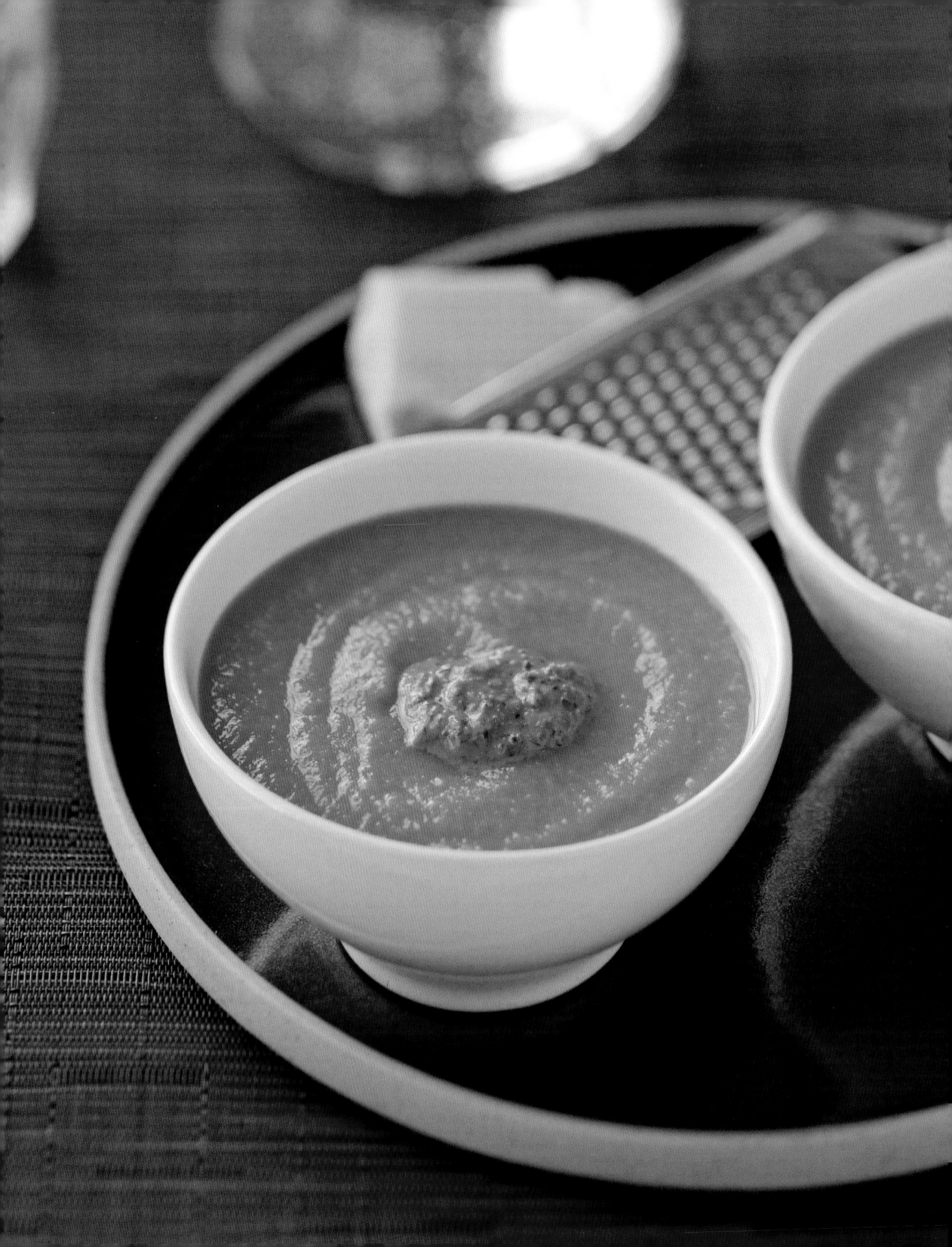

Roasted Red Roma Tomato Soup

For many people, tomato soup is a familiar and beloved comfort food. In this version, the soup benefits from roasting the tomatoes in the oven to lessen their acidity and add sweetness. Just be aware that some tomatoes are juicier than others; if they're very juicy, you may need to drain some of the juice into a bowl during the roasting process. Using the pan juices as the broth creates supercharged scrump-dilly-iciousness! Plus, the roasted tomatoes blend beautifully (and colorfully) with the carrots. This soup is equally delicious served hot, at room temperature, or chilled. SERVES 6

- 4 pounds Roma tomatoes, halved
- 2 tablespoons extra-virgin olive oil
- Sea salt
- 1 onion, diced small
- 3 carrots, scrubbed and diced small
- 1 clove garlic, chopped
- Up to 2 cups Magic Mineral Broth (page 54) or store-bought vegetable stock, as needed
- 1/4 teaspoon agave nectar (optional)
- Parsley Basil Drizzle, for garnish (page 187; optional)
- Grated organic Parmesan cheese, for garnish (optional)

Preheat the oven to 400°F.

Gently squeeze the tomatoes by hand to remove excess seeds, then put them in a bowl and toss with 1 tablespoon of the olive oil and 1/2 teaspoon of salt until evenly coated. Place the tomatoes, cut side down, in a single layer on sheet pans and roast for 20 to 30 minutes, until their skins are just browning and the juices are bubbly. Let cool for 5 minutes, then lift off the skins with a fork.

Meanwhile, heat the remaining 1 tablespoon olive oil in a soup pot over medium heat, then add the onion and a pinch of salt and sauté until golden, about 4 minutes. Add the carrots, garlic, and 1/4 teaspoon of salt and continue to sauté until the carrots are just tender, about 5 minutes.

In a blender, puree the tomatoes with their juice and the carrot mixture until smooth.

(continued, next page)

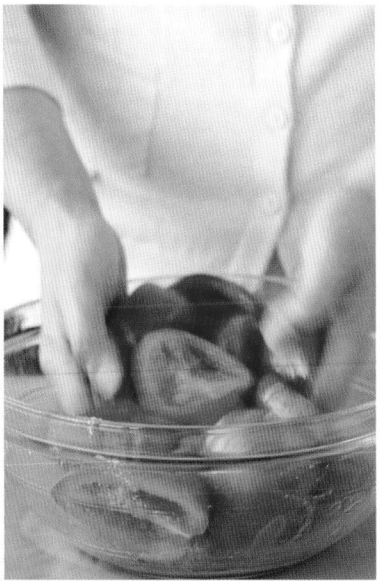

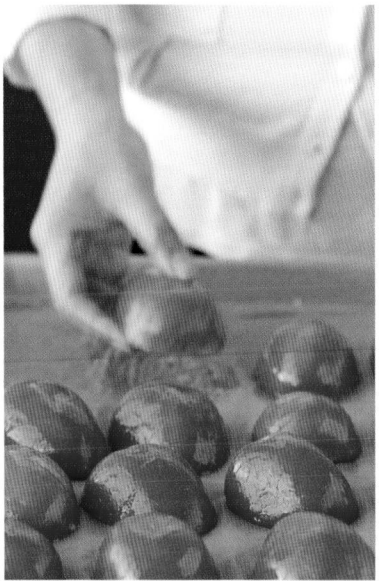

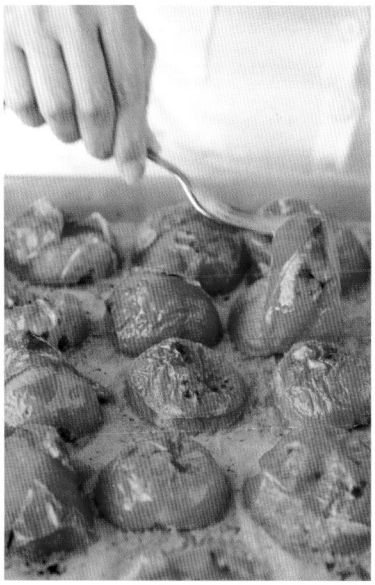

You may need to add some broth at the end of the blending process depending on the juiciness of the tomatoes. Add 1 cup at a time until you have the desired thickness.

Return the soup to the pot and gently reheat over medium-low heat. Stir in another 1/4 teaspoon of salt, then do a FASS check. Tomatoes can sometimes be acidic, so you may want to add a bit of agave nectar and another pinch of salt.

Serve topped with the Parsley Basil Drizzle and a sprinkling of Parmesan cheese (if using).

Variation: If fresh tomatoes aren't available, you can substitute two 28-ounce cans of plum tomatoes.

PREP TIME: 20 minutes · COOK TIME: 35 minutes

STORAGE: Store in an airtight container in the refrigerator for 5 days, or in the freezer for 2 months.

PER SERVING: Calories: 135; Total Fat: 5.4 g (0.8 g saturated, 3.4 g monounsaturated); Carbohydrates: 21 g; Protein: 4 g; Fiber: 6 g; Sodium: 280 mg

Cooling Cucumber Avocado Soup

Avocado lovers will go ga-ga over the taste and those with swallowing difficulties or mouth sores will delight in the texture. Those of you into cool or room-temperature soups will embrace the clean, fresh feel of this blend. Avocados are one of those great superfoods, full of good fats and vitamins. They're fun to work with, and all of the great shades of green in this soup are like preparing a beautiful watercolor that you can eat. SERVES 6

- 2 cups water
- 2 pounds English cucumbers, peeled, seeded, and cut into chunks
- 2 ripe avocados, pitted and peeled
- 3 tablespoons freshly squeezed lime juice
- 1/4 teaspoon agave nectar
- Sea salt
- Pinch of cayenne
- 1 tablespoon finely chopped fresh mint
- 1 tablespoon finely chopped fresh cilantro

Pour 1 cup of the water into the blender, then add the cucumbers, avocados, lime juice, agave nectar, 1/4 teaspoon of salt, and the cayenne. Blend until extremely smooth, gradually adding more water until you reach the desired consistency. Taste and adjust the amount of salt, adding as much as 3/4 teaspoon more.

Chill for at least 2 hours, then stir in the mint and cilantro just before serving.

PREP TIME: 15 minutes · COOK TIME: 2 hours in the refrigerator

STORAGE: Store in an airtight container in the refrigerator for up to 2 days.

PER SERVING: Calories: 95; Total Fat: 7.2 g (1 g saturated, 4.5 g monounsaturated); Carbohydrates: 8 g; Protein: 2 g; Fiber: 4 g; Sodium: 105 mg

REBECCA'S NOTES English cucumbers, which are usually wrapped in plastic in the produce section of the grocery store, really make a difference in this recipe. They're less watery than standard cucumbers and will add more substance to the soup.

Rockin' Black Bean Soup

A staple of Latin cuisine, this black bean soup rocks because it's a nutritional powerhouse. Black beans are rich in protein and dietary fiber, and recent studies link black bean consumption to reduced rates of pancreatic, breast, and prostate cancers. Cooking the beans with kombu, an easy to find dried Japanese seaweed that breaks down the bean's sugars, eases gas and bloating while softening the bean's exterior. As for taste, I guarantee your taste buds will say "more, please!" SERVES 6

- 2 cups black beans
- 2 tablespoons extra-virgin olive oil
- 2 cups diced yellow onions
- Sea salt
- 1 cup finely diced red bell pepper
- 1 1/2 teaspoons seeded and finely diced jalapeño pepper
- 1 tablespoon minced garlic
- 1 1/2 teaspoons dried oregano
- 1/2 teaspoon ground cumin
- 1/4 teaspoon ground cinnamon
- 8 cups Magic Mineral Broth (page 54)
- 4 cloves garlic, smashed
- 1 6-inch strip of kombu
- 1 cinnamon stick
- 1 bay leaf
- 3 corn tortillas, for garnish
- 1/4 cup fresh cilantro, chopped, for garnish
- Avocado Cream (page 178), for garnish

REBECCA'S NOTES You can use canned organic black beans, but make sure you give them the spa treatment first: Rinse, spritz with lemon juice, and sprinkle with salt. Add cooked beans just after sauteing the vegetables.

Place the beans in a pan or bowl with water to cover and soak overnight, or for at least 8 hours.

Heat the olive oil in a soup pot over medium heat, then add the onions and a pinch of salt and sauté until the onions are translucent, about 4 minutes. Add the bell pepper, jalapeño, minced garlic, oregano, cumin, cinnamon, and 1/4 teaspoon of salt and sauté for 1 minute. Pour in 1/2 cup of the broth to deglaze the pot and cook until the liquid is reduced by half.

Add the remaining 7 1/2 cups broth, along with the black beans, smashed garlic, kombu, cinnamon stick, and bay leaf. Bring to a boil over high heat, then simmer, partially covered, for 1 hour.

Test a bean, and once they are at least halfway cooked, add another 1/4 teaspoon salt. (If too much salt is added too early, it will inhibit the softening of the beans.) Continue to simmer for another 30 minutes, until the beans are nice and soft.

Meanwhile, preheat the oven to 350°F. Cut the corn tortillas into strips and arrange them in a single layer on a sheet pan. Bake for 5 minutes, until slightly golden.

Using a slotted spoon, fish out and discard the kombu, cinnamon stick, and bay leaf, then remove half of the cooked beans and set aside. Puree the remaining beans and the broth in a blender, in batches if need be, blending until the beans are as smooth as velvet.

Return the soup to the pot over low heat, stir in the reserved beans, and gently reheat. Do a FASS check, and if it needs a little extra pop, add another 1/4 teaspoon of salt and 2 teaspoons of lime juice.

Serve garnished with the tortilla strips, a sprinkling of cilantro, and a dollop of the Avocado Cream.

PREP TIME: 15 minutes (after soaking the beans overnight)

COOK TIME: 1 hour 45 minutes

STORAGE: Store in an airtight container in the refrigerator for up to 5 days or in the freezer for up to 2 months.

PER SERVING: Calories: 390; Total Fat: 5.6 g (0.8 g saturated, 3.4 g monounsaturated); Carbohydrates: 70 g; Protein: 16 g; Fiber: 11 g; Sodium: 300 mg

Spiced Sweet Potato Soup

Thank heavens that sweet potatoes are no longer relegated just to Thanksgiving. For years bodybuilders, who follow strict eating regimens to repair their muscles after workouts, have feasted on sweet potatoes because of their outstanding nutritional content, ease of digestion, and pleasant flavor. Chock-full of beta-carotene, vitamin A, and other body boosters, sweet potatoes are also extremely anti-inflammatory, which may protect against cancer growth. As a cook, I like sweet potatoes because they make a wonderful creamy canvas for warming spices such as cinnamon and ginger. This soup is an especially great meal for people with a lingering metallic taste in their mouth due to chemotherapy. It's delicious served with a dollop of Apricot Pear Chutney (page 175). SERVES 6

- 3 pounds sweet potatoes, peeled and diced into 1-inch cubes
- 2 tablespoons unrefined virgin coconut oil, melted, or olive oil
- 1/2 teaspoon sea salt
- 1/4 teaspoon ground cinnamon
- 1/4 teaspoon ground allspice
- 1/8 teaspoon ground cardamom
- 1/8 teaspoon freshly grated nutmeg
- 6 to 8 cups Magic Mineral Broth (page 54)

REBECCA'S NOTES These roasted spiced sweet potatoes are fantastic on their own. Consider making half a recipe of soup and saving the remaining sweet potatoes for a delicious side dish or a quick and easy snack.

Want an easy way to melt coconut oil without dirtying up an extra pan or using the microwave? Place a small ramekin filled with coconut oil in a bowl filled with a small amount of very hot water (don't use too much water, or it might overflow into the ramekin). The oil will turn to liquid before your eyes.

Preheat the oven to 400°F and line a baking sheet with parchment paper.

Toss the sweet potatoes with the coconut oil until they're evenly coated. In a small bowl, combine 1/4 teaspoon of the salt with the cinnamon, allspice, cardamom, and nutmeg and stir until well combined. Sprinkle the spice mixture over the potatoes and toss again until evenly coated.

Place the sweet potatoes in a single layer on the prepared pan and roast for 40 minutes, until tender.

Pour 1/3 cup of the broth into a blender, add one-third of the roasted potatoes, and blend until smooth, adding more liquid as needed. Transfer to a soup pot over low heat and repeat the process two more times. Stir in any remaining broth, along with the remaining 1/4 teaspoon salt, before serving.

PREP TIME: 10 minutes · COOK TIME: 55 minutes

STORAGE: Store in a covered container in the refrigerator for 5 to 7 days or in the freezer for up to 2 months.

PER SERVING: Calories: 280; Total Fat: 4.8 g (4 g saturated, 0.3 g monounsaturated); Carbohydrates: 57 g; Protein: 5 g; Fiber: 9 g; Sodium: 465 mg

"Food and friends enabled me to have joy in my life while going through cancer treatment. I loved going to cooking classes where I could laugh and escape from 'cancer world.' And then there was the generosity extended by friends and family who brought over nourishing meals when I didn't feel like cooking. The best gift of all was a big pot of soup awaiting me on my doorstep!"

—Jennifer O., breast cancer survivor

Summer's Best Zucchini Soup

I like the way nature balances her books. In summertime, everyone gets hot and loses water. So what does Mother Nature do? She produces an abundance of summer squash, which happens to be full of water, making it an ideal vegetable to combat dehydration. I think of zucchini as the perfect party guest. It's mild and mixes well with a crowd. The key with zucchini is good prep, so that the flesh stays somewhat firm and tasty. SERVES 8

- 2 tablespoons extra-virgin olive oil
- 1 cup finely diced yellow onion
- Sea salt
- 2 cloves garlic, chopped
- 1 Yukon gold potato, peeled and diced small
- 6 1/2 cups Chicken Magic Mineral Broth (page 55), Magic Mineral Broth (page 54), or store-bought organic stock
- 3 1/2 pounds zucchini, quartered lengthwise, then cut crosswise into 1/2-inch pieces
- 1 teaspoon dried oregano
- Pinch of red pepper flakes
- 1 cup grated zucchini
- 3 teaspoons freshly squeezed lemon juice
- Pistachio Cream (page 181), for garnish
- 1 tablespoon chopped fresh parsley, for garnish
- 1 tablespoon chopped fresh mint, for garnish

Heat the olive oil in a sauté pan over medium heat, then add the onion and a pinch of salt and sauté until golden, about 5 minutes. Add the garlic, potato, and 1/4 teaspoon of salt and continue to sauté for about 8 minutes, until the potatoes begin to get tender, adding 1 tablespoon of broth if they begin to stick or the pan gets too dry. Add the diced zucchini, oregano, red pepper flakes, and another 1/4 teaspoon of salt and sauté for 4 minutes. Pour in 1/2 cup of the broth to deglaze the pan and cook until the liquid is reduced by half. Remove from the heat.

Pour 2 cups of the broth into a blender, add one-third of the zucchini sauté, and blend until smooth. Transfer to a soup pot over low heat, and repeat the process two more times. Stir in the grated zucchini and lemon juice, then taste and adjust the seasoning if needed until you have achieved yum.

Serve garnished with the Pistachio Cream, parsley and mint.

Variation: For a luscious curried zucchini soup, omit the oregano and add 1 teaspoon of curry powder and 1/4 teaspoon of cumin. In place of the Pistachio Cream, parsley, and mint, garnish with a dollop of Sweet and Savory Yogurt (page 189) or Tomato Mint Chutney (page 176). Yum!

PREP TIME: 10 minutes · COOK TIME: 20 minutes

STORAGE: Store in an airtight container in the refrigerator for up to 3 days or in the freezer for up to 2 months.

PER SERVING: Calories: 130; Total Fat: 4.1 g (0.7 g saturated, 2.6 g monounsaturated); Carbohydrates: 23 g; Protein: 4 g; Fiber: 5 g; Sodium: 175 mg

Velvety Red Lentil Dahl

I was working at the Chopra Center for Wellbeing when the only living woman Indian saint stopped in. Her entourage laid down some pretty strict rules: No talking to the saint. No approaching the saint. And whatever you do, don't touch the saint. But after eating her bowl of dahl, this little imp of a holy woman motioned me over and then . . . proceeded to kiss me on the forehead! The Chopra folks (and I guess the saint as well) like their dahl chunky, and I love it that way too, but it's just as enjoyable blended and smooth. Blend the dahl a bit if you want something a little easier to swallow or digest. Small amounts of this dahl are wonderful for someone who isn't particularly hungry, as the cumin is an appetite stimulant. SERVES 6

- 2 tablespoons unrefined virgin coconut oil or extra-virgin olive oil
- 1 1/2 teaspoons cumin seeds
- 1 1/2 teaspoons black or brown mustard seeds
- 1 onion, diced small
- 1 tablespoon minced fresh ginger
- 2 teaspoons turmeric
- 2 teaspoons ground cumin
- Sea salt
- 2 cups chopped tomatoes, or 1 14-ounce can diced tomatoes, drained
- 8 cups Magic Mineral Broth (page 54)
- 2 cups red lentils, rinsed well
- 1 cinnamon stick
- 1 teaspoon freshly squeezed lime juice
- 1/2 teaspoon agave nectar or maple syrup
- 1/4 cup finely chopped fresh cilantro or mint, for garnish
- Tomato Mint Chutney (page 176), for garnish

REBECCA'S NOTES If you're in the mood for a heartier meal, skip the blender and just eat the dahl atop brown basmati rice, topped with a dollop of chutney. Or, blend half of the dahl until smooth, then add the unblended dahl to your velvety mixture.

Heat the coconut oil in a soup pot over medium heat. Add the cumin and mustard seeds and sauté until they begin to pop, then quickly add the onion, ginger, turmeric, ground cumin, and a pinch of salt and sauté for about 3 minutes. Add the tomatoes and 1/4 teaspoon of salt and sauté for 2 minutes more. Pour in 1/2 cup of the broth to deglaze the pan and cook until the liquid is reduced by half.

Add the red lentils and stir well, then add the remaining 7 1/2 cups broth and the cinnamon stick. Bring to a boil over high heat, then lower the heat, cover, and simmer for about 30 minutes, until tender.

Add another 1/4 teaspoon of salt and simmer, for another 5 minutes. Remove the cinnamon stick and stir in the lime juice and agave nectar.

In a blender, puree the soup in batches until very smooth, adding additional broth or water if you'd like a thinner soup.

Return the soup to the pot and gently reheat. Serve garnished with the chopped cilantro and a dollop of Tomato Mint Chutney.

PREP TIME: 15 minutes (with canned tomatoes) · COOK TIME: 45 minutes

STORAGE: Store in an airtight container in the refrigerator for 5 days or in the freezer for 2 months.

PER SERVING: Calories: 365; Total Fat: 7 g (4.1 g saturated, 0.6 g monounsaturated); Carbohydrates: 58 g; Protein: 20 g; Fiber: 14 g; Sodium: 300 mg

WHO KNEW? Add Spice for Life We know what fresh spices can do for the flavor of a dish, but as it turns out, they can also have a powerful impact on cancer. Integrative oncologist Donald Abrams especially likes turmeric, and so do many of his colleagues. At the American Society of Clinical Oncology's annual meeting in 2006, an entire morning was devoted to the cancer-fighting benefits of turmeric, specifically in regard to antitumor properties with colon cancer and possibly pancreatic cancer. Turmeric may also help with other chronic diseases. "Turmeric is a good spice," says Abrams. "We think it's one of the reasons that there's so little Alzheimer's disease in India and also less cancer than we'd expect in a nation of that size." A spice with a mind-body connection? Works for me.

Creamy Broccoli and Potato Soup

A lot of people have only had a close-up encounter with broccoli as raw crudités or boiled until it's gray and limp, which is unappetizing and often difficult to digest. Here, sautéing the broccoli in olive oil, infusing it with broth, and then blending releases all of its sweetness and cancer-fighting properties and helps everything go down nice and easy. SERVES 6

- 2 tablespoons extra-virgin olive oil
- 1 cup finely diced onion
- 2 cloves garlic, chopped
- 2 cups peeled and finely diced Yukon gold potatoes
- 1/2 teaspoon sea salt
- 3/4 pound broccoli
- 4 1/2 cups Chicken Magic Mineral Broth (page 55), Magic Mineral Broth (page 54), or organic store-bought stock
- 3 shavings of nutmeg
- Shredded organic Cheddar cheese, for garnish (optional)

WHO KNEW? The Best Offense Is a Good Defense
Here's a reason to eat organic that I bet you've never heard before: Compared to their commercially raised cousins, organics are natural-born fighters. And here's the really cool part; they're able to pass their survival skills on to those who eat them. Dr. Donald Abrams, director of integrative oncology at UCSF Medical Center, explains: "If a vegetable is grown indoors or in a hothouse, it doesn't have to do anything to protect itself from its environment. Whereas if you grow, say, a tomato organically outdoors, it needs to protect itself from insects and other predators and from sunshine. So it produces chemicals to protect itself. And it turns out, for the most part, that those are the phytonutrients that are beneficial to people." A little symbiotic survival: that's what I call a win-win!

Heat the olive oil in a large sauté pan over medium heat, then add the onion and sauté until lightly golden, about 3 minutes. Stir in the garlic and then the potatoes, along with a generous 1/4 teaspoon of the salt. Sauté until the potatoes are just tender, about 5 minutes.

Meanwhile, cut the broccoli florets into bite-size pieces. Trim and peel the stems and cut them into bite-size pieces as well. Pour in 1/2 cup of broth to deglaze the pan, turn down the heat to medium-low, and cook until the liquid is reduced by about half. Add the broccoli and the remaining 1/4 teaspoon salt, cover, and cook until the broccoli is bright green and just tender, 3 to 4 minutes.

Pour 2 cups of the remaining broth into a blender, add half of the broccoli mixture, and blend until smooth. Pour the mixture into a soup pot, then repeat the process with the remaining 2 cups broth and the remaining vegetables. Stir in the nutmeg.

Gently reheat the soup over low heat, then do a FASS check. You may want to add additional salt, a grinding of pepper, and about 1/2 teaspoon of lemon juice.

Serve garnished with a sprinkle of the cheese.

Variation: For even more yum, replace the sautéed garlic with roasted garlic. To roast garlic, preheat the oven to 325°F. Cut the top off a head of garlic, place it on a square of parchment paper, and drizzle 1 teaspoon of olive oil over the garlic. Wrap the garlic in the parchment paper and then in a slightly larger piece of aluminum foil. Bake for 45 minutes, until golden brown. The aroma will tell you when it's ready. Once the garlic is cool, squeeze the pulp out into a small bowl. Add 1 teaspoon when blending this soup, and refrigerate the remainder in an airtight container for later use. Roasted garlic makes a yummy addition to many savory dishes, especially Roasted Red Roma Tomato Soup (page 69), and Navy Bean and Sun-Dried Tomato Dip (page 131).

PREP TIME: 20 minutes · COOK TIME: 20 minutes

STORAGE: Store in an airtight container in the refrigerator for 4 days.

PER SERVING: Calories: 155; Total Fat: 5.1 g (0.8 g saturated, 3.4 g monounsaturated); Carbohydrates: 26 g; Protein: 4 g; Fiber: 4 g; Sodium: 330 mg

CHAPTER 4

Vital Vegetables

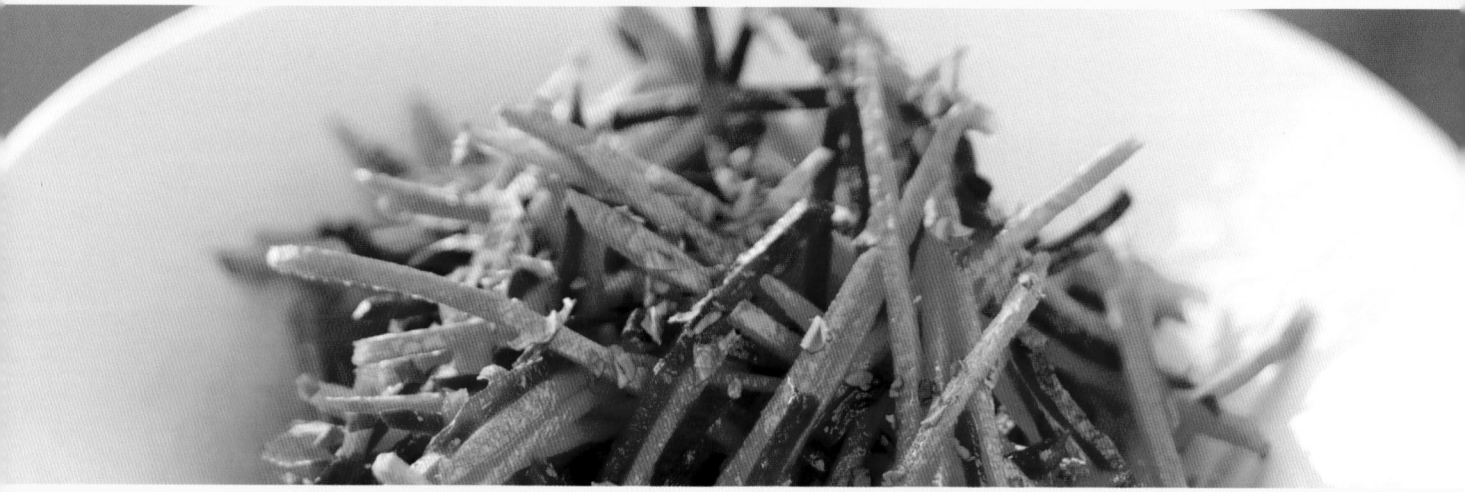

78 *Basil Broccoli*

80 *Baby Bok Choy with Yam and Ginger*

81 *Green Beans with Brazil Nuts and Basil*

83 *Cucumber, Jicama, and Mango Salad*

84 *Emerald Greens with Orange*

86 *Gregg's Stuffed Acorn Squash with Quinoa, Cranberries, and Swiss Chard*

88 *Kale with Carrots*

89 *Kale with Sweet Potatoes and Pecans*

90 *Mashed Cinnamon Butternut Squash*

91 *Mixed Greens with Edamame, Radish, and Avocado*

92 *Warm Napa Cabbage Slaw*

93 *Purple Peruvian Smashed Potatoes*

93 *Warm and Toasty Cumin Carrots*

95 *Hungarian Roasted Root Vegetable Potpie*

97 *Stir-Fried Baby Bok Choy with Shiitake Mushrooms*

98 *Shredded Carrot and Beet Salad*

Vegetables talk to me—really! Oh, they were shy at first, and who can blame them? It takes time to learn their hidden language, which they only speak when they're really, really fresh. What do canned vegetables have to say to us, in terms of taste and nutrition? Not much. If they speak at all, they're likely to sound like Marlon Brando in *The Godfather*—a barely discernible mumble. But when they're at their peak of flavor, nutrition, and color (which, not surprisingly, all happens at the same time), my God! It sounds like a cacophony at the farmers' market: "Pick me! Pick me! Please!" It reminds me of a Southern coming-out ball, with the farmers playing the role of proud parents as they show off with great pride the beautiful children they've raised.

Vegetables have always spoken to my need for visually stimulating foods. I think that is a sense that's often overlooked, but if you think about people whose appetite is on a precipice, lovely *looking* fruits and vegetables can entice them off the ledge and back to the table. Getting folks to enjoy vegetables is often all about changing a long-established skeptical mind-set. I maintain that taste is the ultimate long-term motivator, but you may need a great warm-up act to get people pumped up for the show, in this case by speaking to the senses they engage—sight and smell—before they ever take their first bite. Light up those senses, and victory, by which I mean a diet filled with scrumptious, nutritious fruits and veggies, is suddenly within anyone's grasp.

A lot of my friends laugh at my enthusiasm over vegetables. I like to tell them that while soups bring out my warm, loving side, vegetables bring out my passion. Maybe it's because they're so breathtakingly alive. Vegetables are bursting with phytochemicals that do everything from protect our bodies from daily wear and tear to combat cancer. Is it any wonder that nature is practically screaming to eat these beautiful plant nutrients? Steaming, roasting, sautéing, baking . . . there are so many quick and simple ways to make these delights delicious, and it's so important that people in treatment get the incredible bounty of anticancer properties that veggies willingly offer up, with their heartfelt thanks.

How do I know?

They told me so.

Basil Broccoli

Sometimes creating recipes is like dating. You have to know when to hold 'em and when to fold 'em. I recently broke up with a chopped broccoli dish because we had no chemistry. It just wasn't happening. I might have been depressed if not for another broccoli suitor that swept me off my feet. This guy—well, as mom likes to say, he cleans up nice. Maybe it's the company he keeps as well; surrounding himself with fresh basil, red bell peppers, a little lemon . . . they're a sprightly crowd, fun to hang with, and healthy, too, full of anti-inflammatories and other anticancer properties. SERVES 4

1 bunch of broccoli

Sea salt

2 tablespoons extra-virgin olive oil

1 tablespoon finely chopped garlic

Pinch of red pepper flakes

1/2 cup diced red bell pepper or cherry tomatoes

1 tablespoon freshly squeezed lemon juice

2 teaspoons lemon zest

1/4 cup fresh basil, finely chopped

REBECCA'S NOTES No skimping on the basil! Not only does it contain powerful antioxidant properties, basil combined with the broccoli and the peppers or tomatoes really takes the flavor over the top.

The combination of the bright green of the broccoli and the red of the bell peppers is beautiful, making this dish a feast for the eyes. Be sure to add the lemon juice and zest just before serving, as the lemon will dampen the color of the broccoli if it sits for more than a few minutes.

Bring a large pot of water to a boil. Cut the broccoli florets off the stalks, then peel the stems and cut them into bite-size pieces. Add a pinch of salt and the broccoli florets and stems to the pot of water and blanch for 30 seconds. Drain the broccoli, then run it under cold water to stop the cooking process; this will retain its lush green color.

Heat the olive oil in a sauté pan over medium heat, then add the garlic and red pepper flakes and sauté for 30 seconds, just until aromatic. Add the bell pepper and a pinch of salt and sauté for an additional minute. Stir in the broccoli florets and 1/4 teaspoon of salt and sauté for 2 minutes; the broccoli should still be firm. Gently stir in the lemon juice, lemon zest, and basil and serve immediately.

PREP TIME: 10 minutes · COOK TIME: 5 minutes

STORAGE: Store in an airtight container in the refrigerator for 5 to 7 days.

PER SERVING: Calories: 125; Total Fat: 7.7 g (1.1 g saturated, 5.4 g monounsaturated); Carbohydrates: 13 g; Protein: 5 g; Fiber: 5 g; Sodium: 125 mg

CULINARY RX Talk about a one-two punch. It turns out that, in tandem, some vegetables have a synergistic effect, pumping up each other's ability to fight cancer. When researchers combined tomato and broccoli, their ability to shrink prostate tumors in mice was significantly higher than what either vegetable could accomplish on its own. Now, if they can only find a similar link between mashed potatoes and gravy . . .

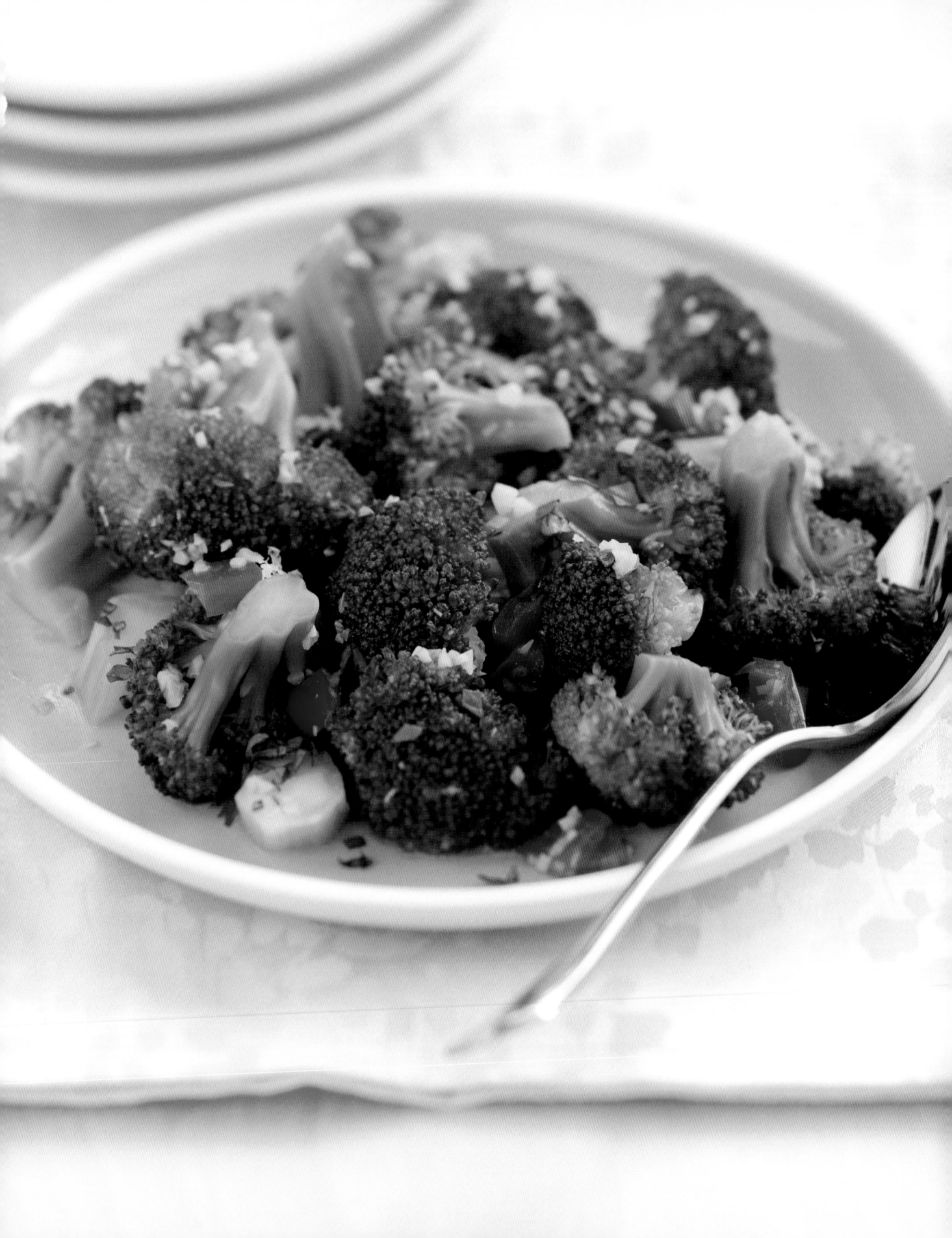

Baby Bok Choy with Yam and Ginger

As much as I love to cook, I also really enjoy watching other cooks go through their creative process. Recently I was at a conference at the Commonweal Retreat Center, where I was able to observe one of my favorite cooks, Claire Heart. She brought out this dish, and the first thing I noticed was that it had bok choy. Now that's a great vegetable, but it tends to be bitter. She completely solved that problem by pairing it with yams to create a dish that tasted like a vegetarian Chinese Thanksgiving. It was a completely unique and delicious pairing. The colors blew me away as well. I went home and decided to play around with her concept, adding a little ginger for zing and digestion and a few more Asian-style flavors. Thank you, Claire! SERVES 6

- 4 heads baby bok choy
- 2 tablespoons light sesame oil
- 2 scallions, white part only, thinly sliced
- 2 tablespoons minced fresh ginger
- 1 cup peeled and finely diced garnet yam
- Sea salt
- 2 tablespoons mirin (optional)
- 1 tablespoon tamari
- 1 tablespoon freshly squeezed lime juice
- 1/4 teaspoon toasted sesame oil

Trim the bases off the bok choy and discard. Trim the leaves from the stems and cut both crosswise into bite-size pieces, keeping the stems and leaves separate.

Heat the light sesame oil in a sauté pan over medium heat, then add the scallions and ginger and sauté for 30 seconds. Add the yam and a pinch of salt and sauté for an additional minute. Add the bok choy stems, mirin, and tamari and sauté for 2 minutes more. Add the bok choy leaves, lime juice, 1/4 teaspoon of salt, and the toasted sesame oil. Cook until the bok choy is just wilted, about 2 minutes, then do a FASS check and add a squeeze of lime if desired. Serve immediately.

PREP TIME: 15 minutes · COOK TIME: 5 minutes

STORAGE: Store in a covered container in the refrigerator for 3 days.

PER SERVING: Calories: 150; Total Fat: 6 g (0.9 g saturated, 2.2 g mono-unsaturated); Carbohydrates: 19 g; Protein: 9 g; Fiber: 6 g; Sodium: 595 mg

"During the really rough times, the doctors told me to eat whatever I could. I had always wanted doctors to say that to me. After lots of blended meals, I now appreciate the texture of food almost as much as the taste."
—Terri T., oral cancer survivor

Green Beans with Brazil Nuts and Basil

Green bean recipes are a little like socks; everybody has a few. I came across a website that boasted 471 green bean recipes. By the time I linked to it a second later, they were up to 472, so clearly it's a popular vegetable. This dish is dairy-free and delicious. Instead of a common cheese topping, I use finely ground Brazil nuts, which you'll swear taste like Parmesan cheese. Why Brazil nuts? Because they're an amazing source of selenium, a mineral that some scientists believe lessens chemo's toxic effects on healthy cells. SERVES 6

Sea salt
1 pound green beans, trimmed
2 tablespoons extra-virgin olive oil
2 tablespoons chopped shallot
Freshly ground black pepper
Freshly squeezed lemon juice
2 tablespoons finely ground Brazil nuts or walnuts
2 tablespoons finely chopped fresh basil
1/2 teaspoon lemon zest

Bring a generous amount of water (about 8 cups) to a boil. Add 1/4 teaspoon of salt and the green beans and cook until tender but still crisp, 3 to 6 minutes. Drain the green beans, then run them under cold water to stop the cooking process.

Heat the olive oil in a large sauté pan over medium heat, then add the shallot and a pinch of salt and sauté until translucent, about 1 minute. Stir in the beans, add 1/4 teaspoon of salt, and cook, stirring occasionally, until heated through, about 2 minutes. Remove from the heat and add several grinds of pepper, a spritz of the lemon juice, and the nuts. Toss with the basil and lemon zest before serving.

Variation: If you don't have Brazil nuts, Maple-Glazed Walnuts (page 141) make a great substitute.

PREP TIME: 15 minutes · COOK TIME: 10 minutes
STORAGE: Store in an airtight container in the refrigerator for 2 days.
PER SERVING: Calories: 320; Total Fat: 8.3 g (1.1 g saturated, 4.1 g monounsaturated); Carbohydrates: 47 g; Protein: 18 g; Fiber: 12 g; Sodium: 110 mg

CULINARY RX Nuts may suppress the growth of cancers because they contain the antioxidants quercetin and kaempferol. Brazil nuts have especially powerful anticancer properties, as each one contains 80 micrograms of selenium, a trace mineral that may fight prostate cancer.

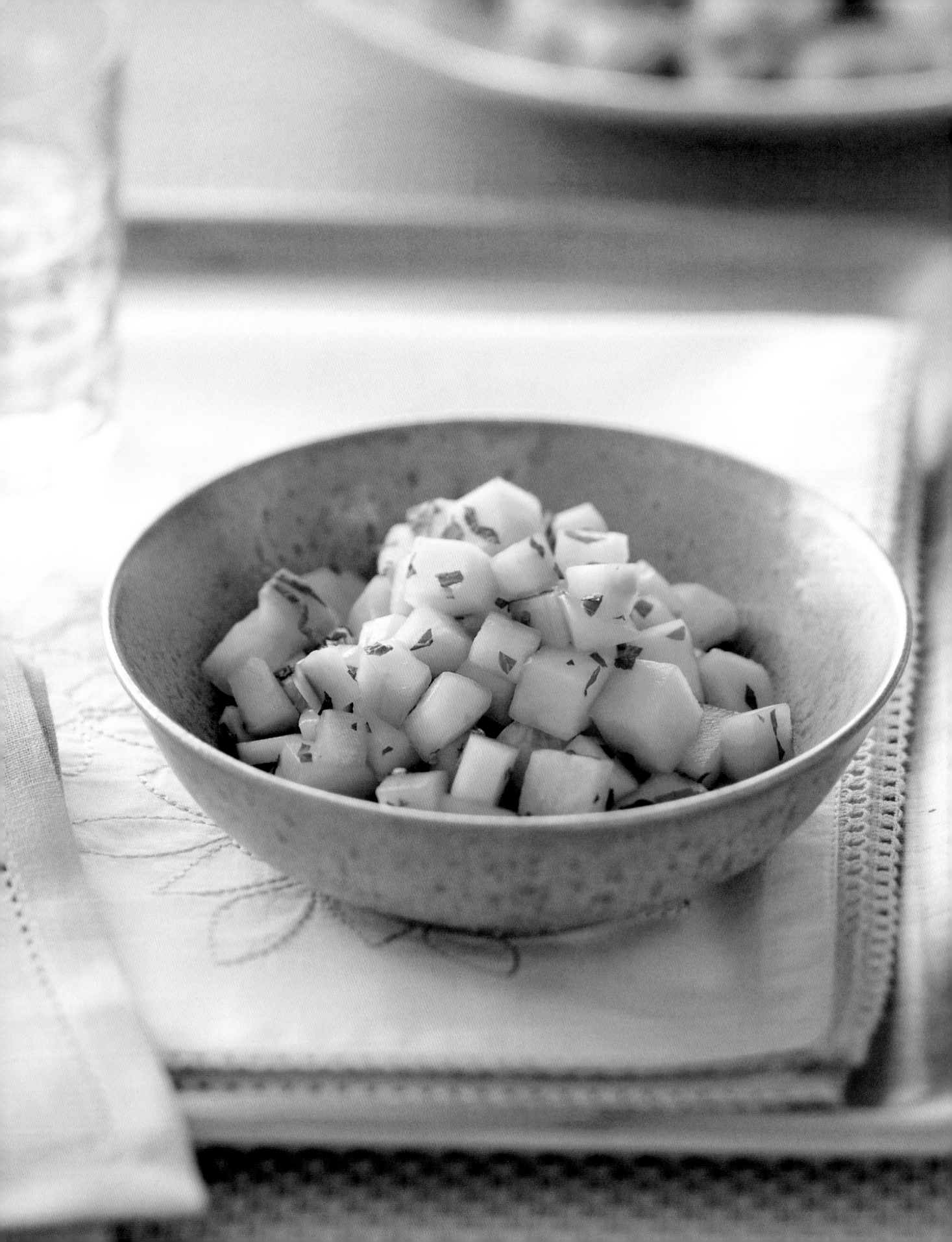

Cucumber, Jicama, and Mango Salad

While the concept of sweet-and-sour dishes is generally appealing, the execution often leaves something to be desired. Sweet-and-sour is like a seesaw; if it tilts too far in either direction, you could be thrown off balance, mangling your taste buds in the process. In this recipe I use a very light hand on both sides; the sour is a delicate brown rice vinegar, the sweet a gentle agave nectar. They dance together nicely on the tongue, more like ballet than Irish clogging. For folks who like a crunchy texture or who want to avoid fat, this one's a winner. SERVES 6

- 1/4 cup brown rice vinegar
- 1/4 cup water
- 2 tablespoons agave nectar
- 1/2 teaspoon freshly squeezed lime juice
- 1/4 teaspoon sea salt
- 1 large English cucumber, peeled
- 1 cup peeled and diced jicama, in 1/2-inch cubes
- 1 cup diced mango, in 1/4-inch cubes
- 3 tablespoons coarsely chopped fresh mint

Combine the vinegar, water, agave nectar, lime juice, and salt in a small saucepan over medium heat and bring to a gentle boil. Cook until the liquid is clear and slightly thickened, about 2 minutes. This should yield 1/4 cup of liquid. Refrigerate the dressing for 15 minutes.

Quarter the cucumber lengthwise, remove the seeds, and slice crosswise into 1/2-inch pieces. Combine the cucumber, jicama, mango, and the cooled vinegar mixture in a bowl and stir well, then stir in the chopped mint.

PREP TIME: 10 minutes · COOK TIME: 15 minutes

STORAGE: Store in an airtight container in the refrigerator for 5 to 6 days.

PER SERVING: Calories: 60; Total Fat: 0.2 g (0 g saturated, 0 g monounsaturated); Carbohydrates: 14 g; Protein: 0 g; Fiber: 2 g; Sodium: 100 mg

REBECCA'S NOTES If you're feeling intimidated by chopping up a jicama or want to save time, many markets have precut jicama available in the refrigerated area of the produce section.

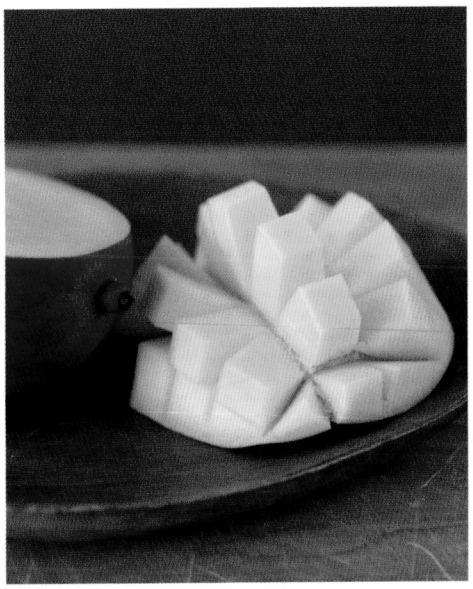

Emerald Greens with Orange

For a lot of people, working with greens is reminiscent of a high school science project. I used to feel that way too. I remember the first time I brought home a bunch of Swiss chard. I laid those big, leafy stalks on my counter and thought to myself, "Should I just put these in a vase and stare at them? Or should I wait until summer and fan myself with them?" The truth is, for many of us, our aversion to greens goes back to childhood because kids are very sensitive to bitter tastes and, many greens, if not prepared properly, can be bitter. However, all it takes to remove that bitter taste is a very simple fix: a quick bath in olive oil and a little heat. Sautéeing chard in olive oil—or any green, for that matter—makes the flavor and consistency much more palate friendly. Adding orange to the mix makes these greens especially yummy, and that's a great thing because greens and the phytochemicals they contain are a must-have for maintaining health. SERVES 4

- 2 tablespoons extra-virgin olive oil
- 1 teaspoon minced garlic
- Pinch of red pepper flakes
- 2 tablespoons dried cranberries
- 1/4 cup freshly squeezed orange juice
- 6 cups stemmed and chopped Swiss chard, in bite-size pieces
- 1/4 teaspoon sea salt
- 1/2 teaspoon orange zest
- 1/4 teaspoon maple syrup

REBECCA'S NOTES The flavor of this dish is greatly intensified by reducing the liquid in the pan. Take the time to perform this step. Your taste buds will be rewarded.

One trick to preparing greens is ripping them off their tough stems. This makes them easier to eat and digest. You can chop the chard stems into small pieces and add them to the pan earlier so they have a chance to cook more.

Heat the olive oil in a large sauté pan over medium heat, then add the garlic, red pepper flakes, cranberries, and orange juice and sauté for 30 seconds, just until aromatic. Add the chard, salt, and zest and sauté until the color of the chard begins to darken and intensify. Use a slotted spoon to transfer the greens to a bowl, then bring the liquid in the pan to a boil. When the liquid shrinks in from the sides of the pan and thickens a bit, stir the greens back in, then stir in the maple syrup. Do a FASS check. You may want to add another pinch of salt. Serve immediately.

Variation: To make this a real jewel of a dish, omit the cranberries and sprinkle 2 tablespoons of gorgeous ruby red pomegranate seeds over the greens just before serving.

PREP TIME: 10 minutes · COOK TIME: 10 minutes

STORAGE: Store in an airtight container in the refrigerator for 5 to 7 days.

PER SERVING: Calories: 90; Total Fat: 7.2 g (1 g saturated, 5 g monounsaturated); Carbohydrates: 7 g; Protein: 1 g; Fiber: 1 g; Sodium: 260 mg

"How did my diet change? I was already eating healthy before treatment, but I got to be more organic than I was before. I looked for the darkest (most nutrient-rich) greens and the cleanest, most hormone- and toxin-free fish and meats."
—Ty H., cancer survivor

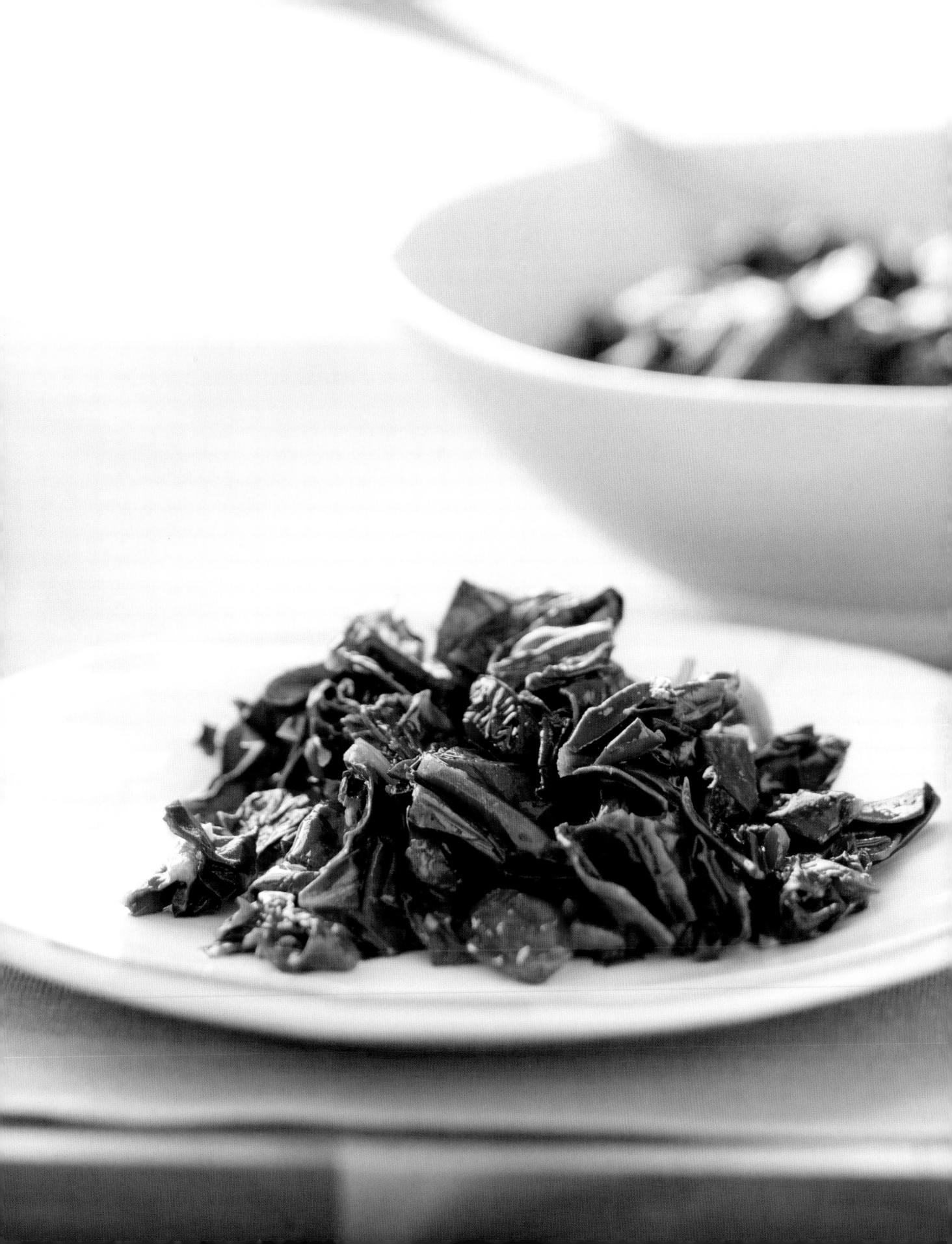

Gregg's Stuffed Acorn Squash with Quinoa, Cranberries, and Swiss Chard

When a confirmed, dyed-in-the-wool meat eater starts claiming a vegetable dish is his favorite meal of all time, that's when I know I'm onto something. I made this for my husband, Gregg, and he went absolutely ga-ga over it. (And no, Gregg's not one of those guys who would say it's great just because I made it. He's an honest food critic.) I've noticed that a lot of people who avoid vegetables gravitate to this dish. It could be because it's colorful or comes in its own bowl, but I really think it's because the hearty taste elicits a comfort food response. Squash has so many things going for it. It's easy to digest and has numerous qualities—anti-inflammatory, antioxidant, immunity-boosting—that make it a boon for anyone dealing with cancer. Squash is also a natural vessel for all sorts of wonderful fillings. And if you aren't in the mood for roasting squash, this quinoa pilaf makes for a yummy dish all on its own. SERVES 4

SQUASH

4 acorn squash

2 tablespoons extra-virgin olive oil

1/4 teaspoon sea salt

1/4 teaspoon ground allspice

1/4 teaspoon ground ginger

1/4 teaspoon ground cinnamon

Pinch of red pepper flakes

FILLING

1 cup quinoa

1 tablespoon plus 2 teaspoons extra-virgin olive oil

1 tablespoon finely diced shallot

3 tablespoons finely diced fennel

1/4 teaspoon ground cumin

1/4 teaspoon ground coriander

2 cups Magic Mineral Broth (page 54) or water

1/2 teaspoon sea salt

2 cloves garlic, minced

Pinch of red pepper flakes

1/2 cup dried cranberries or raisins

6 cups stemmed and chopped Swiss chard or kale, in bite-size pieces

Fresh squeezed lemon juice

Preheat the oven to 350°F and line a sheet pan with parchment paper.

To make the squash, cut the tops off the squash and scoop out the strings and seeds. Also cut the pointy ends off the bottoms of the squash so they'll stand up once they're stuffed.

Stir the olive oil, salt, allspice, ginger, cinnamon, and red pepper flakes together in a bowl. Use a brush to spread the spice mixture over the inside of the squash. Place the squash, top side down, on the prepared pan and roast for 20 to 25 minutes, until tender. Check after 20 minutes by touching the top of a squash with your finger. If it's soft, transfer the squash from the oven and cover with foil until you're ready to fill them.

Meanwhile, make the filling. Put the quinoa in a fine-mesh sieve and rinse well under running cold water.

Heat the 2 teaspoons of olive oil in a saucepan over medium heat. Add the shallot and fennel and sauté until soft, about 3 minutes. Stir in the cumin and coriander, then stir in the quinoa. Stir in the broth and 1/4 teaspoon of the salt, cover, and bring to a boil, then lower the heat and simmer for 15 to 20 minutes, until the quinoa has absorbed all of the liquid. Remove from the heat, and fluff with a fork.

While the quinoa is cooking, heat the 1 tablespoon of olive oil in a large sauté pan over medium heat, then add the garlic, red pepper flakes, and cranberries. Stir for 10 seconds, then add the kale and the remaining 1/4 teaspoon salt. Sauté until the greens are tender, about 5 minutes for kale, or 3 minutes for chard. Remove from the heat and stir in a squeeze of the lemon juice.

To assemble the dish, spoon the quinoa mixture into the squash, then top each squash with a scoop of the greens.

PREP TIME: 25 minutes · COOK TIME: 45 minutes

STORAGE: Store in an airtight container in the refrigerator for 3 days or in the freezer for 1 month.

PER SERVING: Calories: 530; Total Fat: 16.3 g (2.3 g saturated, 9.9 g monounsaturated); Carbohydrates: 93 g; Protein: 11 g; Fiber: 13 g; Sodium: 650 mg

WHO KNEW? Taking Care of Yourself during Treatment When it comes to taking care of yourself during treatment, here's why it's important to walk the talk. Numerous studies show that the more patients do to improve their quality of life—exercise, having a support group, reducing or managing stress, eating well, and so on—"the better they're going to respond to treatment," says Keith Block, a doctor who has extensively studied cancer and supportive treatments. Passive patients don't do nearly as well, says Block, noting that "25 to 35 percent of all patients undergoing conventional treatment drop out . . . and patients who drop out or miss therapies don't do as well."

Shopping for Organics

Why go organic? Where do I begin?! Taste, color, nutrient-density—organic food is superior in all these areas. Why would you opt for food raised with commercial pesticides, additives, and artificial color and flavoring if you have a better choice? Best of all, the groundswell toward eating organic in the last few years has made them less expensive and more widely available. Growers who meet the standards of the Federal Organic Foods Production Act and receive state or federal certification can label their foods as organic, but they're not the only entities providing organic foods. Small farmers who sometimes don't want to incur the cost or time involved in meeting the requirements of the federal organic act also grow organic foods, including hormone- and chemical-free poultry and meats. You'll find these purveyors most often at farmers' markets, where they often enjoy chatting about the foods they've raised.

If you can't afford to buy all organic produce, I recommend you steer clear of the most compromised items. The Environmental Working Group (www.ewg.org), a nonprofit that conducts research and publishes information on the effects of environmental factors on health, recommends avoiding the following nonorganically raised produce:

Peaches	Celery	Cherries	Pears
Apples	Nectarines	Lettuce	Spinach
Sweet Bell Peppers	Strawberries	Grapes (imported)	Potatoes

The following non-organically raised fruits and vegetables have the least amount of pesticide residue:

Onions	Pineapples	Asparagus	Cabbage
Avocados	Mangoes	Kiwi Fruit	Broccoli
Sweet Corn (frozen)	Sweet Peas (frozen)	Bananas	Eggplant

For a pocket guide and more comprehensive pesticide food list, visit www.foodnews.org

For the latest science and news about organics, visit the Organic Center: www.organic-center.org

For more information on organic foods, visit the Organic Trade Association: www.ota.com

Kale with Carrots

We've come a long way with greens since those days when the produce section in the grocery store consisted primarily of iceberg lettuce. First we started seeing more romaine, then—gasp!—mesclun, and now there are endless varieties of field greens, baby greens, micro greens, and even micro sprouts. That's not a bad thing, of course, but it can be a little intimidating when you stare at the produce and say, "Hmm . . . what's that?" Which brings us to kale. People sometimes steer away from kale because it's slightly bitter, but a yin-yang approach will bring it into balance—in this case, using carrots and ginger to neutralize kale's slight bitterness. Greens really are vital for maintaining health during treatment, and this recipe will help you learn to love the taste. For a decadently delicious touch, sprinkle Maple-Glazed Walnuts (page 141) over the greens just before serving. SERVES 4

- 4 cups stemmed and chopped curly kale, in bite-size pieces
- 2 tablespoons extra-virgin olive oil
- 1 red onion, cut into half moons
- Sea salt
- 2 carrots, peeled and diced small
- 3 cloves garlic, minced
- 1 teaspoon minced fresh ginger
- 2 tablespoons freshly squeezed lemon juice

REBECCA'S NOTES The longer the lemon just sits on the greens, the more the greens will lose their beautiful color. Wait to add the lemon juice until just before serving.

No curly kale at the market? No worries! Any kale will do, or substitute spinach, Swiss chard, collard greens, mustard greens, or any other leafy green.

Cover the kale with cold water and set aside. Heat the olive oil in a large, deep sauté pan over medium-high heat, then add the onion and a pinch of salt and sauté for 3 minutes. Decrease the heat to low and cook slowly until the onions are caramelized, about 20 minutes.

Increase the heat to medium, add the carrots, garlic, ginger, and a pinch of salt and sauté for 3 to 4 minutes, until the carrots are tender. Drain the kale and add it to the pan along with a scant 1/4 teaspoon of salt. Sauté until the greens turn bright green and wilt, about 3 minutes. Test the greens, you may need to add 1 tablespoon of water and continue cooking, covered, until they become just a little more tender, 2 to 3 minutes. Drizzle on the lemon juice and stir gently. Serve immediately.

PREP TIME: 5 minutes · COOK TIME: 30 minutes

STORAGE: Store in a covered container in the refrigerator for 3 days.

PER SERVING: Calories: 120; Total Fat: 7.6 g (1.1 g saturated, 5 g monounsaturated); Carbohydrates: 14 g; Protein: 3 g; Fiber: 3 g; Sodium: 125 mg

WHO KNEW? Every Veggie Counts! Oncology nurse Theresa Koetters says she's noticed that while some people in her treatment center claim not to like vegetables, asking a few direct questions often makes them realize that this just isn't true. Koetters recalls a man who just wrinkled up his nose at the idea of eating veggies: "So I said 'what about peas and corn and beans and broccoli and kale and beets and squash, and . . .' I went down a whole list and he said, 'Oh yeah, I like that, and that, and that.' I said, 'Okay, now you've got five vegetables that you can start adding a couple of times a day, or every other day—anything is going to be more than what you're doing now.' We talked about baby steps and incremental improvements." One small pea pod for a man, one giant leap into the produce aisle. . .

Kale with Sweet Potatoes and Pecans

If there's a safe haven in the vegetable kingdom, it's sweet potatoes. In fact, I bet that if every kid's introduction to veggies were a sweet potato, it would knock down parental stress over healthy eating by at least 50 percent. I mean, what's not to love? Sweet taste, beautiful color, and fantastic nutrition, not to mention a creamy texture that allows you to introduce chopped greens in a nonthreatening manner. Here, I've added kale, which has some outstanding anticancer properties, and ginger, which aids digestion, for a little zip. SERVES 4

- 2 tablespoons extra-virgin olive oil or unrefined virgin coconut oil
- 1 teaspoon minced fresh ginger
- 1 cup peeled and finely diced sweet potato or garnet yam
- 1/8 teaspoon ground cinnamon
- 1/4 cup Magic Mineral Broth (page 54) or water
- 3 cups cleaned, stemmed, and chopped dinosaur kale, in bite-size pieces
- 1/4 teaspoon sea salt
- 2 tablespoons golden raisins
- 1/4 teaspoon maple syrup
- 2 tablespoons ground pecans, for garnish

Heat the oil in a large sauté pan over medium heat, then add the ginger and sauté for 30 seconds, just until aromatic. Add the sweet potato, cinnamon, and broth and sauté for about 1 minute. Add the kale, salt, and raisins and sauté until the kale is a darker shade of green and the sweet potatoes are tender, about 5 minutes. Stir in the maple syrup, then do a FASS check and add another pinch of salt if desired.

Serve garnished with the ground pecans.

Variation: The ground pecans have the same texture as a sprinkling of finely grated cheese. If you'd like something more crunchy, place 1/4 cup of pecans on a baking sheet and toast at 350°F for 7 to 10 minutes, until aromatic and slightly browned. Chop coarsely before sprinkling on this beautiful dish.

PREP TIME: 15 minutes · COOK TIME: 10 minutes

STORAGE: Store in a covered container in the refrigerator for 5 days.

PER SERVING: Calories: 160; Total Fat: 10.1 g (1.3 g saturated, 6.6 g monounsaturated); Carbohydrates: 17 g; Protein: 3 g; Fiber: 3 g; Sodium: 200 mg

CULINARY RX Kale is like a twenty-four-hour pharmacy unto itself. It possesses a variety of phytochemicals that attack different cancers. In one large study, women who ate diets rich in kaempferol (found in kale and other green vegetables such as broccoli, leeks, and spinach) were 40 percent less likely to develop ovarian cancer. Kale has similar effects on the development of bladder and breast cancers. Kale is also rich in numerous antioxidants that promote immune system wellness.

Mashed Cinnamon Butternut Squash

To the uninitiated, winter squash can be a bamboozling vegetable. Sure, it tastes delicious, but being so hard and often so funny-looking, it's a bit intimidating whole. The first time I got one home, I felt like I was working with a tree stump. How was I going to get to all of that delicious flesh in the middle? Machete? Chainsaw? Actually, a good sharp chef's knife is all you need, and if you don't want to go there, most supermarkets now sell precut squash. I don't mind the work, because of the wonderful reward—a succulent, sweet, yum-alicious treasure that, when pureed and roasted, tastes like candy. Really! If you've ever worked with a pumpkin, taking on squash isn't all that different. Only there's no trick here, just treat. (Personally, I'm a fan of cutting squash in half lengthwise then prebaking it so I can easily scoop out the middle, but that's just me.) SERVES 4

- 1 butternut squash, peeled and cut into 1-inch cubes
- 2 tablespoons extra-virgin olive oil
- 1/4 teaspoon ground cinnamon
- 1/4 teaspoon ground ginger, or 1 teaspoon grated fresh ginger
- Sea salt
- 1/4 teaspoon maple syrup
- 1/8 teaspoon freshly grated nutmeg

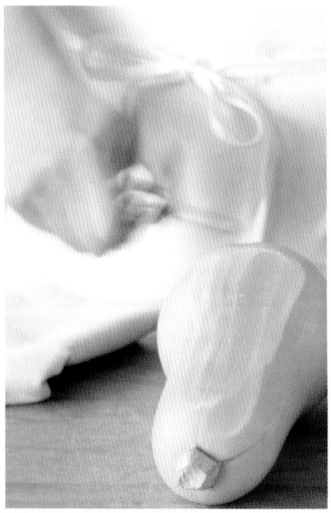

Preheat the oven to 400°F and line a baking sheet with parchment paper.

Toss the squash with the olive oil, cinnamon, ginger, and 1/4 teaspoon of salt until the squash is well coated, then spread it in a single layer on the prepared pan. Roast for 25 to 30 minutes, until soft and tender.

Transfer the squash to a food processor, add the maple syrup, nutmeg, and a pinch of salt, and process until smooth and creamy. Do a FASS check. If you think it needs a little extra punch, try adding 1 teaspoon of fresh lemon juice.

Variation: If you don't feel like dealing with a butternut squash, replace it with 3 carrots and 3 parsnips, chopped into 1-inch pieces.

PREP TIME: 15 minutes · COOK TIME: 35 minutes

STORAGE: Store in an airtight container in the refrigerator for 3 days.

PER SERVING: Calories: 160; Total Fat: 7.2 g (1.1 g saturated, 5 g monounsaturated); Carbohydrates: 25 g; Protein: 2 g; Fiber: 4 g; Sodium: 155 mg

"I found the following things helped me get through treatment: Regular acupuncture treatments, getting out in nature as often as possible, and arranging my chemo for Fridays so I could have the weekend to recover before going to work on Monday. Keeping my work schedule as regular as possible made me feel normal."
—Diana C., two-time breast cancer survivor

Mixed Greens with Edamame, Radish, and Avocado

Some soy lovers might be surprised that their beloved bean goes by another name—edamame—which is the fresh, green, undried form, with all of its nutrients intact. Here, I've taken the edamame out of their furry little pods, and mixed them in with radishes, which have a fresh flavor and just a tad of heat. My friend calls radishes the sorbet of the vegetable set because of the way they brighten the palate and leave it feeling clean and happy. SERVES 4

- 6 cups mixed salad greens
- 1 cup fresh or frozen shelled edamame, mixed with a spritz of fresh lime juice and a pinch of sea salt
- 4 radishes, trimmed and sliced
- 1/2 avocado, spritzed with fresh lime juice and sprinkled with sea salt (so it doesn't discolor)
- 1/4 cup Cilantro-Lime Vinaigrette (page 181)

Combine the greens with the edamame, radishes, and avocado in a large bowl. Add the vinaigrette and toss to combine.

PREP TIME: 15 minutes · COOK TIME: Not applicable

STORAGE: If you must store the salad, don't add the dressing. Store the greens and veggies in an airtight container in the refrigerator for 1 day at most.

PER SERVING: Calories: 160; Total Fat: 11.2 g (1.4 g saturated, 6.7 g monounsaturated); Carbohydrates: 12 g; Protein: 5 g; Fiber: 5 g; Sodium: 200 mg

WHO KNEW? Soy Advice Some people, especially women dealing with breast cancer, have concerns about eating soy. The issue is whether compounds in soy have estrogenic effects that could encourage tumor growth. I put the question to Joel Evans, MD, founder and director of the Center for Women's Health, where he practices integrative obstetrics and gynecology. "Soy is fine in moderation, except for women on tomoxifen," says Evans. "I'm not talking about something small like soy sauce, but major ingredients in a dish. The reason is, soy will knock the tomoxifen drug off the tomoxifen receptor in the body. It's not that it's harming you directly, but it's taking away the benefit of the tomoxifen. You're on it for a reason; if you eat soy, you'll lose that benefit." Evans says that for everyone else, fermented soy is preferable, such as miso and tempeh. He suggests limiting soy to three to five 3-ounce servings per week.

Warm Napa Cabbage Slaw

When I was growing up, coleslaw was pretty one-dimensional. It didn't matter where you went, German deli, Greek diner, it was all pretty much the same: cold cabbage drowned in mayo with a few slivers of carrot for coloring and maybe a few celery seeds. These days, slaw has gotten an extreme makeover, and there are now more versions to choose from. This concoction is both warm and sweet and serves as a great base for salmon, chicken, tofu, or tempeh. Sautéing the onions, red cabbage, and carrots in a little brown rice vinegar, tamari, and ginger makes it easy to eat and mighty flavorful. SERVES 4

- 2 tablespoons brown rice vinegar
- 2 tablespoons tamari
- 1 teaspoon maple syrup
- 1 tablespoon minced fresh ginger
- 1 tablespoon light sesame oil
- 1 cup thinly sliced red onion
- Sea salt
- 2 cups shredded Napa cabbage
- 1 cup shredded red cabbage
- 1 cup peeled and shredded carrots
- 1/4 cup fresh cilantro leaves

Whisk the vinegar, tamari, maple syrup, and ginger together in a bowl.

Heat the sesame oil in a large sauté pan over medium heat, then add the onion and a pinch of salt and sauté until the onions are translucent, about 3 minutes. Add the Napa cabbage, red cabbage, carrots, and a pinch of salt and sauté until the cabbage is slightly wilted, about 2 minutes. Stir in the vinegar mixture and cook until the liquid is reduced by half and coats the vegetables. Remove from the heat and stir in the cilantro.

Variation: Add some protein to this dish by stirring in 1 1/2 cups of shredded roasted chicken, tofu, or tempeh when you add the vinegar. This is a delicious addition and can turn a side dish into an entire meal.

PREP TIME: 10 minutes · COOK TIME: 10 minutes

STORAGE: Store in an airtight container in the refrigerator for 3 to 5 days.

PER SERVING: Calories: 85; Total Fat: 3.7 g (0.5 g saturated, 1.5 g monounsaturated); Carbohydrates: 11 g; Protein: 2 g; Fiber: 2 g; Sodium: 610 mg

REBECCA'S NOTES You may be wondering how to take on cabbage, the bocce ball of vegetables. Place the cabbage on a cutting board with the stem side down. Using a sharp chef's knife, cut the cabbage in half from top to bottom. Use the tip of your knife to remove the core. To shred cabbage by hand, hold the cabbage on the cutting board at an angle and give it a shave by making a thin slice down the flat (cut) side of the cabbage.

Purple Peruvian Smashed Potatoes

Potatoes get a bad rap as being one big carbo load with little or no nutrition. That's a shame, because it's not true of all varieties, especially not purple Peruvian potatoes. Smashing, as the name suggests, uses muscle to get what you need, instead of lots of butter and milk like typical mashed potatoes. A hand mixer will do, but I prefer my mom's old potato masher from 1953. As you pulverize all of those inner starches, you'll produce a fluffy texture, a lot of flavor, and, with these potatoes, a gorgeous and unusual color. SERVES 4

- 1 pound purple Peruvian potatoes, peeled and cut into 1/2-inch cubes
- 1/4 cup Magic Mineral Broth (page 54), Chicken Magic Mineral Broth (page 55), or store-bought organic stock
- Sea salt
- 3 tablespoons extra-virgin olive oil
- 2 tablespoons finely chopped chives
- 2 tablespoons finely chopped fresh parsley

Pour 4 inches of water into a large saucepan or soup pot. Put a steamer basket in the pot and bring the water to a boil. Put the potatoes into the steamer basket and steam until tender, about 10 minutes.

Remove the steamer basket and pour out the water. Put the potatoes into the pot, add the broth, and gently warm over low heat. Add 1/2 teaspoon of salt and the olive oil, then smash with a potato masher. Stir in the chives, parsley, and a generous pinch of salt and serve right away.

PREP TIME: 10 minutes · COOK TIME: 15 minutes

STORAGE: Store in an airtight container in the refrigerator for 3 days.

PER SERVING: Calories: 190; Total Fat: 10.7 g (1.5 g saturated, 7.5 g monounsaturated); Carbohydrates: 24 g; Protein: 2 g; Fiber: 2 g; Sodium: 310 mg

Warm and Toasty Cumin Carrots

Toasting cumin releases its aromatic, flavorful, and incredibly healthy oils. As the seeds heat up, they begin popping like popcorn, which is how you know they're done. SERVES 4

- 1/2 teaspoon cumin seeds
- 2 tablespoons extra-virgin olive oil
- 1 teaspoon minced fresh ginger
- 1 1/2 cups peeled and sliced carrots, cut 1/4 inch thick
- 1/4 teaspoon sea salt
- 2 tablespoons water
- 1 teaspoon freshly squeezed lemon juice
- 1 teaspoon maple syrup
- Chopped fresh parsley, for garnish

Toast the cumin seeds in a dry sauté pan over medium heat, shaking the pan back and forth until they start to pop and become aromatic. Immediately add the olive oil and ginger and sauté for 1 minute. Stir in the carrots and salt, then turn down the heat to medium-low, add the water, cover, and cook for about 2 minutes, until just barely tender. Stir in the lemon juice and maple syrup. Garnish with the parsley and serve immediately.

PREP TIME: 10 minutes · COOK TIME: 5 minutes

STORAGE: Store in an airtight container in the refrigerator for 5 to 7 days.

PER SERVING: Calories: 85; Total Fat: 7.2 g (1 g saturated, 5.1 g monounsaturated); Carbohydrates: 6 g; Protein: 0 g; Fiber: 1 g; Sodium: 180 mg

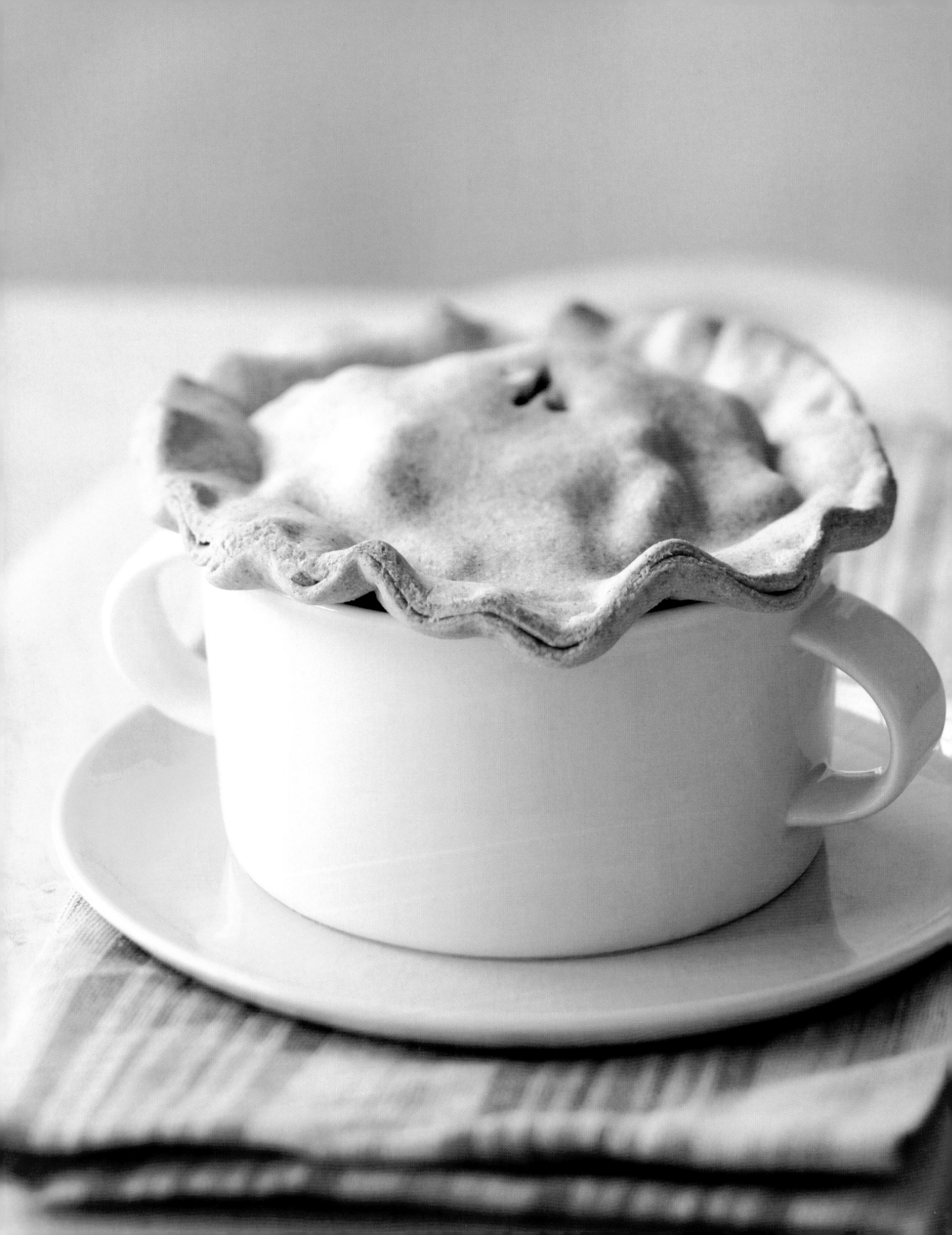

Hungarian Roasted Root Vegetable Potpie

Pretty much everyone has a neighbor or friend (kind of a June Cleaver type) who loves to cook and also somehow manages to be a CEO and raise three Rhodes scholars while spending three hours a day (minimum) in the kitchen. This is the recipe you give that person when she says, "Oh, I'd so like to make something for you." This is a labor of love, and while not quite as physically intensive as, say, coal mining, it takes a bit of effort. But it's worth it, because the recipe is big enough to be made in ramekins so it can serve as six little meals, and it stores well, too. SERVES 6

SPELT CRUST

- 1 1/4 cups whole wheat pastry flour
- 1 cup spelt flour
- 2 teaspoons baking powder
- 1/2 teaspoon sea salt
- 1/2 cup water
- 1/4 cup extra-virgin olive oil
- 1 teaspoon maple syrup

ROOT VEGETABLES

- 1 teaspoon paprika
- 1/2 teaspoon ground allspice
- 1/2 teaspoon ground cinnamon
- 1/2 teaspoon sea salt
- 3 tablespoons extra-virgin olive oil
- 1 1/2 cups peeled and diced turnip, in 1/2-inch cubes
- 1 3/4 cups peeled and diced parsnips, in 1/2-inch cubes
- 1 cup peeled and diced rutabaga, in 1/2-inch cubes
- 1 1/2 cups peeled and diced sweet potato, in 1/2-inch cubes
- 1 1/2 cups peeled and diced kabocha or butternut squash, in 1/2-inch cubes
- 1 cup peeled and diced French fingerling potatoes or red potatoes, in 1/2-inch cubes

SAUTÉ

- 2 tablespoons extra-virgin olive oil
- 1 large onion, diced small
- Pinch of sea salt
- 1 teaspoon caraway seeds
- 1 1/2 cups peeled and finely diced carrots
- 1 1/2 cups finely diced celery
- 1 cup thickly sliced cremini or baby portobello mushrooms

SAUCE

- 2 tablespoons organic clarified butter or extra-virgin olive oil
- 2 tablespoons unbleached all-purpose flour
- 1 1/2 cups Magic Mineral Broth (page 54)
- Pinch of sea salt
- Pinch of freshly ground pepper
- 1 generous shaving of nutmeg

(continued, next page)

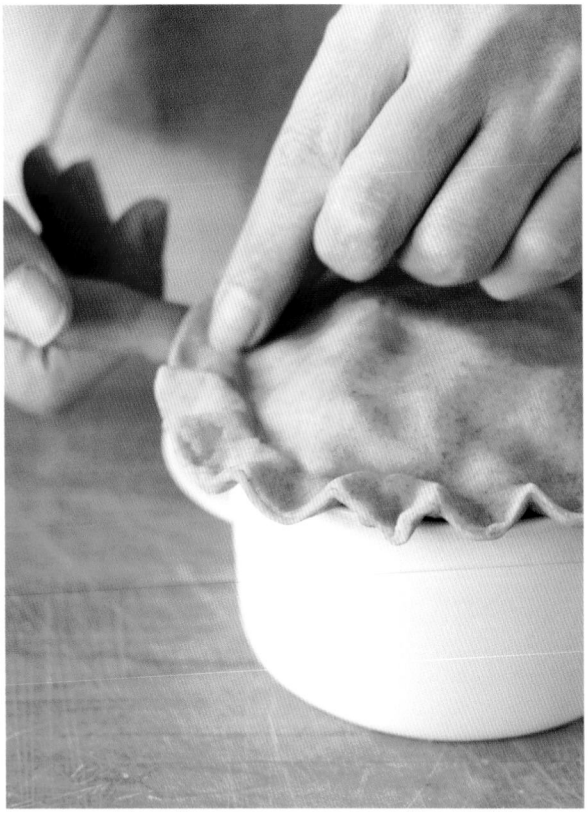

To make the crust, combine the whole wheat flour, spelt flour, baking powder, and salt in a food processor and process for 10 seconds to mix. Separately, whisk the water, olive oil, and maple syrup together, then pour over the flour mixture and pulse just until the dough comes together. Gather the dough and form it into a round flat disk, or if making individual potpies, form it into 6 disks. Wrap in plastic wrap and refrigerate for at least 30 minutes.

Preheat the oven to 400°F and line a large baking sheet with parchment paper.

To make the root vegetables, combine the paprika, allspice, cinnamon, and salt in a large mixing bowl. Slowly pour the extra-virgin olive oil into the bowl, whisking all the while, to make a smooth paste. Add the turnip, parsnips, rutabaga, sweet potato, squash, and potatoes and toss until evenly coated. Spread the vegetables in a single layer on the prepared pan (using two pans if need be). Bake for 25 to 30 minutes, until tender. Remove the vegetables and lower the oven temperature to 350°F.

Meanwhile, make the sauté. Heat the olive oil in a large sauté pan over medium heat, then add the onion, salt, and caraway seeds and sauté until the onions are golden, about 4 minutes. Add the carrots, celery, and mushrooms and sauté for 4 minutes. Transfer the sautéed vegetables to a bowl.

To make the sauce, use the same sauté pan over medium-low heat. Add the clarified butter, and once it melts, whisk in the flour to make a paste. Slowly pour in the broth, whisking all the while, and continue whisking until velvety smooth. Stir in the salt, pepper, and nutmeg. If the sauce is too thick, add a small amount of additional broth.

To assemble the potpie, combine the root vegetables, sautéed vegetables, and sauce and stir until well mixed. On a lightly floured surface, roll the dough out to a circle 2 inches larger than your pie pan, or if using individual 1½-cup ramekins, divide into 6 portions and roll each out to a circle 1 inch larger than the ramekins. Fill the pie pan or ramekins with the vegetable mixture and gently place the dough over the filled dish or ramekins. Fold over the edges of the dough and crimp the edge with your fingers or a fork to seal. Cut a few steam vents in the crust.

Bake for 20 to 30 minutes, until the crust is golden brown and the juices are bubbling. Serve hot.

Variation: Root Vegetable and Chicken Potpie: Substitute 1½ cups of diced cooked chicken for one of the root vegetables. Fold the chicken in when you combine the root vegetables, sautéed vegetables, and sauce. If the mixture is too dry, add another ½ cup of broth.

PREP TIME: 45 minutes · COOK TIME: 1 hour 15 minutes

STORAGE: Store in a covered container in the refrigerator for 5 days or in the freezer for 3 months.

PER SERVING: Calories: 530; Total Fat: 26.9 g (6.1 g saturated, 15.1 g monounsaturated); Carbohydrates: 68 g; Protein: 9 g; Fiber: 11 g; Sodium: 770 mg

Stir-Fried Baby Bok Choy with Shiitake Mushrooms

I love Asian fare, but I can also see why people stay away from it in their own kitchens. It can be a bit daunting, especially all of those veggies with exotic names that most of us didn't grow up with and don't have the faintest idea how to prepare. That's a shame, because most of them have a load of body-supporting phytochemicals. Here I've combined two powerhouses, bok choy and shiitake mushrooms. I prefer baby bok choy, as bok choy gets more bitter as it matures. SERVES 6

- 4 heads baby bok choy
- 2 tablespoons light sesame oil
- 2 scallions, white parts only, thinly sliced
- 2 tablespoons minced fresh ginger
- 2 cloves garlic, minced
- 1/2 pound shiitake mushrooms, stemmed and sliced 1/4 inch thick
- Sea salt
- 2 tablespoons water
- 1 tablespoon tamari
- 1 tablespoon freshly squeezed lime juice
- 1 1/2 teaspoons toasted sesame oil
- 1 tablespoon toasted sesame seeds

REBECCA'S NOTES To toast seeds or nuts, preheat the oven or toaster oven to 350°F and line a baking sheet with parchment paper.

Spread the seeds or nuts in an even layer on the prepared pan and toast until aromatic and slightly browned, 5 to 7 minutes. Check frequently, as they can burn easily.

Trim the bases off the bok choy and discard. Trim the leaves from the stems and cut both crosswise into bite-size pieces, keeping the stems and leaves separate.

Heat the light sesame oil in a sauté pan over medium heat, then add the scallions, ginger, garlic, shiitake mushrooms, and a pinch of salt and sauté for 30 seconds. Add the water, tamari, and the bok choy stems and sauté for 2 minutes. Add the bok choy leaves, lime juice, toasted sesame oil, and a pinch of salt and sauté until the bok choy is just wilted, about 2 minutes. Taste and add another squeeze of lime if you like. Sprinkle with the toasted sesame seeds and serve immediately.

PREP TIME: 15 minutes · COOK TIME: 5 minutes

STORAGE: Store in a covered container in the refrigerator for 3 days.

PER SERVING: Calories: 150; Total Fat: 7.8 g (1 g saturated, 2.6 g monounsaturated); Carbohydrates: 16 g; Protein: 10 g; Fiber: 6 g; Sodium: 585 mg

WHO KNEW? 'Shroom Sagacity Mushrooms, long a staple of healthy eating in Asian diets, are a bit of a yin-yang affair. They can have powerful anticancer effects, but they must be properly prepared. Integrative oncologist Donald Abrams notes that "people are often not aware that white button mushrooms, their brown cousins, the cremini, and their giant cousins, the portobello, really need to be cooked. Putting sliced white button mushrooms in a salad is really something we should avoid, because they may in fact contain hydrazine, a cancer-causing compound that's neutralized when it's cooked." Abrams adds that he loves shiitake and maitake mushrooms for his patients, as both are good immune enhancers.

Shredded Carrot and Beet Salad

One of my favorite gatherings is the Food as Medicine conference, which brings together hundreds of nutritionally minded physicians, nurses, and other wellness professionals. I cook for the attendees, and while they often kindly tell me how much they learn from me, it definitely goes both ways. In fact, this recipe was inspired by Dr. Joel Evans, who is attracted to nutrition from both a scientific and an aesthetic viewpoint and loves to speak about the colors of food having a tangible relation to their healing qualities. There is a school of thought—and increasing scientific evidence—that the more vibrant the color, the more nutrition there is to be found in a food. As an ode to Joel, I set out to create the most colorful salad I could, using purple beets, orange carrots, and fresh mint. If I'd had a vegetable crisper instead of a box of crayons as a kid, this salad would have been the result. You can substitute lemon or lime juice for the orange juice. SERVES 4

- 2 tablespoons freshly squeezed orange juice
- 2 teaspoons freshly squeezed lemon juice
- 2 teaspoons extra-virgin olive oil
- 1/2 teaspoon minced fresh ginger
- 1/4 teaspoon sea salt
- 1 cup peeled and shredded carrot
- 1 cup peeled and shredded red beet
- 2 tablespoons chopped fresh mint

Whisk the orange juice, lemon juice, olive oil, ginger, and salt together until thoroughly combined. Put the carrots in a mixing bowl, drizzle with half of the dressing, and toss until evenly coated. Place the carrots on one side of a shallow serving bowl. Put the beets in the mixing bowl, drizzle with the remaining dressing, and toss until evenly coated. Place the beets in the serving bowl next to the carrots for a beautiful contrast of red and orange. Top with the chopped mint before serving.

PREP TIME: 10 minutes · COOK TIME: Not applicable

STORAGE: Store in an airtight container in the refrigerator for 3 to 5 days.

PER SERVING: Calories: 50; Total Fat: 2.5 g (0.4 g saturated, 1.7 g monounsaturated); Carbohydrates: 7 g; Protein: 1 g; Fiber: 2 g; Sodium: 195 mg

WHO KNEW? Strength in Numbers When it comes to antioxidants, including the carotenoids so prevalent in orange fruits and vegetables, experts pretty much sing the same song: Generally speaking, the right way to go is to cast a wide net instead of focusing on a single antioxidant. (This is their way of saying don't turn into a rabbit and consume so many carrots that you turn orange from a beta-carotene megadose.) Nutritionist Suzanne Dixon notes, "Individual, isolated carotenoids don't tend to provide a whole lot of benefit. You should get the whole food, preferentially. Getting a lot of different carotenoids in the diet, I believe, is a very, very good biomarker of general healthy eating behavior. Those people tend to do better in terms of disease risk across the board."

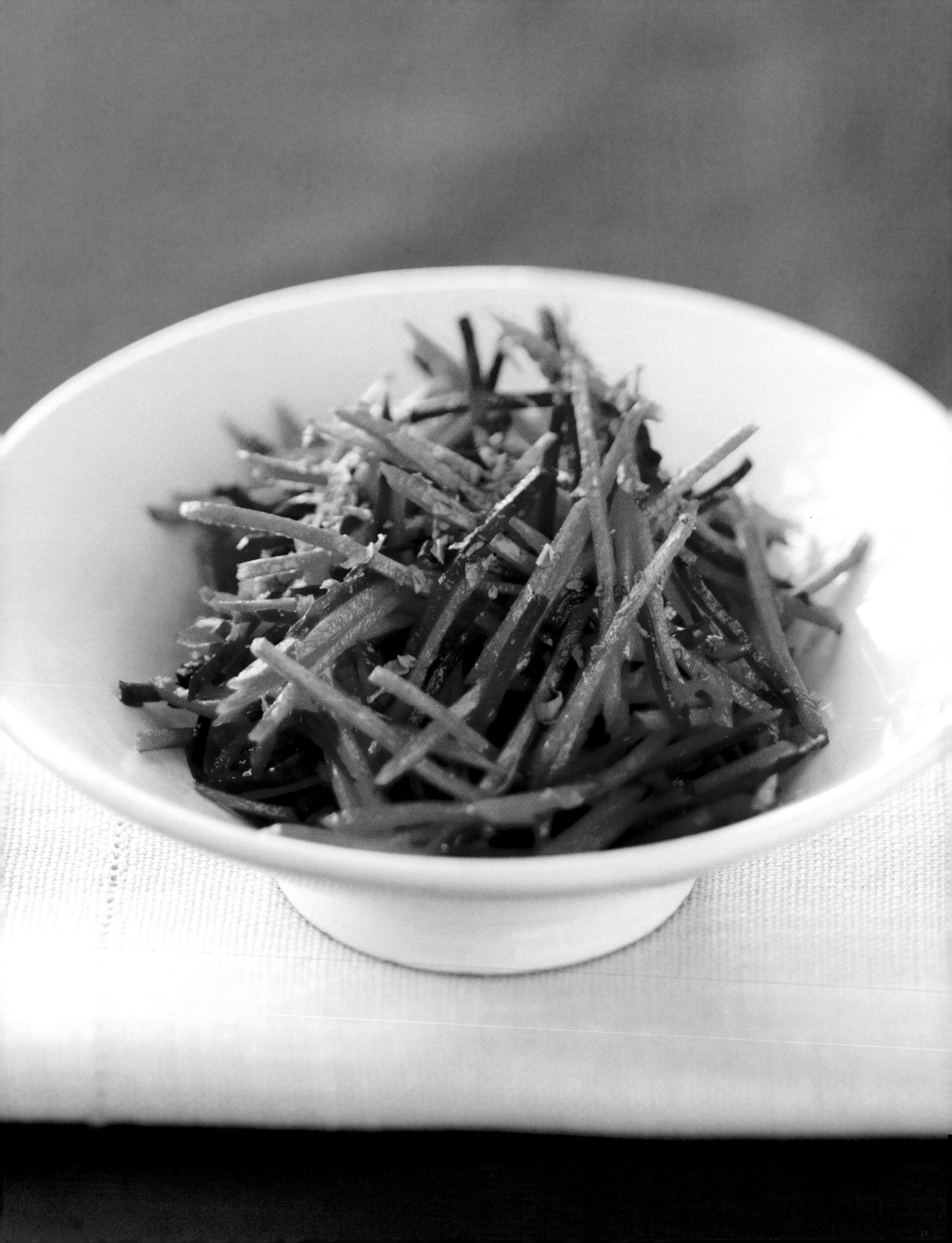

CHAPTER 5

Protein-Building Foods

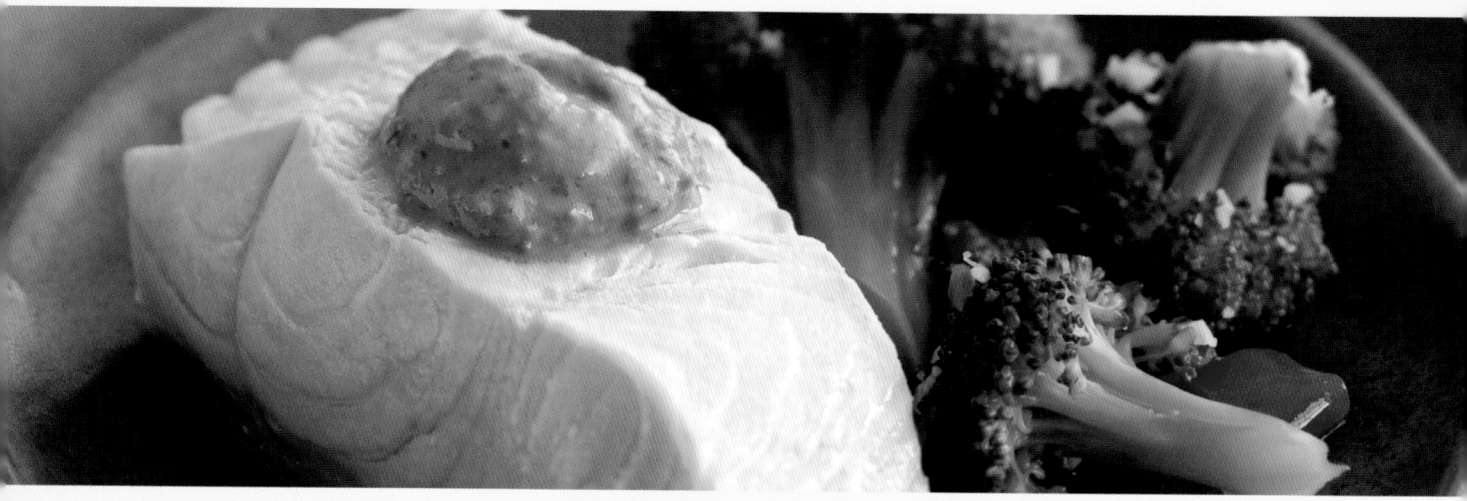

102 *Easy Eggs in a Cup*

104 *Curried Chicken Salad*

105 *Chicken and Broccoli Stir-Fry with Cashews*

106 *Cozy Comfy Chicken and Rice*

107 *Tuscan Farro and Bean Salad*

109 *Lemon Mustard Salmon Salad*

110 *Master Recipe for Cooking Beans*

111 *My Family's Favorite Chicken*

112 *Middle Eastern Chickpea Burgers*

114 *Nana's Egg Salad*

115 *Poached Eggs with Basil Lemon Drizzle*

117 *Orange Ginger Roasted Chicken*

118 *Triple-Citrus Ginger Black Cod*

121 *Poached Salmon with Moroccan Pesto*

123 *Baked Citrus Halibut with Tomato Sauce*

Proteins are the Incredible Hulks of nutrients. Everyone needs protein to repair their body, but that goes doubly so for people in treatment. The cancer experts I consulted say that chemotherapy and other treatments that break down cells and tissues can make the body need 50 to 70 percent more protein just to get back to equilibrium. That sounds like a big number, but fortunately protein is easy to get into your diet. Eggs, fish, chicken, beans, and seafood all deliver much-needed protein, and all are included in recipes throughout this chapter.

Each of these proteins also has unique qualities. Nutritionally, eggs are considered nearly a perfect protein, as though nature decided every part of the egg would be devoted solely to aiding protein production in the body. It's like putting ultra-premium gas in your car. Chicken is similarly efficient in feeding your body's protein engine (heck, it made the egg, didn't it?). Veggie sources of protein—beans, legumes, seeds—each contain combinations of the nine essential amino acids that make up a complete protein, so you have to mix 'em up (for example, have some nuts at noon and a chickpea burger later in the day) to properly utilize those protein makers. Fish protein—notably from cod, which is generally easy to digest—has been shown to increase insulin sensitivity in humans, which may be helpful for people receiving chemotherapy and/or steroids that may increase blood sugar and promote insulin resistance. While recipes throughout the book were designed to combine foods to provide a broad spectrum of the amino acids the body needs to rebuild itself during treatment, those in this chapter are more concentrated sources of essential amino acids.

The great news is that even though you need more protein during treatment, with protein-dense meals you don't have to eat nearly as much to get those essential amino acids. Four ounces of fish or meat has anywhere between 29 and 39 grams of protein, which is almost half the protein a healthy 120-pound woman needs. These recipes jack up the protein while piling on the taste. The chicken and fish recipes you'll find in the following pages have another thing in common that's beneficial for people in treatment: They're all marinated or tenderized, which brings out a ton of flavor and also breaks the proteins down a bit, making them easier to eat and digest. Marinating also adds moisture, which people dealing with dry mouth or throat issues will appreciate.

I'm going to get on my soapbox now, which is important because I'm only a stitch over five feet and I really want you to see me. I'm going to beg, plead, and cajole you to buy wild fish and organic eggs and chicken. I fully understand these products can cost a bit more, but they're worth every penny for someone in treatment. Commercial farm-raised chickens are often treated excessively with antibiotics and some cattle are injected with hormones. That's the last thing you need to ingest. As for fish, those that are caught in the wild generally have much better omega-3 fatty acid profiles; this may play a role in lessening inflammation, which many researchers think may be related to cancer's ability to become resistant to some chemotherapy treatments.

Easy Eggs in a Cup

Baked or shirred (pronounced "sheared") eggs have been around forever. In this recipe, baking eggs over a little sautéed spinach with some feta cheese and a shaving of nutmeg creates a dish that looks and tastes beautiful. Just the sight of these eggs nestled in colorful ramekins is enough to bring even the most reluctant eater back to the table. To further enhance the yum factor, serve topped with Basil Lemon Drizzle (page 177). SERVES 4

1 tablespoon extra-virgin olive oil

1/2 cup finely diced red onion

1 teaspoon minced garlic

4 cups tightly packed baby spinach, washed and dried

Sea salt

Pinch of freshly grated nutmeg

1/4 cup crumbled organic feta cheese (optional)

4 organic eggs

Pinch of freshly ground pepper

REBECCA'S NOTES To avoid a watery end product, make sure the spinach is well dried prior to adding it to the sauté pan. Spinach naturally gives off moisture when it cooks, so you don't want to add even more by cooking it when it's wet. A salad spinner works miracles on drying spinach quickly and efficiently.

For a time-saver, buy prewashed organic bagged spinach from the market.

Preheat the oven to 375°F.

Heat the olive oil in a sauté pan over medium heat, then add the onion and sauté until translucent, about 3 minutes. Stir in the garlic and sauté for an additional 30 seconds, then stir in the spinach and a pinch of salt and cook until wilted and tender, about another 30 seconds. Remove from the heat and stir in the nutmeg.

Lightly grease 4 small ramekins with olive oil. For each ramekin, spoon in one-fourth of the spinach mixture, then sprinkle on 1 tablespoon of the cheese. Gently crack 1 egg on top of the cheese, then sprinkle the pepper and a pinch of salt over all 4 ramekins.

Bake for 12 to 14 minutes, until very little liquid remains and moves around when you shake the ramekins.

Let cool for 3 minutes, then run a knife or an offset spatula around the inside edge of each ramekin to loosen the eggs. Using your knife or spatula to help support the eggs, carefully transfer to a plate and serve immediately.

PREP TIME: 10 minutes · COOK TIME: 20 minutes

STORAGE: Store in an airtight container in the refrigerator for 2 days.

PER SERVING: Calories: 120; Total Fat: 8.5 g (2.1 g saturated, 4.4 g monounsaturated); Carbohydrates: 5 g; Protein: 7 g; Fiber: 1 g; Sodium: 185 mg

WHO KNEW? **Dehydration** Most people think dehydration only happens when you're walking, running, or sweating and don't drink enough water. Actually, when you're in treatment, you can get dehydrated without moving a muscle. Chemotherapy consumes protein like a V-8 Mustang goes through High-test gasoline. When protein levels drop, fluids and nutrients get pulled out of the blood via osmosis (see, we knew high school biology would come in handy). Dehydration can lead to fatigue, cramps, and worse. Vegans and people on macrobiotic diets need to be especially careful to get enough protein during treatment.

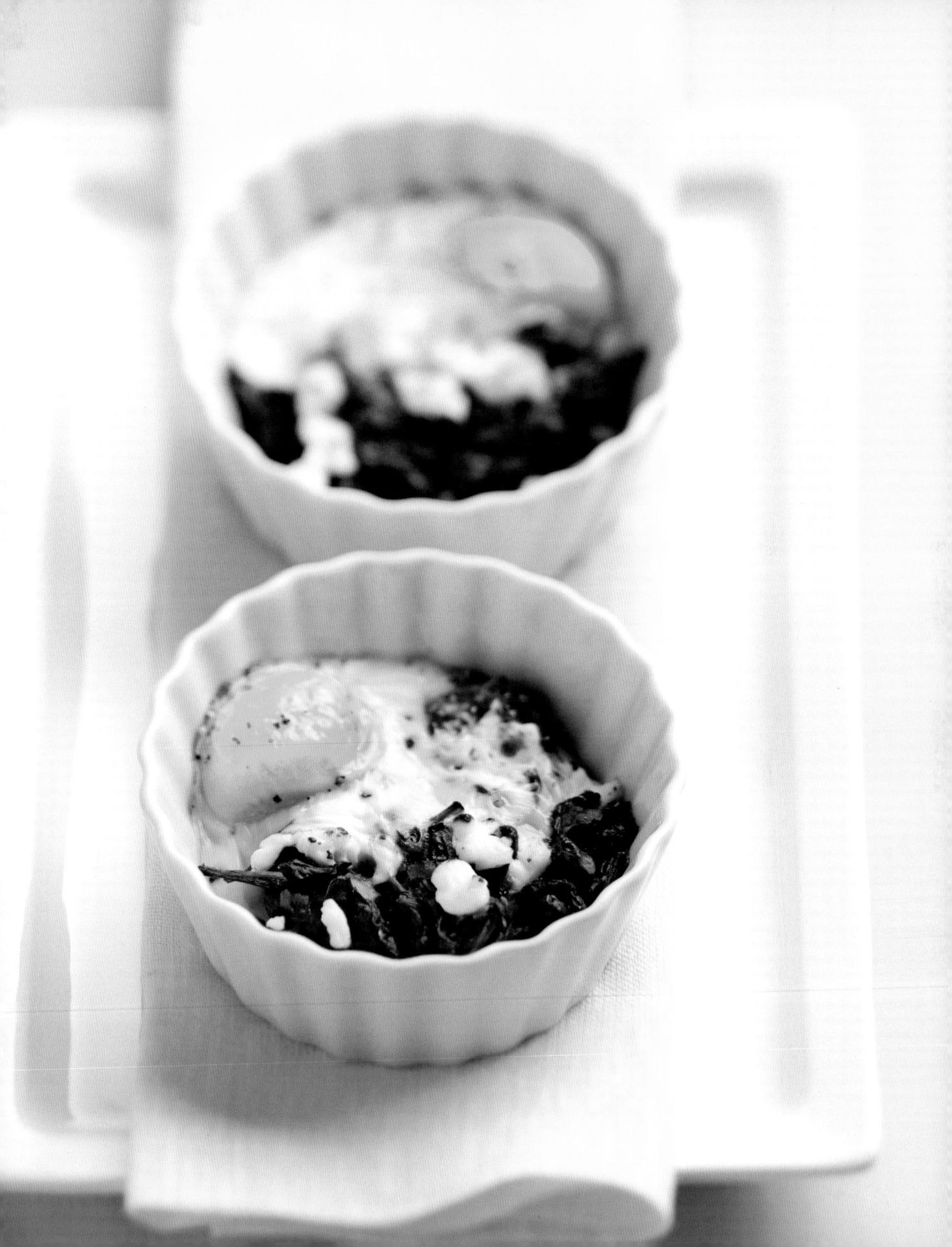

Curried Chicken Salad

This salad was inspired by one of those gorgeous, colorful Bollywood flicks that offer a feast of singing, dancing, and romance. I love Indian food, as it was my first real introduction to all things curry. Only much later did I learn that turmeric, a typical spice in curries that gives them a yellow tint, has tremendous antitumor and anti-inflammatory properties. And to think, I loved it just for its taste! Here, I was hankering for a swirl of flavors with an Indian feel. The chicken makes a great starting point because it's full of protein and amenable to all sorts of accessorizing. In this case, the mango and raisins play delightfully off the curry spices. SERVES 6

- 1 1/2 pounds roasted organic chicken
- 1 firm ripe mango, diced into 1/4-inch pieces
- 1/4 cup raisins or currants
- 1/4 cup minced scallions, green part only
- 2 stalks celery, diced small
- 1/2 cup organic plain Greek-style yogurt
- 1/4 cup mayonnaise
- 1 tablespoon freshly squeezed lime juice
- 1 tablespoon curry powder
- 1/2 teaspoon ground ginger
- 1/2 teaspoon sea salt
- 6 butter lettuce leaves, washed and dried
- 1/4 cup slivered toasted almonds (see page 97), for garnish
- 1/4 cup chopped fresh cilantro, for garnish (optional)

Chop the chicken into 1/2-inch pieces and put them in a bowl. Stir in the mango, raisins, scallions, and celery. Separately, whisk the yogurt, mayonnaise, lime juice, curry powder, ginger, and salt together. Add the yogurt mixture to the chicken and stir gently until thoroughly combined. Serve atop the lettuce leaves, garnished with the almonds and cilantro.

Variations: If you don't have a mango or aren't a mango lover, this salad is wonderful with diced Fuji apples.

Making pita pocket sandwiches is a fantastic way to get much-needed nutrients into your body and fill your belly while you're running errands, waiting for a doctor's appointment, or otherwise on the go. Place a pita on a flat work surface and cut a 2-inch section off the top using a knife. With the pita lying flat, put in 1/4 cup of salad greens, then carefully spread 1/2 cup of the chicken salad on top of the greens, making certain to spread it around the entire cavity of the pita.

PREP TIME: 15 minutes · COOK TIME: Not applicable

STORAGE: Store in an airtight container in the refrigerator for 3 days.

PER SERVING: Calories: 300; Total Fat: 11.3 g (3.1 g saturated, 3.8 g monounsaturated); Carbohydrates: 15 g; Protein: 34 g; Fiber: 2 g; Sodium: 375 mg

REBECCA'S NOTES Save time by using store-bought organic roast chicken or, better yet, the leftovers from Orange Ginger Roasted Chicken (page 117).

Chicken and Broccoli Stir-Fry with Cashews

There's something about a chicken and broccoli stir-fry that screams "Chinese take-out!" But given that this is a healthier and tastier recipe than your standard MSG-fest, let's call it "Chinese take-in." The slightly higher fat content in dark meat makes for a flavorful, moist dish, so people with throat or mouth issues may find it a lot easier to chew and swallow. (That said, you can substitute an equivalent amount of breast meat if you like.) The sauce is thickened with kudzu root, a phenomenal anticancer plant, which is a lot more desirable than the cornstarch of questionable quality found in most carry-out fare. Plus, the blend of tamari, lime juice, ginger, and maple syrup in the sauce is so delicious that you'll be able to take that Chinese restaurant off the speed dial. SERVES 6

Juice of 1 lime
1/2 teaspoon sea salt
4 organic skinless, boneless chicken thighs, cut into bite-size pieces
2 teaspoons kudzu root powder
1/4 cup cold water
1/2 cup tamari
1/4 cup water
6 tablespoons maple syrup
2 1/2 tablespoons freshly squeezed lime juice
2 tablespoons brown rice vinegar
3 teaspoons minced garlic
3 teaspoons minced fresh ginger
Pinch of cayenne
1 teaspoon toasted sesame oil
1/2 pound broccoli
2 tablespoons light sesame oil
1/2 cup toasted cashews (see page 97)

REBECCA'S NOTES For a vegetarian version, use tofu or tempeh in place of the chicken.

Stir the lime juice and salt together. Add the chicken to the blend and marinate for 20 minutes in the refrigerator.

Whisk the kudzu with the 1/4 cup cold water until completely dissolved, making a slurry.

Stir the tamari, 1/4 cup water, maple syrup, lime juice, vinegar, 2 teaspoons of the garlic, 2 teaspoons of the ginger, and the cayenne together in a small saucepan over medium-high heat and bring to a boil. Lower the heat and simmer, uncovered, until the sauce begins to thicken and is reduced in volume by one-third, about 4 minutes. Stir in the slurry while whisking continuously, then stir in the toasted sesame oil and remove from the heat.

Meanwhile, cut the broccoli florets into bite-size pieces. Trim and peel the stems and cut them into bite-size pieces as well, keeping them separate from the florets.

Heat a wok or large, heavy sauté pan over high heat for 2 minutes. Add the light sesame oil and swirl to coat the pan. Add the remaining 1 teaspoon each of the garlic and ginger and stir-fry for 1 to 2 minutes, until aromatic. Stir in the chicken and toss or stir constantly for 2 minutes. Add the broccoli stalks and stir-fry until bright green, then add the broccoli florets and continue stir-frying until bright and vibrant, about 2 minutes. Pour in the sauce and stir-fry for another 30 seconds, tossing constantly.

Serve immediately, garnished with the cashews.

PREP TIME: 25 minutes · COOK TIME: 10 minutes

STORAGE: Store in an airtight container in the refrigerator for 4 days.

PER SERVING: Calories: 250; Total Fat: 12.8 g (2.3 g saturated, 6 g monounsaturated); Carbohydrates: 24 g; Protein: 13 g; Fiber: 1 g; Sodium: 415 mg

Cozy Comfy Chicken and Rice

This has always been my personal comfort dish, a meal I made from leftovers after roasting a chicken on the weekend. One day a friend was in the kitchen when I was making it, and she started asking innocuous questions: "Say, how much of the shallot are you using?" "Was that a half cup of olives?" I was so busy cooking that I didn't really pay attention to what she was doing with the answers. She figured out the recipe and started making it for friends, who loved it and wanted the recipe too. I guess I wasn't meant to hold onto this one. That's okay. It's really, really good, and I hope you get as much pleasure out of it as I do. SERVES 4

- 2 1/4 cups Chicken Magic Mineral Broth (page 55) or store-bought organic chicken stock
- 1/4 teaspoon finely chopped saffron threads
- 1 tablespoon extra-virgin olive oil
- 2 tablespoons finely diced yellow onion
- Sea salt
- 1 tablespoon finely diced shallot
- 1 cup jasmine rice, rinsed
- 1 1/4 cups chopped or shredded roasted organic chicken
- 3 tablespoons chopped olives
- 1 to 2 tablespoons diced pimiento peppers
- Spritz of fresh lemon juice
- 1/2 cup chopped fresh flat-leaf parsley, for garnish

Bring the broth to a boil in a large saucepan. (If it's been frozen give it a spritz of lemon juice.) Pour the broth into a small heatproof bowl, add the saffron, and let it infuse the broth. Using the same saucepan, heat the olive oil over medium-high heat, then add the onion and a pinch of salt and sauté until soft, about 2 minutes. Add the shallot and 1/4 teaspoon of salt and sauté until just golden, about 1 minute. Add the rice and stir until mixed well, about 1 minute to slightly toast the rice.

Stir in the broth and 1/4 teaspoon of salt and give the rice a quick stir. Bring the rice to a boil, then lower the heat, cover, and simmer for 12 minutes.

Stir in the chicken, olives, pimiento, and lemon juice. Cover, remove from the heat, and let stand for 12 minutes.

Fluff with a fork, then serve garnished with the parsley.

Variations: For those who would rather avoid chicken, try this as a rice dish using Magic Mineral Broth . . . it's delicious!

Not everyone is into pimientos and olives. I've been assured by a close friend that this dish is delicious without them.

PREP TIME: 15 minutes · COOK TIME: 30 minutes

STORAGE: Store in an airtight container in the refrigerator for 5 days.

PER SERVING: Calories: 225; Total Fat: 6.2 g (1.2 g saturated, 3.7 g monounsaturated); Carbohydrates: 26 g; Protein: 16 g; Fiber: 2 g; Sodium: 320 mg

REBECCA'S NOTES Sautéing the rice with the onion and shallot gives this dish a little more depth of flavor.

As a time-saver, you can purchase an already roasted organic chicken from the store for this dish.

My favorite type of olives for this dish is an Italian variety called Cerignola. They're more buttery and mellow than many varieties. If you can't find them, kalamata olives are also wonderful here. Just make sure you give them a good rinse before adding them to the dish.

Tuscan Farro and Bean Salad

Here's a great example of what I call culinary architecture, which entails building on a great foundation. In this case, I'm playing off what Middle Easterners call tabouli, a wonderful salad with a fantastic fresh taste that's incredibly easy to make (and impossible to mess up). The base of any tabouli is a grain, lemon juice, parsley, and mint. That's our building block. Then we add the ornamentation, which always emphasizes both form and function. The beans create a complete protein, the pleasing crunch (and a whole bunch of antioxidants) comes from pepper, while olives add a little healthy salt. Like any powerful piece of architecture, it's the combination of simplicity and tasteful elegance that makes this salad so enjoyable and memorable. SERVES 6

- 1 cup cooked cannellini beans (see page 110)
- 2 cups Simple Tuscan Farro (page 148)
- 1/4 cup finely diced red bell pepper
- 3 tablespoons pitted kalamata olives, rinsed and sliced thin
- 1 cup finely chopped and loosely packed fresh flat-leaf parsley
- 1 cup finely chopped and loosely packed fresh mint
- Zest of 1 lemon
- 1/4 cup freshly squeezed lemon juice
- 1/4 cup extra-virgin olive oil
- 1/2 teaspoon sea salt
- 2 ounces organic feta cheese, crumbled (optional)

REBECCA'S NOTES This is a particularly nice vegetarian dish that provides complete protein while also being high in fiber and low in fat. Because of the low fat and high fiber content, it would appeal to breast and prostate cancer patients.

Put the beans, farro, bell pepper, olives, parsley, mint, lemon zest, lemon juice, olive oil, and salt in a large bowl and stir until thoroughly combined. Chill for 1 hour.

Before serving, do a FASS check. You may need to add another pinch of salt or a dash of lemon juice.

Serve with the feta cheese sprinkled over the top.

Variations: Play with the taste of this salad. If you're a tomato fan, add 1 cup of halved cherry tomatoes. If you'd like some more crunch, add 1/4 cup of diced celery. Get creative and have fun!

If you have trouble finding farro or don't have any on hand, brown rice or a wild rice blend makes a wonderful substitute.

You can certainly substitute canned beans in this recipe. Use about half of a 15-ounce can and, as usual, drain and rinse, then refresh the beans with a spritz of fresh lemon juice and a pinch of sea salt.

PREP TIME: 15 minutes · COOK TIME: Not applicable

STORAGE: Store in an airtight container in the refrigerator for 5 to 7 days.

PER SERVING: Calories: 255; Total Fat: 11.1 g (1.6 g saturated, 7.9 g monounsaturated); Carbohydrates: 32 g; Protein: 8 g; Fiber: 6 g; Sodium: 580 mg

"My family, especially my husband, who is the cook in our house, has been so supportive. We have changed our diet to mostly whole foods and eat very little meat."
—Marie E., breast cancer survivor

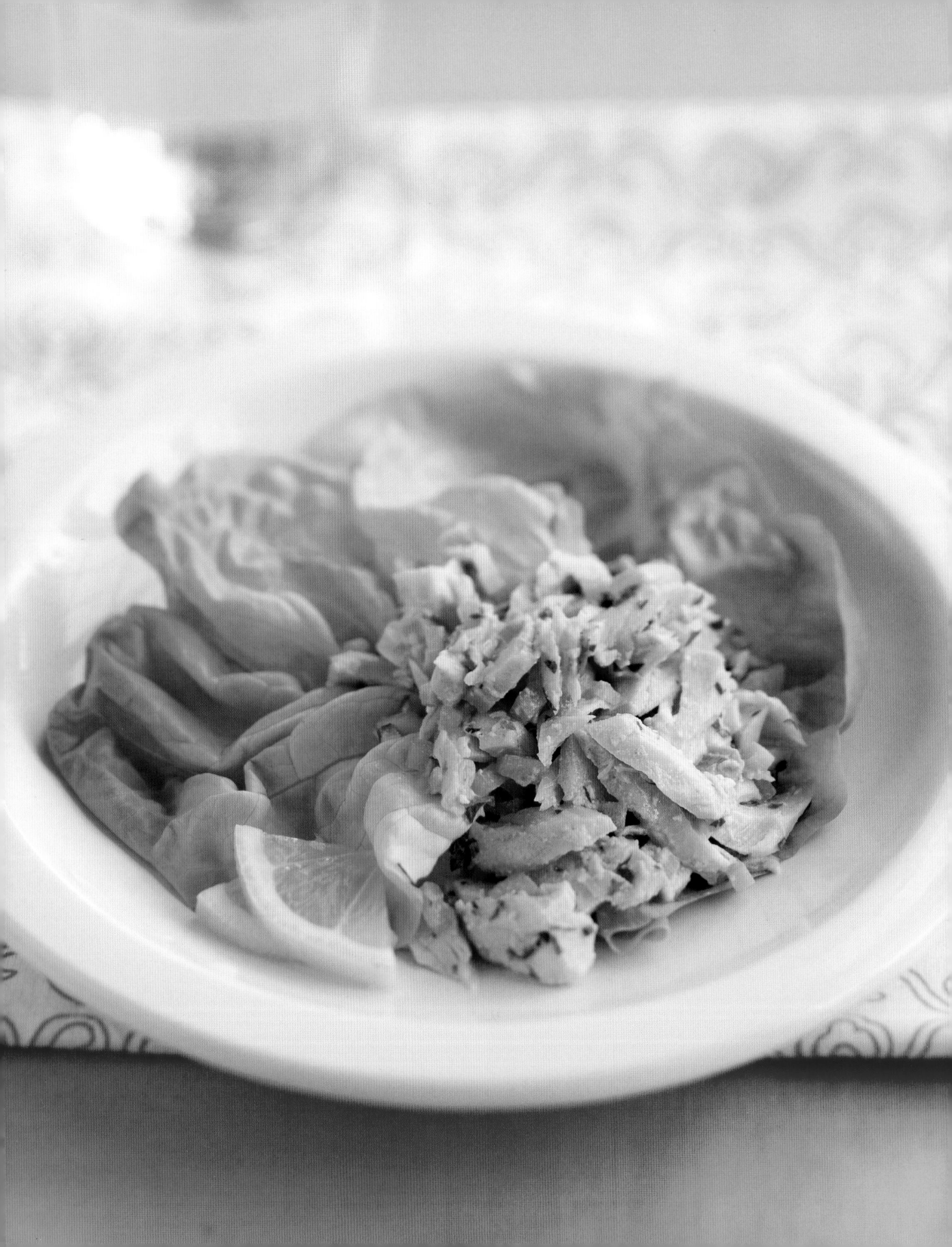

Lemon Mustard Salmon Salad

All salmon are not created equal. This recipe features wild Alaskan sockeye. It's the "wild" part that's really important. Wild salmon are far higher in omega-3s than their farm-raised brethren, and omega-3s have been linked to a whole host of cancer-fighting benefits. The nice thing is, you don't have to go fishing or even handle a salmon fillet to make this dish; there are great brands of wild sockeye that come in cans (see Resources). That said, of course you can also make this with an equal amount of leftover home-cooked salmon. Either way, this salad is easy to prepare: All it takes is a quick stir with a few choice ingredients, and there you go—a nice, filling dish that's rich in protein, yummy, and versatile. Serve it in a pita, wrap it in a tortilla, or mound it atop salad greens. SERVES 2

- 1 7½-ounce can boneless, skinless, sockeye salmon, drained, or leftover Poached Salmon with Moroccan Pesto (page 121)
- 3 teaspoons Dijon mustard
- 2 teaspoons freshly squeezed lemon juice
- 2 teaspoons extra-virgin olive oil
- Pinch of cayenne
- Pinch of sea salt
- 3 tablespoons finely chopped celery
- 2 tablespoons finely chopped fresh flat-leaf parsley

Put the salmon in a bowl and break it into small pieces with a fork. Stir in the mustard, lemon juice, olive oil, cayenne, salt, celery, and parsley, then do a FASS check. If needed, adjust the flavors with lemon juice and a pinch of salt.

Variations: Add capers or chopped radishes to this dish—they will not disappoint!

Or combine just the salmon and celery with 2 tablespoons of the Basil Lemon Drizzle (page 177) or 1 tablespoon of the Moroccan Pesto (page 186); both are great dressings to try with this salmon recipe.

PREP TIME: 5 minutes · COOK TIME: Not applicable

STORAGE: Store in an airtight container in the refrigerator for 2 days.

PER SERVING: Calories: 180; Total Fat: 8.5 g (0.7 g saturated, 3.4 g monounsaturated); Carbohydrates: 1 g; Protein: 27 g; Fiber: 0 g; Sodium: 670 mg

WHO KNEW? Chemo Resistance and Nutrition You may never have heard of chemo resistance, but believe me, your doctor has. Over time, some cancers become less vulnerable to chemotherapy and start to grow again, which is why physicians may switch treatment regimes over time. There's some evidence that chemo resistance may be linked to inflammation and the ratios of fatty acids in cancer cells. In terms of a nutritional approach, Dr. Keith Block says it may help to keep the diet lower in saturated fats and omega-6s—and higher in omega-3s, which are abundant in fish such as salmon and trout.

Master Recipe for Cooking Beans

Many recipes in this book include beans, because they're a great source of protein, fiber, and other nutrients, so I figured I'd better include a basic recipe for cooking them. I cook beans with kombu, which contains an abundance of glutamic acid, an amino acid that helps break down the starches in the beans and makes them less combustible. Adding lemon juice to the soaking water and skimming off the foam make the beans even easier to digest. SERVING SIZE: ONE CUP OF DRIED BEANS YIELDS ABOUT 2 CUPS COOKED; 1/4 CUP OF COOKED BEANS IS A PERFECT SERVING SIZE FOR MAXIMUM DIGESTIBILITY.

Type of Bean	Cooking Time After Soaking	Pressure-Cooking Time After Soaking	Recommended Additions during Cooking
Chickpeas (garbanzo beans)	1 1/2 to 2 1/2 hours	15 to 20 minutes	Garlic cloves
Red kidney beans and cannellini beans	1 to 1 1/2 hours	10 minutes	Garlic cloves, bay leaf
Navy beans	45 to 60 minutes	4 to 5 minutes	Garlic cloves, bay leaf
Black beans	45 to 50 minutes	15 to 20 minutes	Garlic cloves
Lentils, red (no soaking necessary)	20 to 30 minutes	5 to 7 minutes	Bay leaf, garlic cloves, cinnamon stick
Lentils, green (no soaking necessary)	30 to 45 minutes	6 to 8 minutes	Bay leaf, garlic cloves, cinnamon stick

1 cup dried beans
2 tablespoons freshly squeezed lemon juice
1 6-inch strip of kombu
1 teaspoon sea salt

Rinse the beans well in a strainer, then put them in a bowl or pot with water to cover by 2 inches. Stir in the lemon juice and soak overnight.

Drain the beans and rinse well, then put them in a pot, add water to cover by 3 inches, and add the kombu. Bring to a boil, then lower the heat, skim off any foam from the surface, and gently simmer, covered, for 20 minutes to 2 1/2 hours depending on the bean (see the chart above). Start testing the lentils after 20 minutes and other beans after 45 minutes; when they are tender but still al dente, stir in the salt. (Adding salt too soon retards the cooking process.) Check the beans occasionally to see if more water is needed. During the last 15 minutes, the beans will start to cook faster; test them often to ensure they don't overcook. However, if you plan to store and reheat the beans, leave them slightly undercooked.

Drain the beans and discard the cooking liquid. At this point, you can add them to recipes or store them in an airtight container in the refrigerator or freezer.

PREP TIME: 4 to 12 hours for soaking
COOK TIME: 20 minutes to 2 1/2 hours (see chart)
STORAGE: Store in an airtight container in the refrigerator for 4 days or in the freezer for 1 month.

My Family's Favorite Chicken

My Grandma Doris was a real piece of work. As they said in the old days, "That lady had class!" Doris was allergic to kitchens, so she used to take my brother Jeff and me out to fine restaurants whenever we visited. She loved one French restaurant in particular, where she would always order chicken paillard with potato puree. It seemed so exotic, so chic, that Jeff and I always ordered the same dish and loved it. It wasn't until I was in cooking school years later that I learned it was just a fancy name for pounded chicken with mashed potato. You gotta love the French! But it's still my favorite chicken dish, and it's great for people who are having trouble eating. That's because pounding the chicken flat makes it quick to cook and very easy to chew. SERVES 4

- 4 organic skinless, boneless chicken breast halves
- 2 tablespoons freshly squeezed lemon juice
- 1 tablespoon extra-virgin olive oil
- 1/4 teaspoon sea salt
- 1/4 teaspoon red pepper flakes
- 3 cloves garlic, minced
- 1 tablespoon lemon zest
- 1 tablespoon chopped fresh thyme
- 1/4 cup chopped fresh parsley, for garnish
- Parsley Basil Drizzle (page 187), for garnish (optional)

REBECCA'S NOTES Like snowflakes, no two pieces of chicken are alike. Some will be thicker and require a little extra pounding. Don't get carried away with your mallet though, as the thinner parts of the chicken will tear if they're pounded too much.

Here's a time-saving tip: Ask the butcher to pound the chicken for you. They're usually happy to provide this service.

Place the chicken in several layers of parchment paper and pound each with a meat pounder until nice and thin, approximately 1/4 inch thick.

Combine the lemon juice, olive oil, salt, red pepper flakes, garlic, lemon zest, and thyme and whisk until thoroughly blended. Pour the mixture over the chicken and marinate in the refrigerator for 30 to 60 minutes.

Heat a grill or grill pan to high heat. Remove the chicken from the marinade and pat each breast dry with paper towels. Grill for 1 to 2 minutes on each side, until firm to the touch or the juices run clear. Serve garnished with the parsley and the Parsley Basil Drizzle.

Variations: There are many ways to infuse flavor into chicken. Using this recipe as a template, try marinating the pounded chicken in Cilantro Lime Vinaigrette (page 181) and topping it with the pomegranate variation on Mango and Avocado Salsa (page 185). Or marinate in Zesty Lemon Fennel Vinaigrette (page 182) and top with Basil Lemon Drizzle (page 177) or Moroccan Pesto (page 186).

PREP TIME: 20 minutes (plus 30 to 60 minutes for marinating)
COOK TIME: 15 minutes
STORAGE: Store tightly wrapped in the refrigerator for 2 days.
PER SERVING: Calories: 170; Total Fat: 5 g (0.9 g saturated, 2.9 g monounsaturated); Carbohydrates: 2 g; Protein: 28 g; Fiber: 0 g; Sodium: 225 mg

"My friends organized food and meal delivery when I was in treatment. It came every other day, in a cooler that was placed outside on my porch. If I was up to receiving visitors, I went to the door when I heard the footsteps on the porch."
—Kelly T., breast cancer survivor

Middle Eastern Chickpea Burgers

These chickpea burgers are similar to a Middle Eastern falafel. But the Americanized version of falafel usually resembles carnival food: they're often deep-fried in some unhealthy oil. It makes me want to cry, because falafel done right is so delicious and nutritious. It's all in the blend. Here the secret ingredient is basmati rice, which holds the chickpea mixture together and creates a complete protein. I love the mini-burger concept; the whole wheat bun is like putting falafel in a top hat and tails, and it's perfect for folks who like the taste of beans when they're broken down and combined with heady herbs and spices. Gently pan-seared or baked, these burgers are bountiful bites of health, especially topped with a dollop of Tomato Mint Chutney (page 176). MAKES 17 PATTIES

- 2 cups cooked chickpeas (see page 110), or 1 15-ounce can, drained, rinsed, and mixed with a spritz of fresh lemon juice and a pinch of sea salt
- 1/2 teaspoon sea salt
- 1/2 teaspoon turmeric
- 1/2 teaspoon paprika
- 1/4 teaspoon ground cumin
- 1/4 teaspoon ground coriander
- 1/8 teaspoon ground cinnamon
- 2 teaspoons minced garlic
- 1 teaspoon minced fresh ginger
- 3 tablespoons extra-virgin olive oil
- 2 tablespoons freshly squeezed lemon juice
- 2 1/2 cups cooked brown basmati rice
- 3 tablespoons finely diced red bell pepper
- 1/4 cup loosely packed minced fresh flat-leaf parsley

Preheat the oven to 375°F and line a baking sheet with parchment paper.

Combine the chickpeas, salt, turmeric, paprika, cumin, coriander, cinnamon, garlic, ginger, olive oil, and lemon juice in a food processor and process until smooth and well combined, scraping the sides occasionally. Transfer the mixture to a bowl and fold in the rice, bell pepper, and parsley.

Moisten your hands to keep the mixture from sticking, then shape the mixture into 1/4-inch-thick patties about 2 1/2 inches in diameter. Place them on the prepared pan and bake for 22 to 25 minutes, until the patties start to get dry and crisp on the outside. They will firm up as they cool.

Variations: For a crispy burger, heat 2 teaspoons of olive oil in a skillet over medium heat and cook the patties for about 3 minutes on each side, until golden brown.

Want a delicious dip for fresh, raw veggies? The chickpea and spice puree from the food processor makes a delicious hummus.

PREP TIME: 15 minutes · COOK TIME: 25 minutes

STORAGE: Store in a covered container in the refrigerator for 3 to 5 days. Burgers can also be frozen in cooked or uncooked form for 2 months (see Rebecca's Notes).

PER SERVING: Calories: 100; Total Fat: 3.5 g (0.5 g saturated, 2 g monounsaturated); Carbohydrates: 15 g; Protein: 3 g; Fiber: 3 g; Sodium: 223 mg

REBECCA'S NOTES If you want to cook just a few patties, pop them in your toaster oven. To freeze these burgers, either cooked or uncooked, stack them up with parchment paper between the burgers, then wrap first in plastic wrap, then in foil. The parchment paper makes it easy to remove the desired number of burgers from the bundle. Once thawed, cooked burgers can be reheated at 350°F for 15 minutes, and uncooked burgers can be baked as above, at 375°F for 22 to 25 minutes.

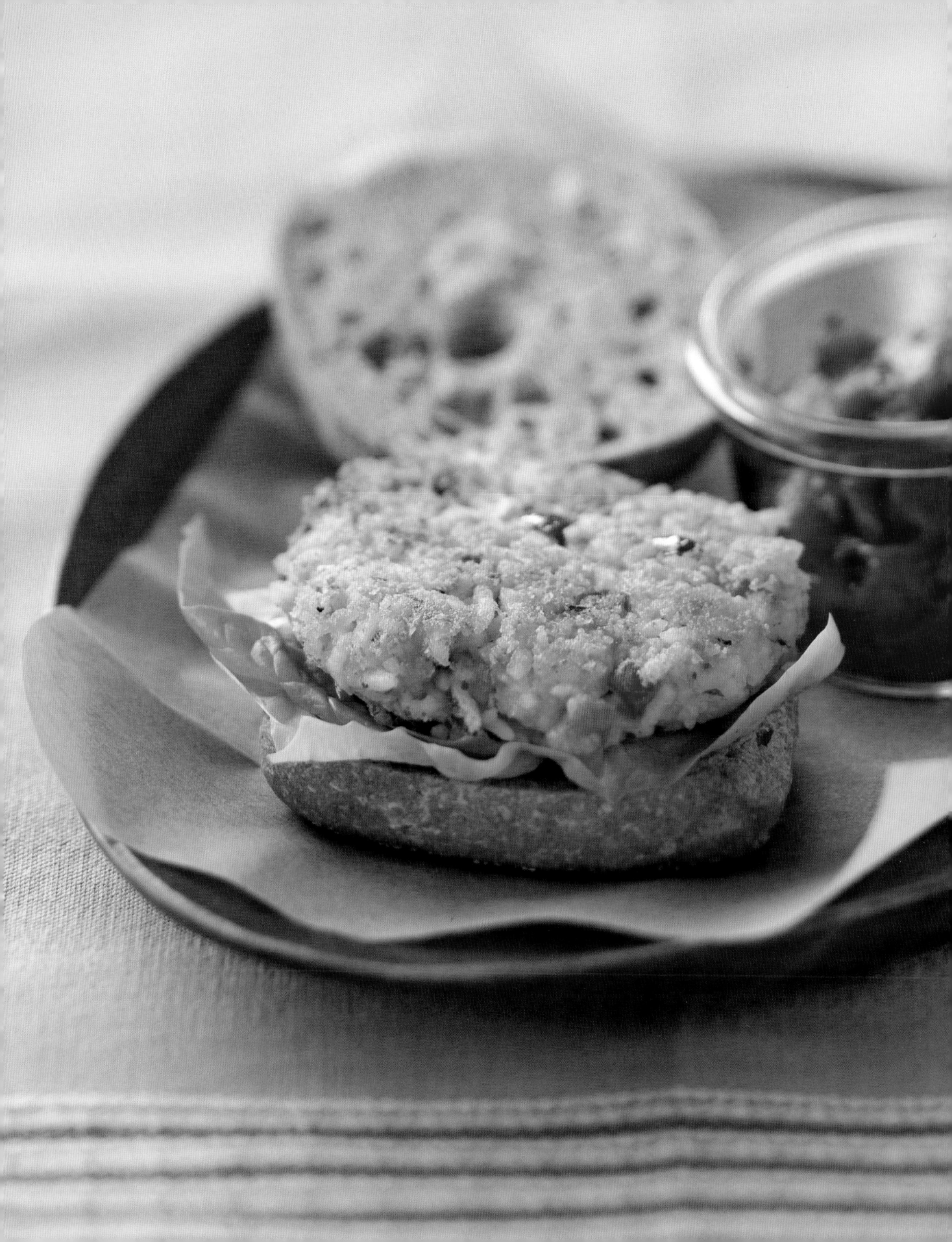

Nana's Egg Salad

Those who are going through treatment often want to eat familiar foods, and for many folks egg salad fits the bill. What I did here was take my nana's egg salad and adapt it a bit so all that great protein was easier to nosh. Instead of the chunks common to German-style egg salad, I opted for a lighter, creamier texture that works great on crackers, in a pita or wrap, or on top of salad greens. Adding a pinch of cayenne and a little lemon gives this egg salad a bit more zip. I have a feeling Nana would approve. SERVES 2

2 organic eggs, hard-boiled
1 teaspoon mayonnaise or Vegenaise
1/4 teaspoon Dijon mustard
1/8 teaspoon sea salt
1/8 teaspoon paprika
Pinch of cayenne
1/4 teaspoon freshly squeezed lemon juice

REBECCA'S NOTES Fresh basil makes a wonderful addition; add about 1 teaspoon, finely chopped.

I learned how to make a perfect hard-boiled egg from my mother, who learned the secret from my culinary hero, Julia Child. Place the eggs in 8 cups of cold water in a high rather than wide pot. Bring the eggs just to a boil, then immediately remove from the heat. Once the water has cooled to the touch, about 15 minutes, the eggs will have a perfectly cooked yolk.

Put the eggs in a mini food processor and pulse just 4 times or so, until they're broken down into small pieces. Alternatively, place them in a bowl and use the back of a fork to break them up. Add the mayonnaise, mustard, salt, paprika, cayenne, and lemon juice and process or stir until combined. Do a FASS check, then add additional salt and lemon juice if needed. Serve immediately.

PREP TIME: 5 minutes · COOK TIME: Not applicable
STORAGE: Store in an airtight container in the refrigerator for 2 to 3 days.
PER SERVING: Calories: 80; Total Fat: 5.5 g (1.6 g saturated, 2 g monounsaturated); Carbohydrates: 1 g; Protein: 6 g; Fiber: 0 g; Sodium: 240 mg

WHO KNEW? Stepping Up Leave it to someone intimately involved with acupuncture and Chinese medicine to have an interesting take on cancer care and where patients can help themselves. Michael Broffman works with many cancer patients at the Pine Street Clinic in Marin County, an area where an unusually high number of women have been diagnosed with breast cancer. Broffman, who coordinates his care with that of area oncologists, explains how eating becomes more important after patients "graduate" from treatment. "The burden of success when a person is going through chemo is more on the chemo than what they're eating. The important thing there is they maintain weight and protein and not become malnourished. Once chemotherapy is over, all of a sudden the burden of success in terms of prevention and reducing risk and recurrence is back in the person's court. If you really deepen your cooking skills and enjoyment of cooking during treatment, that's a good launching pad for starting your prevention program."

Poached Eggs with Basil Lemon Drizzle

Here's all you need to know about poached eggs: Ira Gershwin said his songwriting career wouldn't be complete until he got his beloved poached eggs into one of his songs, which he eventually did ("I'm a poached egg . . . without a piece of toast; Yorkshire pudding . . . without a beef to roast."). I guess Ira felt like so many of us do: sometimes the best little meal is the simplest. In this case, I've enhanced the yum factor by topping this comfort food with Basil Lemon Drizzle. The result is a very light sauce, which the fat from the yolk takes on a trip all around your mouth. Hmm . . . yummmm. SERVES 4

1 tablespoon vinegar
4 organic eggs
Sea salt
Basil Lemon Drizzle (page 177), for garnish

REBECCA'S NOTES Like your yolks more firm? Let them cook for an extra 30 to 60 seconds.

Go the extra mile and prepare this take on eggs Benedict. It's worth it! Put four pieces of sprouted grain bread on a cutting board and use a cookie cutter or the mouth of a large glass to punch out circle shapes. Toast the circles, then drizzle with a bit of extra-virgin olive oil and sprinkle lightly with sea salt. Place a poached egg on top of each piece of toast, then top with 2 teaspoons of Basil Lemon Drizzle.

Pour 6 inches of water into a large saucepan and place over medium-high heat. When it's almost boiling, add the vinegar, then crack each egg open in a small dish and gently slide the egg in the water. Maintain the water temperature at just below a simmer, turning the heat down to low if necessary. Cook until the egg whites are set and the centers are still soft, about 3 minutes. Remove with a slotted spoon and place on a paper towel to drain off excess water.

Serve immediately, sprinkling each egg with a pinch of sea salt and topping with 2 teaspoons of Basil Lemon Drizzle.

PREP TIME: 2 minutes · COOK TIME: 5 minutes
STORAGE: Eat immediately!
PER SERVING: Calories: 70; Total Fat: 5 g (1.6 g saturated, 1.9 g monounsaturated); Carbohydrates: 0 g; Protein: 6 g; Fiber: 0 g; Sodium: 145 mg

WHO KNEW? What's Important Integrative oncologist Debu Tripathy is a world leader in the use of nutrition to treat cancer, especially women with breast cancer. Yet Tripathy's interest in having his patients eat well goes beyond science. "I feel that eating, and nutrition in general, is such an important aspect of life, in illness and health," says Dr. Tripathy, who practices at the University of Texas Southwestern Medical Center. "We put a lot of time and effort into eating well, having fun eating, and eating with family. When people are diagnosed with cancer, the most important thing is that they keep the priorities in their lives straight. If they've used meals as both nourishment and for social reasons, we recommend that they continue to do that. Even putting the health benefits aside, the importance of maintaining an interest in food and meals can't be overlooked."

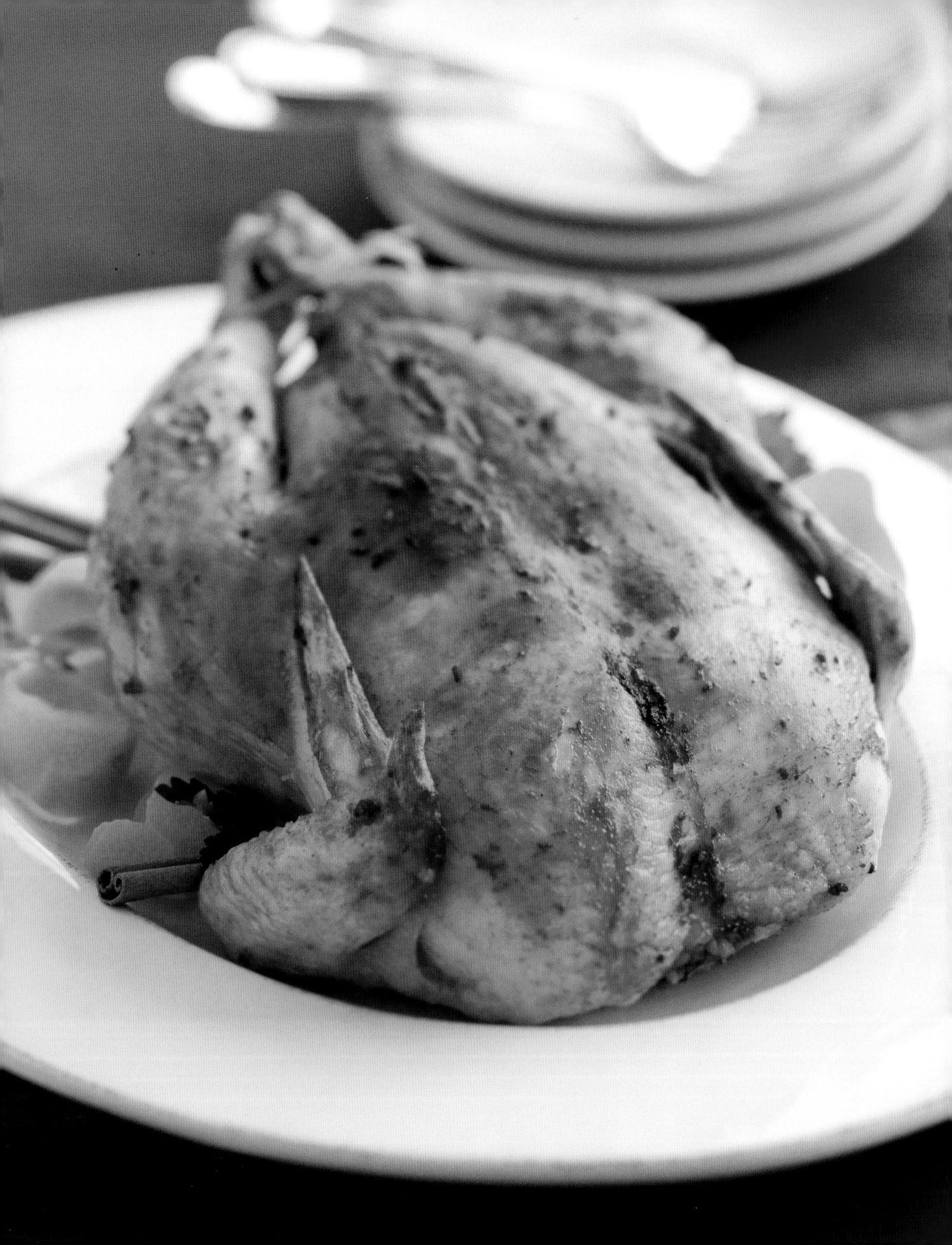

Orange Ginger Roasted Chicken

Roasted chicken is such a staple for many people that I wanted to provide a zippy recipe that would avoid the all-too-frequent pitfall of bland, dry results. Here, I've replaced the common rosemary-thyme rub with ginger, orange zest, and cinnamon, which are also appetite stimulants. Rubbing the spices under the skin, filling the cavity with more aromatics and orange juice, and then roasting the whole shebang makes for one moist, tasty bird! Drizzle with Moroccan Pesto (page 186) or add a dollop of Apricot Pear Chutney (page 175). SERVES 6

- 1 4 1/2- to 5-pound organic chicken
- 1 teaspoon paprika
- 1/4 teaspoon ground coriander
- 1/4 teaspoon ground cinnamon
- 1 1/2 teaspoons sea salt
- 1 orange, zested and juiced, rind reserved
- 1 teaspoon grated fresh ginger, plus 1 finger-length piece of unpeeled fresh ginger, halved lengthwise
- 3 cloves garlic
- 2 cinnamon sticks

REBECCA'S NOTES Leftovers, anyone? Using leftover roasted chicken will save time and add flavor to any recipe calling for roasted or shredded chicken, such as Curried Chicken Salad (page 104), Cozy Comfy Chicken and Rice (page 106), Lemony Greek Chicken Soup (page 60), and Thai It Up Chicken Soup (page 62), or as an addition to Hungarian Roasted Root Vegetable Potpie (page 95).

Use disposable kitchen gloves to handle the bird more easily and keep things sanitary.

Preheat the oven to 400°F.

Pat the chicken dry with paper towels. Stir the paprika, coriander, and cinnamon together, then divide the mixture in half and stir 1 teaspoon of the salt into half. Rub the salted spice mixture all over the outside of the chicken. Sprinkle the remaining 1/2 teaspoon salt inside the chicken.

With your palm facing downward, use your first three fingers to gently lift the skin on both sides of the breast to loosen it from the meat. Rub the remaining spice mixture, the orange zest, and grated ginger under the skin of each breast, massaging them lightly into the meat. Place the garlic, cinnamon sticks, ginger pieces, and orange rind inside the cavity along with half of the orange juice.

Place the chicken on a roasting rack in a glass or ceramic baking dish, breast side up. Roast until a meat thermometer reads 160°F when inserted in the thigh and the juice from the meat runs clear, about 1 hour.

Let the chicken rest for at least 10 minutes before carving. Just before serving, pour the remaining orange juice over the chicken.

Variations: Here are a few other spice blends for a tasty bird:

- In place of the paprika, coriander, and cinnamon, use 1 teaspoon cumin, 1/4 teaspoon ground coriander, and 1/4 teaspoon dried oregano.
- Replace the paprika with anise seeds.
- Replace the oranges with lemons, and in place of the paprika, coriander, and cinnamon, use 1/2 teaspoon dried thyme, 1/4 teaspoon rosemary, and 1/4 teaspoon sage.

PREP TIME: 20 minutes · COOK TIME: 1 hour

STORAGE: Store in a covered container in the refrigerator for 3 to 5 days.

PER SERVING: Calories: 215; Total Fat: 5.1 g (1.3 g saturated, 1.5 g monounsaturated); Carbohydrates: 4 g; Protein: 35 g; Fiber: 1 g; Sodium: 715 mg

Triple-Citrus Ginger Black Cod

Shopping for fish can be intimidating. Maybe it's the fact that half of them are staring at you from behind the counter, as if to say, "Jeez, how did I end up here?" So, if you're going to do them—and yourself—justice, here's how to rustle up a fine, fresh fillet. You need to use your eyes and your nose. Look for a cut where the flesh is moist and glistening, with no flat, brown edges. If the fish looks dull, take a pass. Same goes for any fillet with a fishy or ammonia smell. Don't be shy about asking your fishmonger a few questions, like when the fish came in and from where. Most stores have regular shipments; knowing that schedule in advance can help you plan when to have fish. If black cod were in a band, it would be the bass player: steady, meaty, but not much of a soloist. It benefits from some jazzy front men and especially likes to swing with citrus high notes. You'll find plenty of those riffs in this dish. SERVES 4

- 1/2 cup freshly squeezed orange juice
- 2 tablespoons freshly squeezed lime juice
- 2 tablespoons freshly squeezed lemon juice
- 1 tablespoon extra-virgin olive oil
- Zest of 1 orange
- Zest of 1 lemon
- 1/2 teaspoon minced fresh ginger
- Pinch of cayenne
- 4 3.5-ounce black cod fillets, pinbones removed
- 1/2 teaspoon sea salt
- 1 teaspoon Dijon mustard
- 1/4 cup coarsely chopped fresh flat-leaf parsley or mint

In a small bowl or glass measuring cup, whisk together the orange juice, lime juice, lemon juice, olive oil, orange zest, lemon zest, ginger, and cayenne. Place the cod in a baking dish and season each piece with 1/8 teaspoon of the salt. Pour half of the orange juice mixture over the cod and turn to coat well. Cover and marinate in the refrigerator for 30 minutes.

Preheat the oven to 400°F.

Remove the cod from the refrigerator, uncover, and add 2 tablespoons of water to the bottom of the dish. Bake just until the fillets are tender and an instant-read thermometer inserted into the center of each fillet registers 137°F; it will take 10 to 15 minutes, depending on the thickness of the fillets.

Meanwhile, combine the remaining orange juice mixture and the mustard in a small saucepan over medium heat and simmer until the liquid is reduced by half. Pour the reduction over the fillets, sprinkle with the parsley, and serve immediately.

REBECCA'S NOTES This versatile, delicious marinade is great with other fish, such as sea bass, salmon, and halibut. These flavors also pair nicely with Warm Napa Cabbage Slaw (page 92).

You can also cook the fish on a grill. Wipe the marinade off the fillets and rub them with 1 teaspoon of light sesame oil. Grill over low, even heat for about 4 minutes per side, until the flesh is opaque and flakes easily and the center of each fillet registers 137°F.

PREP TIME: 15 minutes

COOK TIME: 20 minutes (plus 20 minutes to marinate)

STORAGE: Store tightly wrapped in an airtight container in the refrigerator for 1 to 2 days.

PER SERVING: Calories: 130; Total Fat: 4.3 g (0.7 g saturated, 2.6 g monounsaturated); Carbohydrates: 5 g; Protein: 18 g; Fiber: 0 g; Sodium: 370 mg

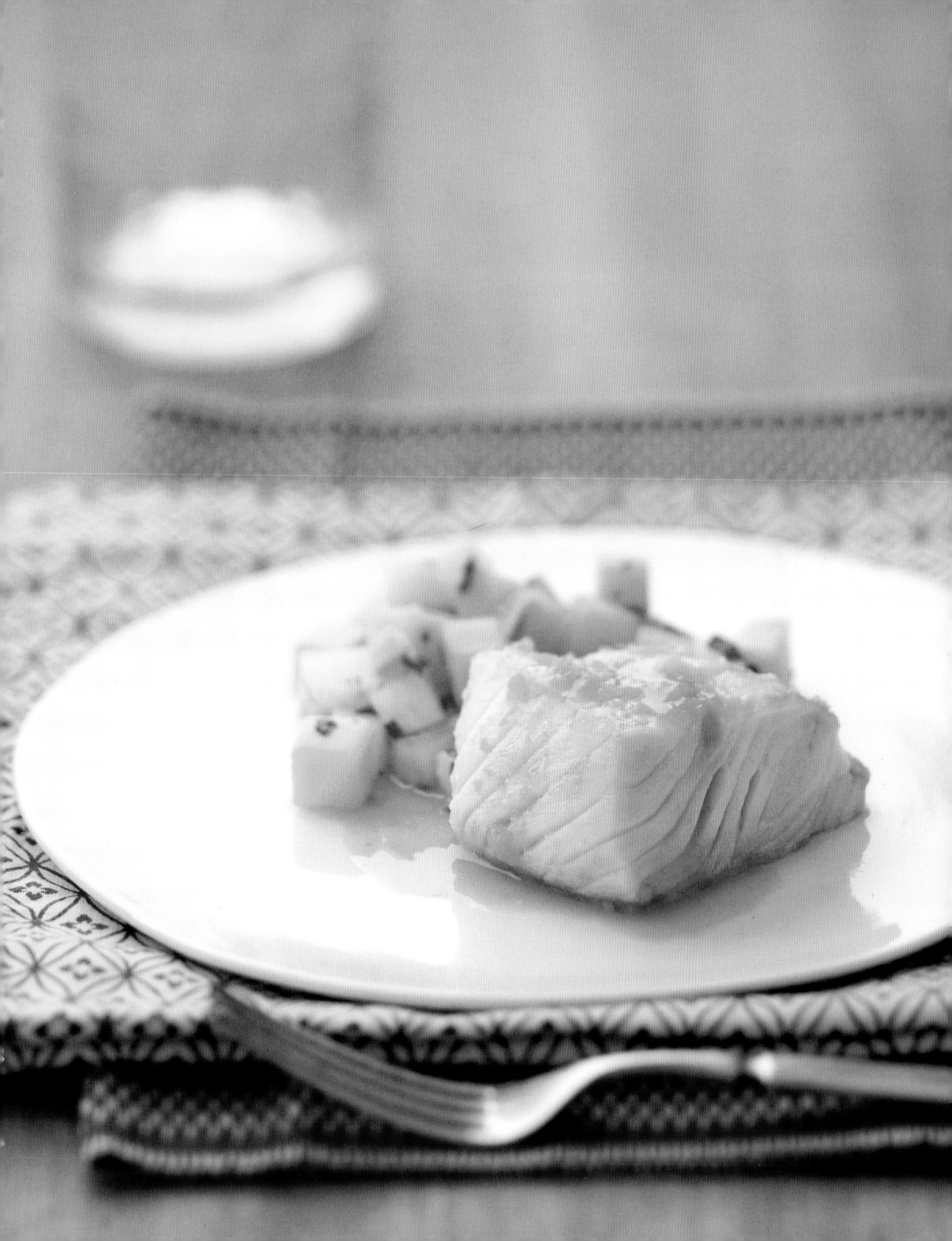

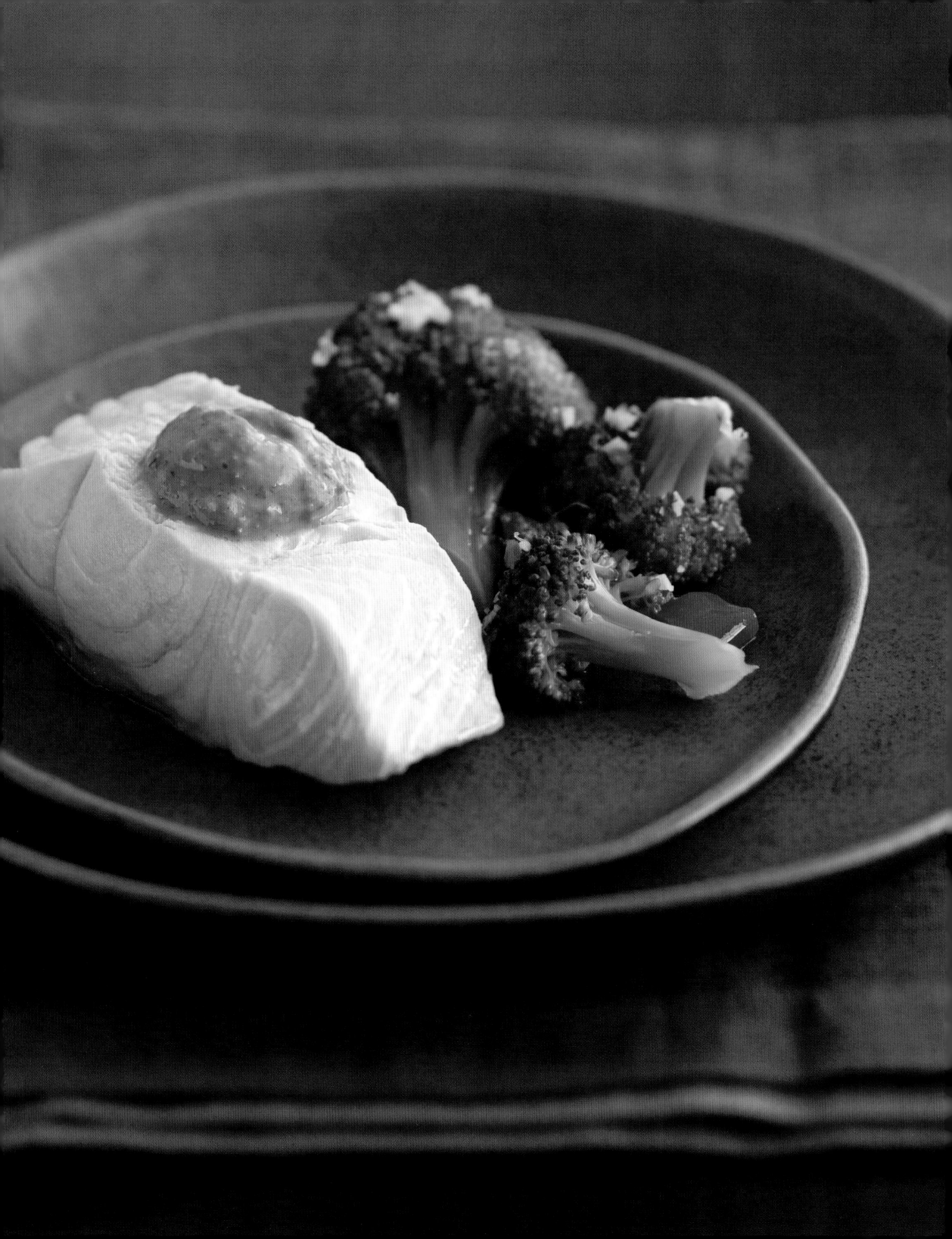

Poached Salmon with Moroccan Pesto

Normally I like to pan-sear or broil salmon, but a lot of my clients have asked for a different way to approach fish. Poaching salmon is the answer. It's a great way to enjoy a fillet without having to endure a lot of cooking smells. Most people associate poaching with eggs, and the concept is the same here. By briefly dunking the fillet in a simmering liquid, it quickly becomes moist and tender. Poaching isn't boiling, and thank goodness, because that kind of long immersion is a sure way to give fish the consistency of a hockey puck. Here, the poaching liquid is Magic Mineral Broth, which infuses the salmon with even more nutrients—and more yum. Moroccan Pesto is a snazzy topping for this dish, but the possibilities are endless. See the variations below for a few more suggestions. SERVES 4

Juice of 1 lemon

1/2 teaspoon sea salt

4 4-ounce salmon fillets, pinbones removed

4 cups Magic Mineral Broth (page 54)

Moroccan Pesto (page 186), for serving

REBECCA'S NOTES Usually it's best to buy your fish the same day you're preparing it. However, life doesn't always work that way. If you must store the fish longer, put it in a resealable plastic bag in the coldest part of your refrigerator, which is usually the back of the bottom shelf. It should hold for an extra two days. Put a note on the fridge to remind you that the fish is there. You know that old saying, "Out of sight, out of mind."

Stir the lemon juice and salt together, then add the salmon and turn to coat thoroughly. Marinate in the refrigerator for 20 minutes.

In a large straight-sided sauté pan or a low-sided pot just wide enough to hold the salmon in a single layer, bring the broth to a slow boil over medium heat. Slide the salmon into the broth and poach for 7 to 9 minutes, just until the fish is tender and an instant-read thermometer inserted into the center of each fillet registers 127°F.

Garnish each with a generous dollop of Moroccan Pesto and serve immediately.

Variations: There are many toppings you can dollop on poached salmon, including Basil Lemon Drizzle (page 177), Olive and Caper Relish (page 186), and Parsley Basil Drizzle (page 187).

PREP TIME: 10 minutes

COOK TIME: 20 minutes (plus 20 minutes to marinate)

STORAGE: Store in an airtight container in the refrigerator for 2 days.

PER SERVING: Calories: 245; Total Fat: 10.9 g (1.7 g saturated, 4.9 g monounsaturated); Carbohydrates: 12 g; Protein: 24 g; Fiber: 2 g; Sodium: 530 mg

WHO KNEW? One Fish, Two Fish, Right Fish, Great Fish! Are you wondering which fish cancer experts like in terms of beneficial nutritional content? Integrative oncologist Donald Abrams, an ardent foodie, suggests the following: "I like fish from deep, cold water. Salmon, albacore tuna, black cod, herring, mackerel, sardines—those are all rich in omega-3 fatty acids."

Best and Worst Fish Choices

BEST CHOICES	WORST CHOICES
Abalone	Caviar (wild)
Anchovies*	Chilean sea bass†
Artic char	Cod, Atlantic
Black cod, Alaskan*	Grouper
Catfish	Halibut, Atlantic
Halibut, Pacific	Marlin†
Herring*	Monkfish
Mackerel, Atlantic*	Orange roughy†
Sablefish, Alaskan*	Rockfish or rock cod
Salmon, wild*	Salmon, Atlantic (farmed)†
Salmon can sockeye*	Shark†
Sardines*	Shrimp (imported)
Scallops, bay (farmed)	Skate
Striped bass (farmed)	Snapper
Tilapia, U.S.	Sturgeon†
	Swordfish†
	Tilefish†
	Tuna, albacore†
	Tuna, bluefin

** = High in omega-3 fatty acids*

† = Highest mercury levels

Sources: The Environmental Working Group, www.foodnews.org, and Oceans Alive, www.oceansalive.org

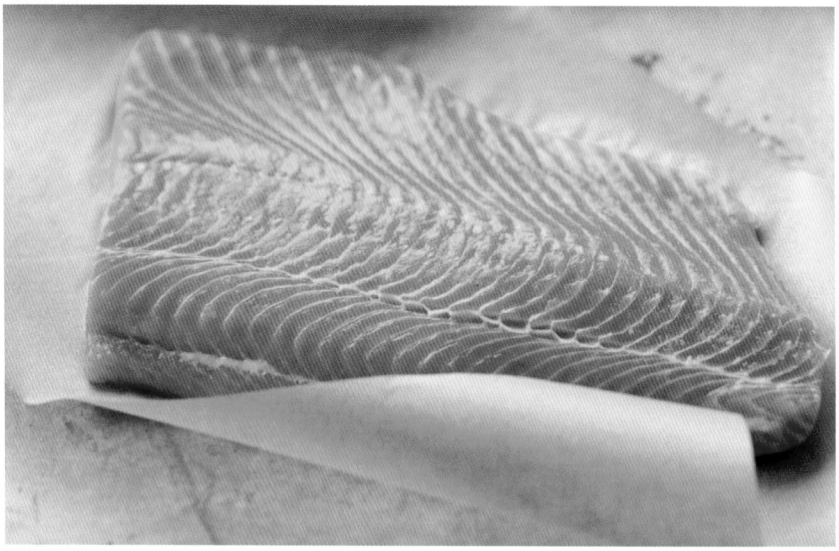

Baked Citrus Halibut with Tomato Sauce

Sometimes creating a recipe is a little like trying to solve a Rubik's cube. You twist it this way and that and get real close to figuring it out, only to realize you're not quite there yet. Such was the case here. Halibut is a great fish for health, but left to its own devices it can be rather bland. So I toyed, I tinkered, and went through more fish than Shamu until—hallelujah!—I got it right. If you aren't in the mood for this southern Italian version, try the south-of-the border variation below. SERVES 4

- 2 tablespoons freshly squeezed lemon juice
- 1/4 teaspoon sea salt
- 4 6-ounce halibut fillets
- 1 teaspoon extra-virgin olive oil
- 1 cup Signora's Tomato Sauce (page 188)
- 1/4 cup Olive and Caper Relish (page 186)

Preheat the oven to 400°F and lightly oil an ovenproof pan large enough to accommodate all of the fillets in a single layer.

Stir the lemon juice and salt together, then coat the halibut in the mixture and refrigerate for 15 minutes.

Pat the fillets dry with paper towels and place them in the prepared pan. Brush each fillet with 1/4 teaspoon of the olive oil and top with 1/4 cup of the tomato sauce.

Bake for 12 to 15 minutes, until the fish is opaque and flakes easily. To be certain the fish is done, push a two-pronged kitchen fork straight down into the flesh. If you feel no resistance, the fish is cooked; if not, return the fish to the oven for another minute or two.

Top each fillet with 1 tablespoon of the relish before serving.

Variation: For a totally different taste sensation, marinate the halibut in Cilantro Lime Vinaigrette (page 181) for 30 minutes. Pat the fillets dry with paper towels. Sprinkle each fillet with a pinch of salt and a pinch of cayenne, and bake as above. Top with a dollop of Mango and Avocado Salsa (page 185) before serving.

PREP TIME: 25 minutes (including marinating) · COOK TIME: 15 minutes
STORAGE: Store in an airtight container in the refrigerator for 2 days.
PER SERVING: Calories: 380; Total Fat: 28 g (4.7 g saturated, 17.4 g monounsaturated); Carbohydrates: 5 g; Protein: 26 g; Fiber: 1 g; Sodium: 450 mg

CULINARY RX Nutritionists tout fish as a great source of omega-3 fatty acids, which studies suggest may be beneficial for people fighting breast and prostate cancer. But recent research suggests that not all fish are created equal, and what people really should be looking at is the ratio of omega-3 to omega-6, as omega-6s may promote cancer growth. This ratio could be at the heart of the benefits of the so-called Mediterranean diet, which some researchers believe is linked to lower cancer rates in Mediterranean countries. The magic ratio of omega-3s to omega-6s appears to be no less than 1 to 1 (and preferably a lot more omega 3s). For example, halibut's ratio is 2.5 to 1 (good), wild king salmon comes in at 5.6 to 1 (better), and fish roe weighs in at 11.1 to 1 (a slam dunk). By contrast, farm-raised catfish has fifty times more omega-6s than omega-3s. A good rule of thumb is to look for wild fish, as opposed to farm-raised, since the feed given to some cultivated fish can be high in omega-6s.

CHAPTER 6

Anytime Foods

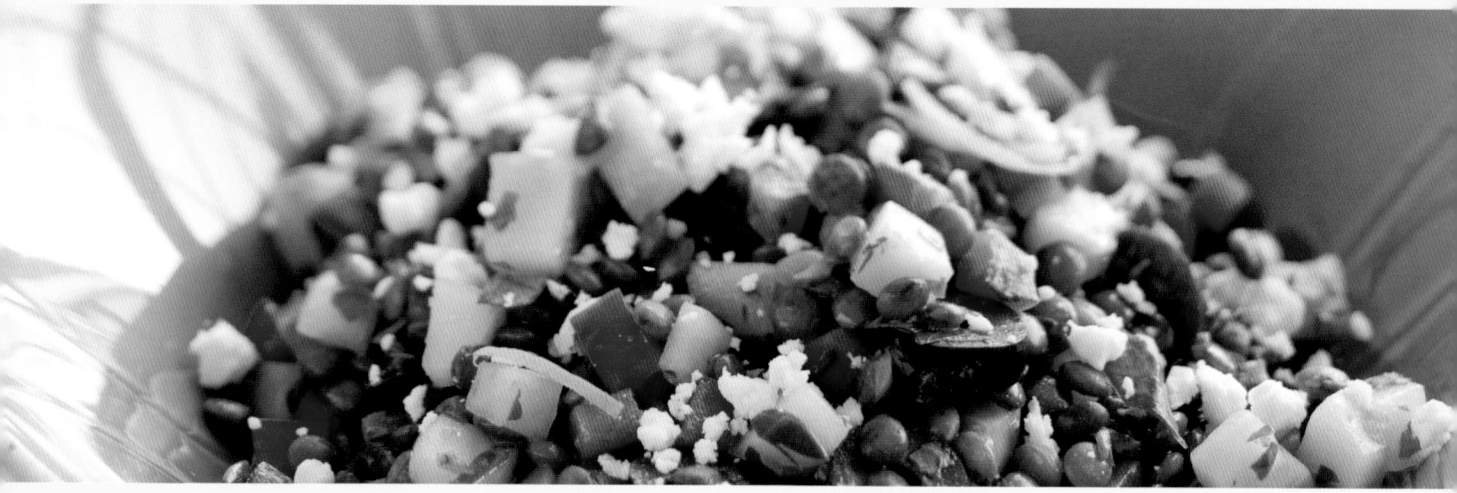

126 *Anytime Bars*

128 *Best Oatmeal Ever*

129 *Beyond Just Good Cornbread*

131 *Edamame Avocado Dip with Wasabi*

131 *Navy Bean and Sun-Dried Tomato Dip*

132 *Cannellini Bean Dip with Kalamata Olives*

132 *Black Bean Hummus*

133 *Curried Hummus*

134 *Creamy Polenta*

135 *Catherine's Magic Green Tea Rice*

136 *Creamy Millet*

138 *Creamiest Buckwheat*

139 *Spiced Toasted Almonds*

141 *Maple-Glazed Walnuts*

142 *Mediterranean Lentil Salad*

145 *Orange Pistachio Couscous*

146 *Roasted Asparagus Pasta with White Beans and Thyme*

147 *Forbidden Rice Salad*

148 *Simple Tuscan Farro*

149 *Quinoa Pilaf*

150 *Rice Paper Moo-Shu Rolls*

153 *Curried Hummus and Vegetable Pinwheels*

People pride themselves on eating at regular intervals, like clockwork, but cancer and associated treatment can often make one's appetite timepiece go kaflooey. Why? Mostly two reasons: Certain cancers—among them throat and stomach cancers—depress appetite, either because they make eating or digestion difficult, or because the cancer itself affects the brain's hunger center. Then there's treatment. Some chemotherapies drive blood sugar down, while certain steroids used to counteract chemo side effects raise blood sugar; the net effect is to again throw off common eating patterns. So those three square large meals you're used to? Well, perhaps you'll be up for that, but as often as not, you'll need to get your nutrition whenever you're hungry, regardless of the hour, or whether you just ate a half-hour ago.

That's why these anytime foods are so important: Whenever you get a craving to eat, you'll want something at hand that you'll find desirable, easily accessible, and nutrient dense. Nutrient dense just means that ounce for ounce, there are no wasted calories; every bite carries a load of the macronutrients you need to get through the day. Remember the story of the tortoise and the hare? Mr. Slow and Steady had the right idea: a small but consistent effort at eating can have wonderful cumulative effects. As you'll see elsewhere in the book, many experts suggest that when you're battling cancer, you try to get in six small meals or snacks a day. The best way to do that is to concentrate not on how much you eat, but how often. The idea is that you want to stay nourished throughout the day, which is where these anytime foods come in. As the name implies, anytime foods are snacks designed to be portable, storable, and accessible anytime the mood hits. Plus, these recipes are nutrient-dense, and of course I plan on blowing your mind with the taste. I'd rather see you take a single satisfying nibble every few hours than try to force yourself to eat when you clearly don't feel like it. That creates a negative association with food, which you can't afford.

I've taken an expansive approach to these anytime foods in the hope that they'll remind you of some of your favorite snacks. Dips, salads, wraps—they're all designed to provide long-lasting energy with each bite. Toasted nuts are really a no-brainer. They're a wonderful nutrient-dense food, and it only takes a bit of prep to turn them into tiny taste sensations. You can eat them straight or use them as a topping for salads, oatmeal, and other dishes. Either way, they'll provide extra nutrition and a big dose of yum. Plus, they're highly portable, earning them a spot on my short list of great to-go foods. They're an ideal snack anytime you're on the road. And speaking of portable, at the end of the chapter you'll find two recipes that I like to think of as "wrap, roll, and carry." These easy and delicious mobile meals are packed with protein.

In a very real sense, I'm trying to engage you in high-performance eating, just like athletes or hikers who eat certain high-energy foods with a sense of purpose. By noshing throughout the day (and at night, if you want; we're talking a twenty-four hour day here for your six meals), you're providing your body with the nutrients it needs and keeping your blood sugar optimal, which can help your mood and health.

Anytime Bars

The whole idea of Anytime Bars is right in the name; you never know when hunger is going to strike, and you want to be ready to take advantage of those moments to nourish yourself. A lot of my clients take these portable packets of pleasure to chemo sessions. It may seem odd that people want to eat during treatment, but many do, and these bars are a delicious, healthy alternative to the bowls of sweets so often found around infusion centers. The great thing about this recipe is that you can change the ingredients to fit your taste preferences. You can even split the batter and make half with currant and cranberries and the other half with walnuts or whatever you'd like. These bars come together very quickly with the food processor, but if you don't have one, you can certainly chop the fruit and nuts by hand. MAKES 25 BARS

- 1 cup raw pecan halves
- 1 cup whole raw almonds
- 2 tablespoons spelt flour
- 2 tablespoons unbleached all-purpose flour
- 2 tablespoons finely ground flaxseeds
- 1/4 teaspoon sea salt
- 1/8 teaspoon baking powder
- 1/8 teaspoon baking soda
- 1/4 cup old-fashioned rolled oats
- 1 cup pitted dates, quartered (preferably Medjool)
- 1 cup unsulfured dried apricots, cut in half
- 1 organic egg
- 5 tablespoons maple syrup
- 1 teaspoon vanilla extract

Preheat the oven to 350°F and line a baking sheet with parchment paper. Lightly oil a 9-inch square pan.

Spread the pecans in a single layer on the prepared baking sheet and toast for 7 to 10 minutes, until aromatic and slightly browned. Watch them carefully, as they can burn easily. Repeat this process for the almonds. Turn down the oven to 325°F.

Combine the spelt flour, all-purpose flour, flaxseeds, salt, baking powder, and baking soda in a food processor and process for 5 seconds to combine. Add the pecans and almonds and pulse 5 times to coarsely chop the nuts. Add the oats, dates, and apricots and pulse 10 to 15 times, until the mixture is well chopped but still coarse.

In a large bowl, whisk the egg, maple syrup, and vanilla together until thoroughly combined. Add the fruit and nut mixture and use your hands to mix thoroughly, being sure to separate any clumps of fruit. Spread the mixture in the oiled baking pan in an even layer and bake for 25 to 30 minutes, until set and golden brown; don't overbake, or the bars will be too dry. Let cool on a wire rack for 5 minutes, then cut into 25 squares. Leave the bars in the pan until completely cool so they'll hold together when you remove them.

Variations: When it comes to changing up the mixture, the only limit is your imagination. Here are a few ideas to get you started:

- Use walnuts instead of pecans.
- Add 1/4 cup dried cranberries, cherries, blueberries, raisins, or currants when mixing together at the end.
- Add 1 tablespoon of grated orange zest when mixing together at the end.
- Add 2 tablespoons of sesame seeds when mixing together at the end.
- Add 1/4 cup of unsweetened shredded coconut when mixing together at the end.
- For a gluten-free version, substitute a gluten-free muffin mix for the spelt flour and all-purpose flour. While oats don't contain gluten, they're often processed alongside wheat, so if your sensitivity to gluten is extreme, be sure to use Bob's Red Mill gluten-free oats (see Resources).

PREP TIME: 15 minutes · COOK TIME: 30 minutes

STORAGE: Store in an airtight container at room temperature for 5 to 7 days or in the freezer for 2 months.

PER SERVING: Calories: 120; Total Fat: 6.5 g (0.6 g saturated, 3.7 g monounsaturated); Carbohydrates: 14 g; Protein: 2 g; Fiber: 2 g; Sodium: 35 mg

WHO KNEW? Just the Flax, Ma'am Flaxseeds have gone under the microscope, and scientists like what they're seeing. In a well-respected study in Montreal, a researcher had biopsies from women who had just been diagnosed with breast cancer but weren't scheduled to undergo surgery for another 8 to 12 weeks. Dr. Jeanne Wallace says that the researcher "sent the women muffins in which she baked flaxseeds or placebo muffins, without flaxseeds." After the women underwent surgery, the researcher compared their postsurgery biopsies to the baseline tissues. "She was able to show that just this flaxseed intervention, over a period of not quite three months, was able to slow the growth rate of the cancer and to reduce estrogen signaling" (which has been linked to some breast cancers). Wallace says flaxseeds are preferable to flax oils, which oxidize easily, making them potentially damaging to health, rather than healing.

Best Oatmeal Ever

Ever notice how in the United States the consistency of most oatmeal falls somewhere between wall plaster and grout? The things we do to those poor oats. There oughta be a law! As a result, we often resort to the culinary equivalent of wallpapering, covering up the abomination with butter and brown sugar. This is a shame, because oatmeal just needs a little love to deliver a heartwarming, nutritious meal. The best oatmeal recipe is akin to a two-part harmony, pairing solid prep with inspiring spices to yield a joyous anytime song. Part of the trick is to soak the oats overnight, so plan ahead. Top this with fruit compote or nuts, and you'll never again wonder why oatmeal isn't used as an industrial adhesive. SERVES 2

- 1 cup rolled or steel-cut oats
- 1 1/2 tablespoons freshly squeezed lemon juice
- 2 cups water
- 1/4 teaspoon sea salt
- 1/4 cup dried cranberries, cherries, raisins, currants, blueberries, or a mixture
- 1/4 teaspoon ground cinnamon
- 1/4 teaspoon ground ginger, or 1 teaspoon grated fresh ginger
- 1/8 teaspoon ground cardamom
- 1 teaspoon maple syrup
- 1/4 cup organic milk or soy milk (optional)
- Chopped toasted almonds or walnuts (see page 97), for garnish (optional)
- Dried Fruit Compote (page 183), Blueberry Compote (page 185), or Seasonal Stewed Fruit (page 184), for garnish (optional)

Place the oats in a pan or bowl with the lemon juice and water to cover and soak overnight.

Drain the oats in a fine-mesh sieve and rinse well under cold running water. Combine the oats, water, and salt in a saucepan and bring to a boil over medium-high heat. Cover, lower the heat, and stir in the dried fruit, cinnamon, ginger, and cardamom. Continue cooking, stirring occasionally, for 10 minutes. The oatmeal will become very creamy as the water evaporates. For less-moist oatmeal, leave the lid off for the last 3 to 4 minutes of cooking. Stir in the maple syrup and milk (if using) and serve garnished with toasted nuts or a dollop of compote if you like.

Variations: Try substituting quinoa for the rolled oats for a nutrition-packed alternative.

PREP TIME: 5 minutes (after soaking the oats overnight)
COOK TIME: 15 minutes
STORAGE: Store in an airtight container in the refrigerator for 3 days.
PER SERVING: Calories: 220; Total Fat: 2.7 g (0 g saturated, 0 g monounsaturated); Carbohydrates: 42 g; Protein: 7 g; Fiber: 5 g; Sodium: 295 mg

REBECCA'S NOTES Our ancestors had it right. Before they cooked their oatmeal, they soaked it overnight in a bowl of water and lemon juice. Why lemon juice? Because its acids help break down the outer shell of the oats. This makes their nutrients more avialable and also gives them a creamier texture. For the best taste and nutrition, go with organic rolled oats or organic steel-cut oats, which are popular in Ireland and Scotland.

Beyond Just Good Cornbread

Cornbread is one of those foods people get mighty opinionated about, as in "Nobody makes cornbread as good as my (momma, grammy, Uncle Phoebus, just fill in the blank)." Not only that, but once someone gets a beloved piece of that cornbread in their hands, well, as one writer said, "If you try to take my cornbread, there will be consequences and repercussions." I think of cornbread a bit like barbecue: Just about every region of the country has its variation, which, as if ordained from above, is simply the best. Cornbread, cornpone, jonnycakes, hush puppies—the names and approaches differ, but not the devotion. My version is California-style, as in how do we keep all of that awesome taste while using healthier ingredients? Using some spelt flour helps, as does using just a bit of organic maple syrup as a sweetener and extra-virgin olive oil in place of butter. The lemon zest allowed me to put the word "beyond" into the title of this recipe. If you'll allow me to play yenta, I'd match the cornbread with the Rockin' Black Bean Soup (page 71). They're a very happy couple. MAKES 16 PIECES

1 cup cornmeal
1/2 cup spelt flour
1/2 cup whole wheat flour
2 teaspoons baking powder
1/2 teaspoon baking soda
1/2 teaspoon sea salt
1 organic egg
1 cup organic buttermilk
1/4 cup maple syrup
1/4 cup extra-virgin olive oil
1 tablespoon lemon zest

Preheat the oven to 400°F and lightly oil an 8-inch square baking pan.

Combine the cornmeal, flours, baking powder, baking soda, and salt and stir with a wire whisk until well combined.

In a small bowl, whisk together the egg, buttermilk, maple syrup, olive oil, and lemon zest until well combined, then pour into the dry ingredients and whisk just until the batter is evenly moistened and no large lumps remain; don't overmix, or the cornbread will be tough and dry.

Scrape the batter into the prepared pan and bake until lightly browned and just beginning to pull away from the edges of the pan, 20 to 25 minutes.

Let cool on a wire rack for about 10 minutes, then cut into 16 squares and serve warm.

PREP TIME: 10 minutes · COOK TIME: 30 minutes

STORAGE: Store tightly wrapped in the refrigerator for 4 days or in the freezer for 2 months.

PER SERVING: Calories: 115; Total Fat: 5 g (1 g saturated, 3 g monounsaturated); Carbohydrates: 16 g; Protein: 3 g; Fiber: 2 g; Sodium: 200 mg

REBECCA'S NOTES Cornbread is one of those foods that's best served warm, so when you pull leftovers out of the fridge, warm them in an oven or toaster oven.

Spelt, the grandmother of wheat, contains less gliadin than conventional wheat. Gliadin is the component of gluten thought to be most responsible for adverse reactions, and many people do indeed find spelt easier to digest. You can use all spelt flour in this recipe, but the texture will be a bit denser. If you really want to be adventurous, try using sprouted flours. The sprouting of the grains makes them even easier to digest and more flavorful. Look in the Resources section for information on where to find these special ingredients.

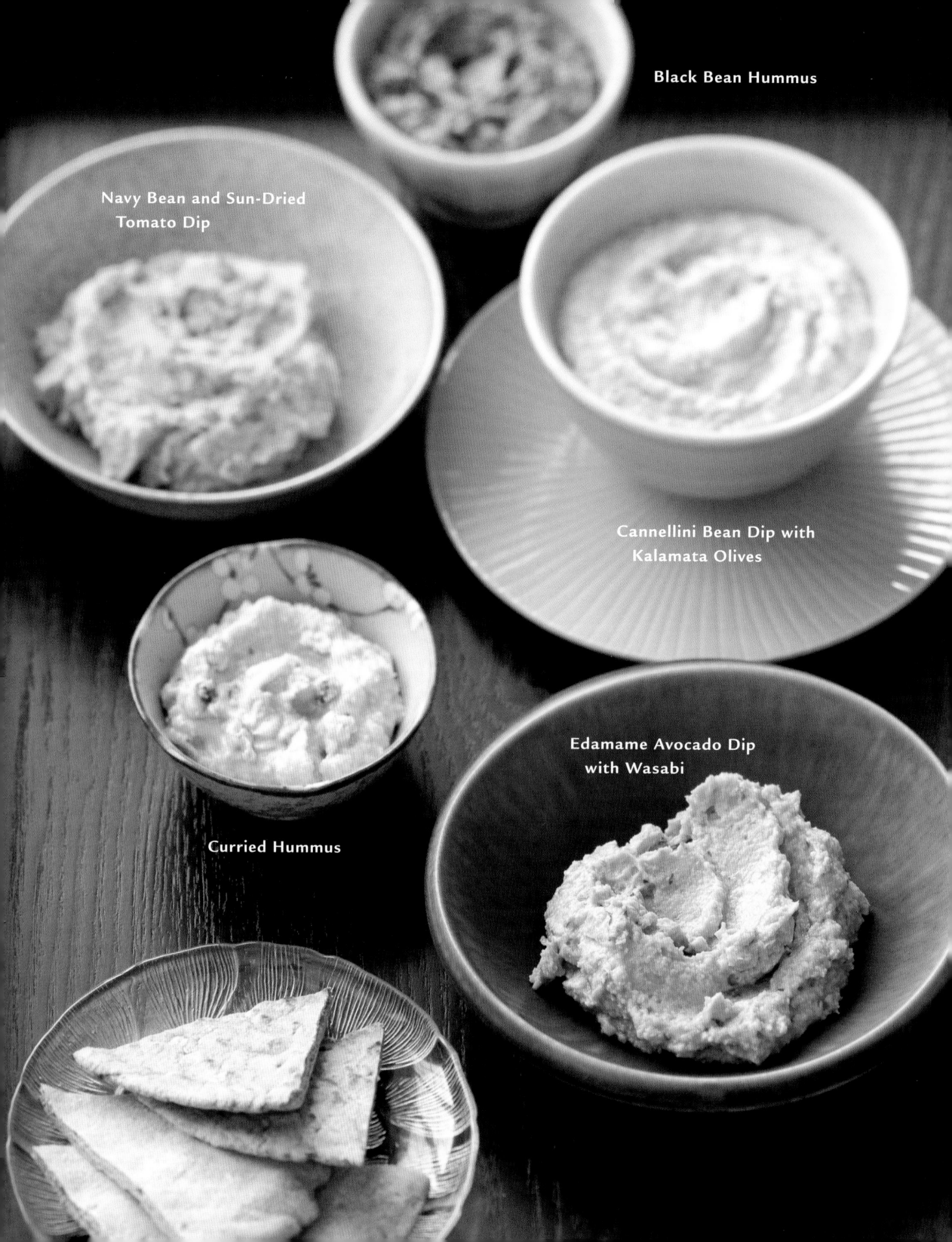
Black Bean Hummus
Navy Bean and Sun-Dried Tomato Dip
Cannellini Bean Dip with Kalamata Olives
Edamame Avocado Dip with Wasabi
Curried Hummus

Edamame Avocado Dip with Wasabi

Wasabi is rich in chemicals that some studies show cause cancer cells to starve. The combination of wasabi and ginger might be a bit much for those with swallowing difficulties, but for everyone else this dip's creamy coolness makes it perfect for slathering on rice crackers or dipping veggies into, especially jicama. SERVES 6

- 1 cup fresh or frozen shelled edamame, mixed with a spritz of fresh lime juice and a pinch of sea salt
- 2 avocados, peeled, pitted, and spritzed with fresh lime juice and a pinch of salt
- 1 teaspoon minced fresh ginger
- 1/2 teaspoon minced garlic
- 1/4 cup water
- 3 tablespoons freshly squeezed lime juice
- 1 tablespoon extra-virgin olive oil
- 1/4 teaspoon sea salt
- 1/4 teaspoon wasabi powder
- 1 tablespoon chopped fresh mint

Combine all of the ingredients in a food processor and process until smooth. Do a FASS check and add additional lime juice or salt if needed.

Variation: You can use frozen peas in place of the edamame. Just blanch them for 1 minute in boiling water, then rinse in cold water before blending. Remember to give them a spritz with lime juice.

PREP TIME: 10 minutes · COOK TIME: Not applicable

STORAGE: Store in an airtight container in the refrigerator for 2 days.

PER SERVING: Calories: 130; Total Fat: 10.3 g (1.3 g saturated, 6.1 g monounsaturated); Carbohydrates: 8 g; Protein: 4 g; Fiber: 5 g; Sodium: 115 mg

REBECCA'S NOTES If you're up for it, go the extra mile and add some additional heat! Another 1/4 teaspoon of wasabi powder will turn up the wow factor in this dip. This gorgeous dip is very versatile. Use it like a condiment, spread on sandwiches or wraps. Yum!

Navy Bean and Sun-Dried Tomato Dip

The creaminess of navy beans makes a great base for spreads and dips, which I've supercharged by adding sun-dried tomatoes. Use it as a sandwich spread, or a dollop on veggies. SERVES 6

- 2 cups cooked navy beans (see page 110), or 1 15-ounce can, drained, rinsed, and mixed with a spritz of fresh lemon juice and a pinch of sea salt
- 1/4 cup oil-packed sun-dried tomatoes, rinsed
- 1/4 cup chopped fresh parsley
- 1/2 teaspoon minced garlic
- 3 tablespoons extra-virgin olive oil
- 2 tablespoons freshly squeezed lemon juice
- 2 tablespoons water
- 1/2 teaspoon sea salt

Combine all of the ingredients in a food processor and process until smooth. Do a FASS check and add another spritz of lemon juice or a pinch of salt if needed.

PREP TIME: 10 minutes · COOK TIME: Not applicable

STORAGE: Store in an airtight container in the refrigerator for 5 to 7 days.

PER SERVING: Calories: 195; Total Fat: 8.2 g (1.1 g saturated, 5.5 g monounsaturated); Carbohydrates: 24 g; Protein: 8 g; Fiber: 9 g; Sodium: 635 mg

Cannellini Bean Dip with Kalamata Olives

The creamy white beans provide a nutritious canvas that blends well with the purplish black kalamatas. The beans are high in protein, which keeps the body in fighting shape during treatment. SERVES 6

- 2 cups cooked cannellini beans (see page 110), or 1 15-ounce can, drained, rinsed, and mixed with a spritz of fresh lemon juice and a pinch of sea salt
- 1/2 teaspoon minced garlic
- 3 tablespoons extra-virgin olive oil
- 2 tablespoons water
- 2 tablespoons freshly squeezed lemon juice
- 1/2 teaspoon sea salt
- Pinch of cayenne
- 1/4 cup pitted kalamata olives, rinsed
- 1/4 cup chopped fresh basil

Combine all of the ingredients in a food processor and process until smooth. Do a FASS check and add a pinch or two of salt if needed to balance out the lemon.

PREP TIME: 10 minutes · COOK TIME: Not applicable

STORAGE: Store in an airtight container in the refrigerator for 5 days.

PER SERVING: Calories: 195; Total Fat: 8.5 g (1.2 g saturated, 6.1 g monounsaturated); Carbohydrates: 22 g; Protein: 8 g; Fiber: 6 g; Sodium: 715 mg

Black Bean Hummus

I used black beans in this recipe because I love their taste and nutritional profile—lots of antioxidants. Because the beans are pureed, you don't get too much bang for your buck. SERVES 6

- 2 cups cooked black beans (see page 110), or 1 15-ounce can, drained, rinsed, and mixed with a spritz of fresh lemon juice and a pinch of sea salt
- 1/2 teaspoon chopped garlic
- 2 tablespoons water
- 1 tablespoon tahini
- 1 tablespoon freshly squeezed lemon juice
- 1/2 teaspoon ground cumin
- 1/4 teaspoon sea salt
- 1/4 teaspoon paprika
- 1/8 teaspoon cayenne
- 1/8 teaspoon ground cinnamon
- 1 tablespoon extra-virgin olive oil
- 1/4 cup finely chopped fresh cilantro (optional)

Combine the beans, garlic, water, tahini, lemon juice, cumin, salt, paprika, cayenne, and cinnamon in a food processor and process until smooth. Add the olive oil and process to combine. Do a FASS check and add a spritz of lemon and an additional pinch of salt if needed. Serve garnished with the cilantro.

PREP TIME: 10 minutes · COOK TIME: Not applicable

STORAGE: Store in an airtight container in the refrigerator for 5 days.

PER SERVING: Calories: 145; Total Fat: 4 g (1 g saturated, 3 g monounsaturated); Carbohydrates: 21 g; Protein: 7 g; Fiber: 9 g; Sodium: 525 mg

REBECCA'S NOTES If you really want to put this dip over the top, place a dollop of Avocado Cream (page 178) on top, or for a quick fix, a few slices of avocado will do.

Curried Hummus

Sometimes I feel like the United Nations is meeting in my kitchen. This time around it's India and Lebanon at the table. It sounds exotic, but this is really just a nice, simple hummus (that's the Lebanese part) with a zingy curry buzz (hello, Sri Lanka). Chickpeas are rich in protein and essential amino acids for keeping the body strong, while the sesame seeds in the tahini have high levels of anticancer phytochemicals; and since the seeds are ground into a paste, they're easy to digest. SERVES 6

- 1/4 cup currants
- 2 cups cooked chickpeas (see page 110), or 1 15-ounce can, drained, rinsed, and mixed with a spritz of fresh lemon juice and a pinch of sea salt
- 2 tablespoons water
- 2 tablespoons freshly squeezed lemon juice
- 1 tablespoon tahini
- 1 tablespoon extra-virgin olive oil
- 1 teaspoon curry powder
- 1 teaspoon ground ginger
- 1/2 teaspoon sea salt

Place the currants in a small bowl of hot water to soak and plump up. Combine the chickpeas, water, lemon juice, tahini, olive oil, curry powder, ginger, and salt in a food processor and process until smooth. Transfer to a mixing bowl and do a FASS check. Add a spritz of lemon if it needs a little extra zing.

Before serving, drain the currants thoroughly and stir them into the hummus.

PREP TIME: 10 minutes · COOK TIME: Not applicable

STORAGE: Store in an airtight container in the refrigerator for 5 to 7 days.

PER SERVING: Calories: 180; Total Fat: 5.7 g (0.7 g saturated, 2.6 g monounsaturated); Carbohydrates: 27 g; Protein: 7 g; Fiber: 7 g; Sodium: 630 mg

REBECCA'S NOTES For a time-saving trick, buy a 16-ounce container of premade organic hummus at the market and add cury powder, ginger, lemon juice, and currants, as above. This is a wonderful way to spice up a store-bought snack.

Creamy Polenta

Polenta is the frequent flier of the cornmeal set. Just about anywhere there's an airport, you're likely to find some version of this staple. Hungarians call it puliszka, *the Turks call it* mamalika, *and us Americans—well, we just call it grits. Polenta is fabulous to work with because it morphs itself amiably into so many settings. I've seen it prepared with tomato sauce, different cheeses, various oils, garlicky greens, you name it. This version is somewhat similar to oatmeal (think thin oatmeal, not the stuff that doubles as wallpaper paste) using Magic Mineral Broth to add taste and nutritional value far beyond what you'd get with plain water.* SERVES 6

- 4 cups Magic Mineral Broth (page 54), Chicken Magic Mineral Broth (page 55), or store-bought organic stock
- 1/2 teaspoon sea salt
- Spritz of fresh lemon juice
- 1 cup polenta
- 2 tablespoons extra-virgin olive oil
- 1/4 cup grated organic Parmesan cheese (optional)

REBECCA'S NOTES For easy polenta cleanup, use cold water to clean the pan, as warm or hot water will make a sticky mush.

Bring the broth to a boil in a saucepan over high heat. Stir in the salt and lemon juice, then very slowly add the polenta in a steady stream, whisking all the while. Immediately decrease the heat to low, switch to a wooden spoon, and stir until smooth. Add the olive oil and stir constantly for about 15 minutes. Stir in the cheese and serve immediately.

Variations: Top your polenta with a serving of Emerald Greens with Orange (page 84), Signora's Tomato Sauce (page 88), simple poached eggs (see page 115), or Basil Lemon Drizzle (page 117).

You can also use Creamy Polenta for a breakfast cereal. Use water in place of the broth, omit the cheese, and add 1/2 teaspoon of maple syrup toward the end. Top with Blueberry Compote (page 185) and Maple-Glazed Walnuts (page 141).

Another variation is to make polenta rounds: Pour the polenta onto a sheet pan and allow it to cool and firm up. Once the polenta is firm, cut it into rounds using a cookie cutter or a glass. Try using polenta rounds instead of toast with a poached egg, or for a nosh with your favorite dollop.

PREP TIME: 5 minutes · COOK TIME: 15 minutes

STORAGE: Store in an airtight container in the refrigerator for 4 days. Polenta circles can be wrapped and frozen in a resealable plastic bag for 1 month.

PER SERVING: Calories: 190; Total Fat: 7 g (1.4 g saturated, 3.3 g monounsaturated); Carbohydrates: 28 g; Protein: 4 g; Fiber: 3 g; Sodium: 535 mg

Catherine's Magic Green Tea Rice

Green tea and rice, baked? At first glance, that may seem more like a ceramic project you'd put into a kiln and pray it comes out right. But look a little closer, and you'll see the insight of my brilliant colleague Catherine McConkie. We fiddled with this dish forever, and then Catherine suggested we bake it. That might seem strange, but baking rice is common in restaurants where large batches are made, and it guarantees perfect texture. It's a slightly longer process, but the baking completely neutralizes the green tea's sometimes astringent flavor, while allowing all of its wonderful nutrients to permeate the rice. SERVES 4

- 1 cup brown basmati rice
- Juice of 1/2 lemon
- 1 cup green tea (brewed for 10 minutes)
- 1 cup Magic Mineral Broth (page 54)
- 1/2 teaspoon sea salt
- 1/4 cup sliced scallions, green part only, cut thinly on a diagonal

WHO KNEW? Copper Calamaties When a well runs dry, it only makes sense to dig a new well if you're looking for life-sustaining water. Similarly, cancer tricks the body into constantly growing new blood vessels so it can have a continuous supply of energy. This process, called angiogenesis, is driven by enzymes that have one nutrient in common: copper. Drive copper levels down, says Dr. Jeanne Wallace, who specializes in cancer and nutrition, and you may slow cancer growth. Her advice? "You don't want to be cooking your food in copper kettles, wearing copper jewelry, taking supplements high in copper, or eating the foods that are elevated in copper, such as organ meats and shellfish." Don't worry about copper pennies; if they were made after 1982, they're really 97.5 percent zinc.

Place the rice in a pan or bowl with the lemon juice and water to cover and soak overnight, or for at least 8 hours.

Preheat the oven to 375°F.

Drain the rice in a fine-mesh sieve and rinse well under running cold water. Put the rice in a 2-quart casserole dish or other baking dish with a fitted lid. Pour the tea and broth over the rice, add the salt, and carefully stir. Cover and bake for 40 to 60 minutes, until the rice is tender and has absorbed all of the moisture. Fluff with a fork, then add the scallions and fluff again.

Variation: If you'd rather cook this dish on the stovetop, here's how: Bring the tea and broth to a boil in a saucepan, then stir in the rice and salt. Lower the heat, cover, and simmer for 25 minutes. Check the rice, and if there are steam holes in the top, it's ready; if not, cook for about 5 minutes more. Remove from the heat, fluff with a fork, then add the scallions and fluff again. This recipe also works well in a rice cooker; just add all of the ingredients and press the cook button.

PREP TIME: 10 minutes (after soaking the rice overnight)

COOK TIME: 40 minutes

STORAGE: Store in an airtight container in the refrigerator for 5 days, or in the freezer for 1 month.

PER SERVING: Calories: 175; Total Fat: 1.1 g (0 g saturated, 0 g monounsaturated); Carbohydrates: 36 g; Protein: 3 g; Fiber: 2 g; Sodium: 330 mg

Creamy Millet

The tall, stalk-like plants that millet comes from are lush, and in the field, the variety sometimes called broom corn millet resembles acre after acre of swaying pussy willows. Whole millet looks a lot like quinoa, and also like quinoa it's both gluten free and a great protein source. It cooks up plump and creamy in this recipe, and with the compote and almonds, it makes for a delightful breakfast or anytime pick-me-up. SERVES 4

- 2 cups freshly squeezed orange juice
- 1 cup water
- 1 cup millet, rinsed well
- 1/2 teaspoon sea salt
- 1/2 teaspoon ground cinnamon
- 1/2 teaspoon ground ginger
- 1/4 teaspoon ground cardamom
- 1/4 teaspoon allspice
- 3/4 cup almond milk (or substitute soy or rice milk)
- 1/4 teaspoon orange zest
- 1 tablespoon unrefined virgin coconut oil
- 1 tablespoon maple syrup
- Blueberry Compote (page 185), Dried Fruit Compote (page 183), or Seasonal Stewed Fruit (page 184), for serving
- 2 tablespoons toasted slivered almonds (see page 97), for serving

REBECCA'S NOTES To reheat the millet after storing in the refrigerator, place the millet and a small amount of almond milk in a saucepan over low heat until warm and creamy, stirring occasionally and breaking up any clumps with the edge of a spoon.

Bring the orange juice and water to a boil in a small saucepan, then stir in the millet, salt, cinnamon, ginger, cardamom, and allspice. Once it returns to a gentle boil, lower the heat, cover, and simmer for 25 minutes.

Pour in the almond milk and stir until incorporated, breaking up any clumps in the millet; the millet should be soft and have the consistency of oatmeal. Stir in the orange zest, coconut oil, and maple syrup.

Serve topped with the blueberry compote and almonds.

Variation: Add 1/2 cup dried cranberries and 1/4 cup unsweetened shredded coconut to the cooked millet.

PREP TIME: 5 minutes · COOK TIME: 30 minutes

STORAGE: Store in an airtight container in the refrigerator for 5 to 7 days.

PER SERVING: Calories: 355; Total Fat: 8.4 g (3.5 g saturated, 2.1 g monounsaturated); Carbohydrates: 64 g; Protein: 8 g; Fiber: 7 g; Sodium: 330 mg

WHO KNEW? Color Coordination When it comes to which fruits have the most antioxidants, integrative oncologist Donald Abrams says intensity of color is often a tip-off: "Among fruits, the heavily pigmented fruits, particularly berries, are rich in antioxidants and phytonutrients that are beneficial to all people, but especially to patients with cancer." As for concerns that eating antioxidants might interfere with treatments that depend upon creating oxidation to knock out cancer cells, Abrams says a little perspective is in order: "I say let's be realistic here. If it comes down to a blueberry versus that beam of radiation, I don't think there's a real chance that the blueberry is going to win." Meaning if you want a blueberry, nosh away.

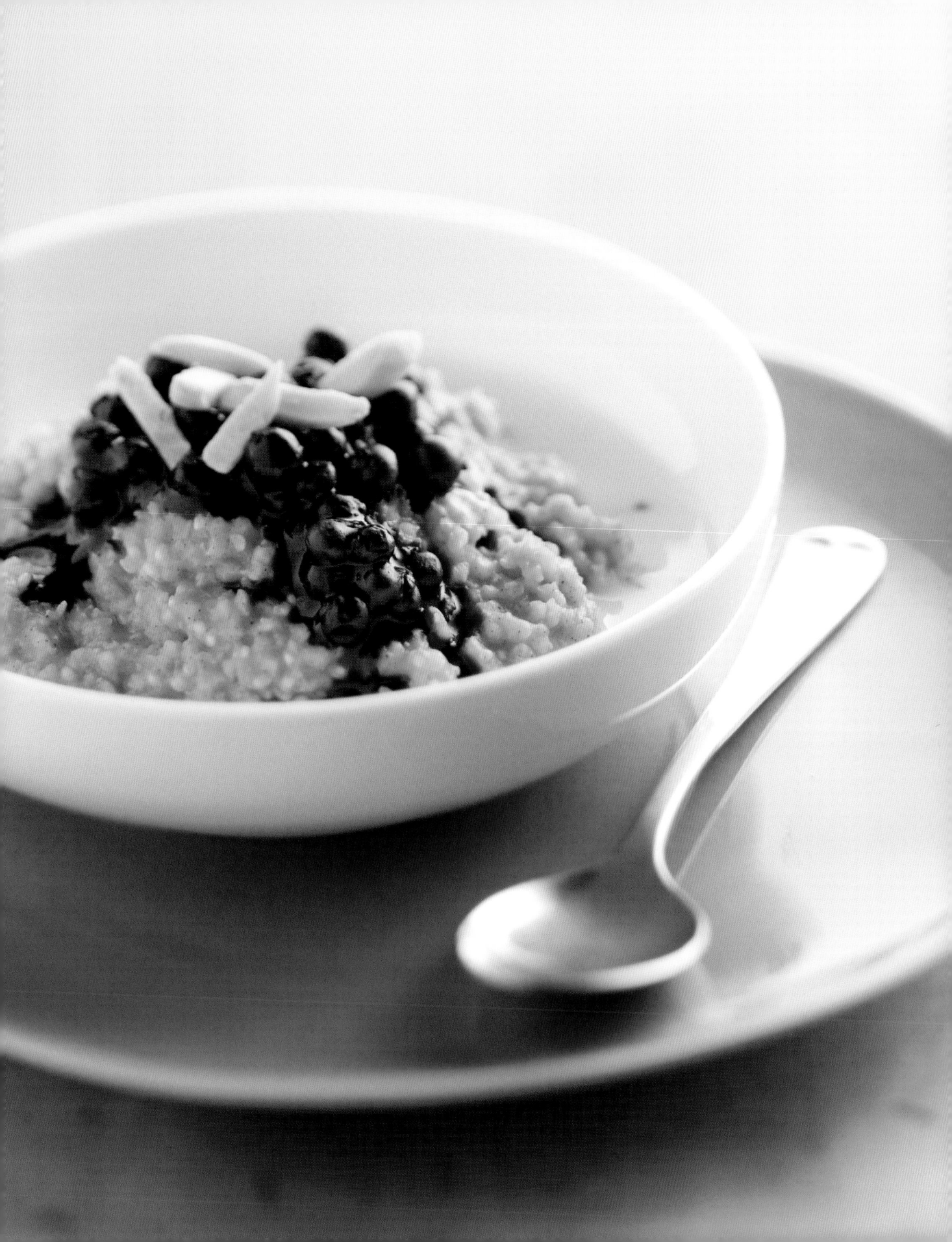

Creamiest Buckwheat

Some people prefer oatmeal, but I've always been a creamy buckwheat fan. It was my mom's go-to food when I didn't feel well as a kid, and ever since, its taste has sent me to a good place. Despite its name, buckwheat doesn't contain a shred of wheat—and it's gluten free. For people whose nutritional status is compromised, that can be really important, because gluten sensitivity can cause stomach problems and intestinal problems, including an inability to properly absorb much-needed nutrients. SERVES 6

- 4 cups water
- 1/4 teaspoon sea salt
- 1 cup cream of buckwheat cereal, rinsed
- 1/2 teaspoon ground ginger
- 1/4 teaspoon ground cinnamon
- 1/8 teaspoon ground cardamom
- Pinch of freshly grated nutmeg
- 1 teaspoon unrefined virgin coconut oil or organic butter
- 1 teaspoon maple syrup
- Dried Fruit Compote (page 183), Blueberry Compote (page 185), or Seasonal Stewed Fruit (page 184), for serving
- 2 tablespoons toasted sliced almonds (see page 97), for serving

Bring the water and salt to a boil in a saucepan, then slowly pour in the buckwheat while stirring constantly. Once it returns to a boil, lower the heat and simmer for 5 minutes, stirring frequently. Stir in the ginger, cinnamon, cardamom, nutmeg, and coconut oil and simmer for 3 minutes more, stirring often to prevent sticking. Serve topped with a few heaping tablespoons of fruit compote and the almonds.

Variations: For added flavor, consider replacing the water with milk, soy milk, rice milk, or almond milk. And if you're reheating the cereal, add enough milk to help "declump" the buckwheat and stir continuously over medium-low heat. It will restore the cereal's creamy consistency.

If you don't have any fruit compote on hand, add about 1/4 cup of dried fruit when you add the spices. Apricots and cranberries are good choices. The fruit will soften nicely during the remainder of the cooking process.

PREP TIME: 5 minutes · COOK TIME: 15 minutes

STORAGE: Store in a covered container in the refrigerator for 2 days.

PER SERVING: Calories: 370; Total Fat: 1.8 g (0.8 g saturated, 0.7 g monounsaturated); Carbohydrates: 77 g; Protein: 6 g; Fiber: 12 g; Sodium: 155 mg

"My appetite at times was pretty poor, so my approach was to eat a little bit every few hours, whether I was hungry or not."
—Betty L., renal cancer survivor

Spiced Toasted Almonds

Sometimes I think that if we could get cars to run off almonds, you wouldn't need more than a handful to go from San Francisco to L.A. Yeah, they have that much energy—twenty nuts are more than enough to get most people I know through a hunger rush—and they're nutrient dense, so the body can put every calorie to work. It's really easy to prep up a whole bunch of these; all it takes is a little olive oil, some seasoning, and a few minutes in the oven and they're ready to rock. I often tell my clients to leave little bowls of these around the house so they're constantly tempted to grab a healthy nibble. MAKES 2 CUPS

2 cups raw almonds
1 teaspoon extra-virgin olive oil
1/2 teaspoon maple syrup
1/4 teaspoon sea salt
1 teaspoon cinnamon
1/4 teaspoon ground ginger

REBECCA'S NOTES When in doubt, take them out! Nuts will continue to cook after they have been removed from the oven.

Preheat the oven to 350°F.

Toss the almonds with the olive oil, maple syrup, salt, cinnamon, and ginger until evenly coated, then spread them evenly on a sheet pan. Bake for 7 to 10 minutes, until aromatic and slightly browned. You know they're done when you can smell them. The almonds will become crispy as they cool.

Variations: While I was scuttling around the Commonweal Retreat Center's kitchen, I came up with the following mix of tasty morsels that everyone seemed to love. To 2 cups of toasted almonds, add 1 tablespoon of dark chocolate chips, 1/4 cup of dried cherries, and 1/4 cup of pumpkin seeds.

If you're looking for a more savory flavor, swap out the cinnamon and ginger for 1/4 teaspoon each of dried rosemary, sage, and thyme.

PREP TIME: 5 minutes · COOK TIME: 10 minutes

STORAGE: Store in an airtight container in the refrigerator for 2 weeks or in the freezer for 2 months.

PER SERVING: Calories: 105; Total Fat: 9.1 g (0.7 g saturated, 5.7 g monounsaturated); Carbohydrates: 4 g; Protein: 4 g; Fiber: 2 g; Sodium: 40 mg

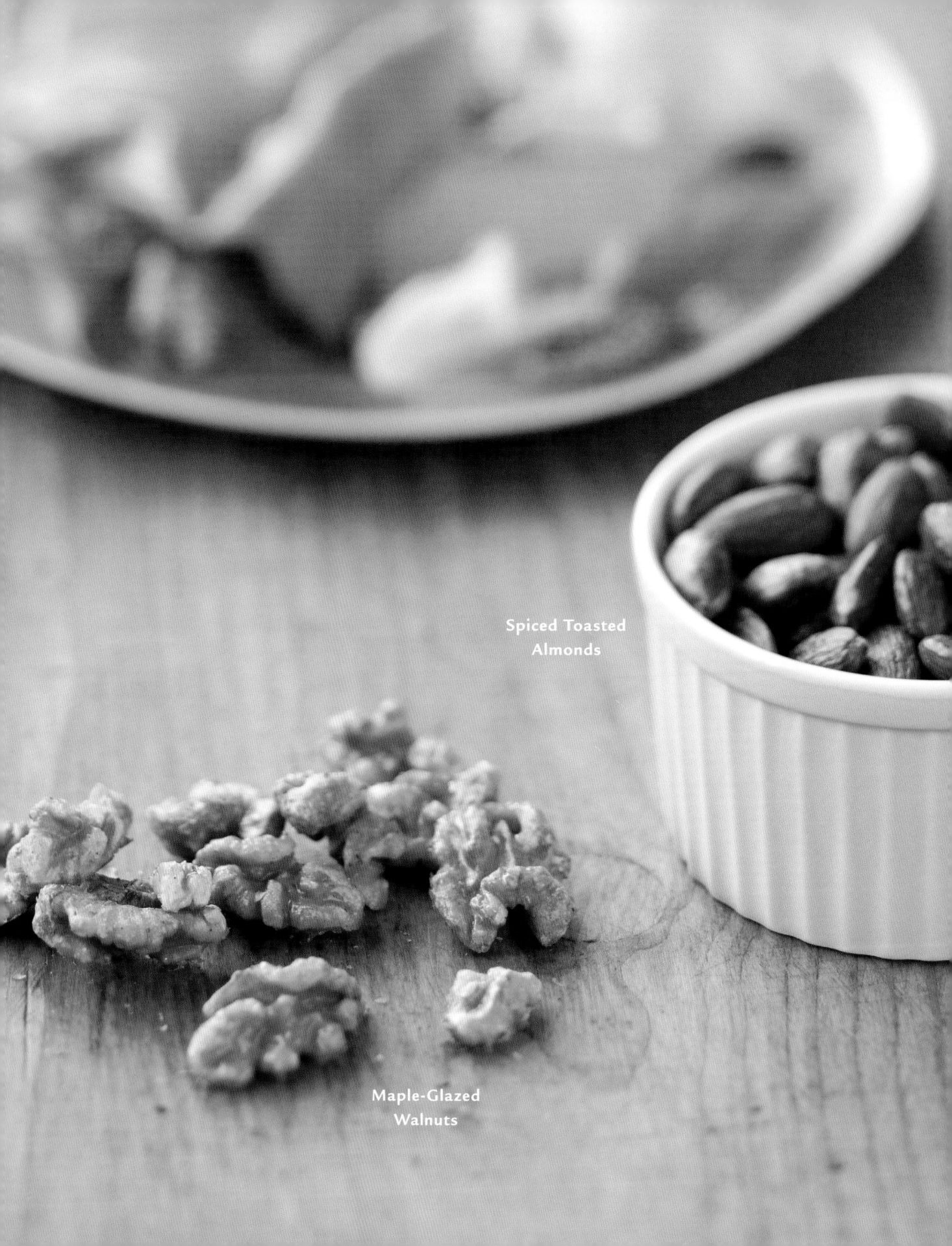
Spiced Toasted
Almonds
Maple-Glazed
Walnuts

Maple-Glazed Walnuts

In Celtic folklore, the walnut tree—and the nuts that fall from it—are associated with an unrelenting passion for all of life's challenges. Maybe that's why I'm so crazy for this treat. Or maybe it's just because I love crunchy maple treats. Someone laughingly said that these delicious nuts are like peanut brittle without the chewy toffee grout. All I know for sure is that this is a delight for those who gravitate toward crispy snacks. Plus, walnuts have so many nutritional benefits. In addition to being high in omega-3s, they're heart-healthy and may even help slow memory loss. So don't be shy about eating these straight up, or sprinkle them on cereal, salad, or anything you like for extra flavor and crunch. MAKES 1/2 CUP

1/2 cup raw walnuts
2 teaspoons maple syrup
Pinch of salt
Pinch of cayenne

Preheat the oven to 350°F and line a sheet pan with parchment paper.

Toss the walnuts with the maple syrup, salt, and cayenne until evenly coated, then spread them evenly on the sheet pan. Bake for 7 to 10 minutes, until aromatic and slightly browned. Let cool to room temperature, then use a metal spatula to loosen the nuts.

Variations: For an extra kick, add some ginger and 1/4 teaspoon of orange zest.

If you'd prefer a savory variation, substitute 1/4 teaspoon of olive oil for the maple syrup.

If you aren't a walnut fan, substitute 1/2 cup sliced almonds or pecans.

PREP TIME: 5 minutes · COOK TIME: 10 minutes

STORAGE: Store in an airtight container in the refrigerator for 2 weeks or in the freezer for 2 months.

PER SERVING: Calories: 90; Total Fat: 8.2 g (0.8 g saturated, 1.1 g monounsaturated); Carbohydrates: 4 g; Protein: 2 g; Fiber: 1 g; Sodium: 75 mg

Mediterranean Lentil Salad

I really should have called this Lentil Inside-Out Salad. Here's why: With most salads, you pour the dressing on at the end and coat the dish from the outside in. But in this salad, the lentils cool off in the fridge in a bath of dressing—in this case olive oil, vinegar, lemon, and cumin. They absorb all of this wonderful flavor, which is heightened by the addition of red bell pepper, kalamata olives, parsley, and mint. This Mediterranean delight is like a vacation to the island of Crete without leaving your home. Le Puy lentils are resilient little things that hold their shape well throughout the cooking process, making them perfect for a salad. SERVES 6

- 1 cup dried lentils, preferably Le Puy green lentils, rinsed well
- 1 clove garlic, peeled and smashed
- 1/4 teaspoon dried oregano
- 2 bay leaves
- 1 cinnamon stick, or 1/4 teaspoon ground cinnamon
- 1/4 cup extra-virgin olive oil
- 1 tablespoon brown rice vinegar
- 2 tablespoons freshly squeezed lemon juice
- 1 teaspoon lemon zest
- 1/2 teaspoon ground cumin
- 1/4 teaspoon sea salt
- 1 red bell pepper, seeded and diced small
- 1 small cucumber, seeded and diced small
- 1/4 cup pitted kalamata olives, rinsed and sliced
- 3 tablespoons chopped fresh mint
- 3 tablespoons chopped fresh flat-leaf parsley
- 2 ounces organic feta cheese, crumbled (optional)

Combine the lentils, garlic, oregano, bay leaf, and cinnamon stick in a saucepan and cover with water or broth by 2 inches. Bring to a boil, then cover, lower the heat, and simmer until the lentils are tender, 20 to 25 minutes. Drain the lentils thoroughly and discard the whole spices.

In a separate bowl, whisk the olive oil, vinegar, lemon juice, lemon zest, cumin, and salt together. Toss the lentils with the vinaigrette, then refrigerate for 20 minutes.

Stir in the bell pepper, cucumber, olives, mint, and parsley and combine, then do a FASS check—and season as needed with another pinch of salt, a few grinds of pepper, or lemon juice. Serve with the feta cheese sprinkled over the top.

PREP TIME: 10 minutes · COOK TIME: 25 minutes

STORAGE: Store in an airtight container in the refrigerator for 3 to 5 days.

PER SERVING: Calories: 210; Total Fat: 11.6 g (1.5 g saturated, 7.8 g monounsaturated); Carbohydrates: 21 g; Protein: 7 g; Fiber: 5 g; Sodium: 195 mg

WHO KNEW? Carpe Diem! For most people going through cancer—even those having a really rough time—there's generally a point between treatment sessions when you'll find yourself feeling a little more energetic and a little less blah. Michael Broffman, an acupuncturist who also utilizes herbs and foods to help numerous cancer patients at his Pine Street Clinic in Marin County, says these good days are a great opportunity for a culinary workout: "We encourage our patients to use those days to take the time to assess their cooking skills, cook something, get a recipe out of a book, start to play with it, go to cooking classes, and deepen their skill sets. That way, once treatment is over, they're well on their way to organizing this on a regular basis."

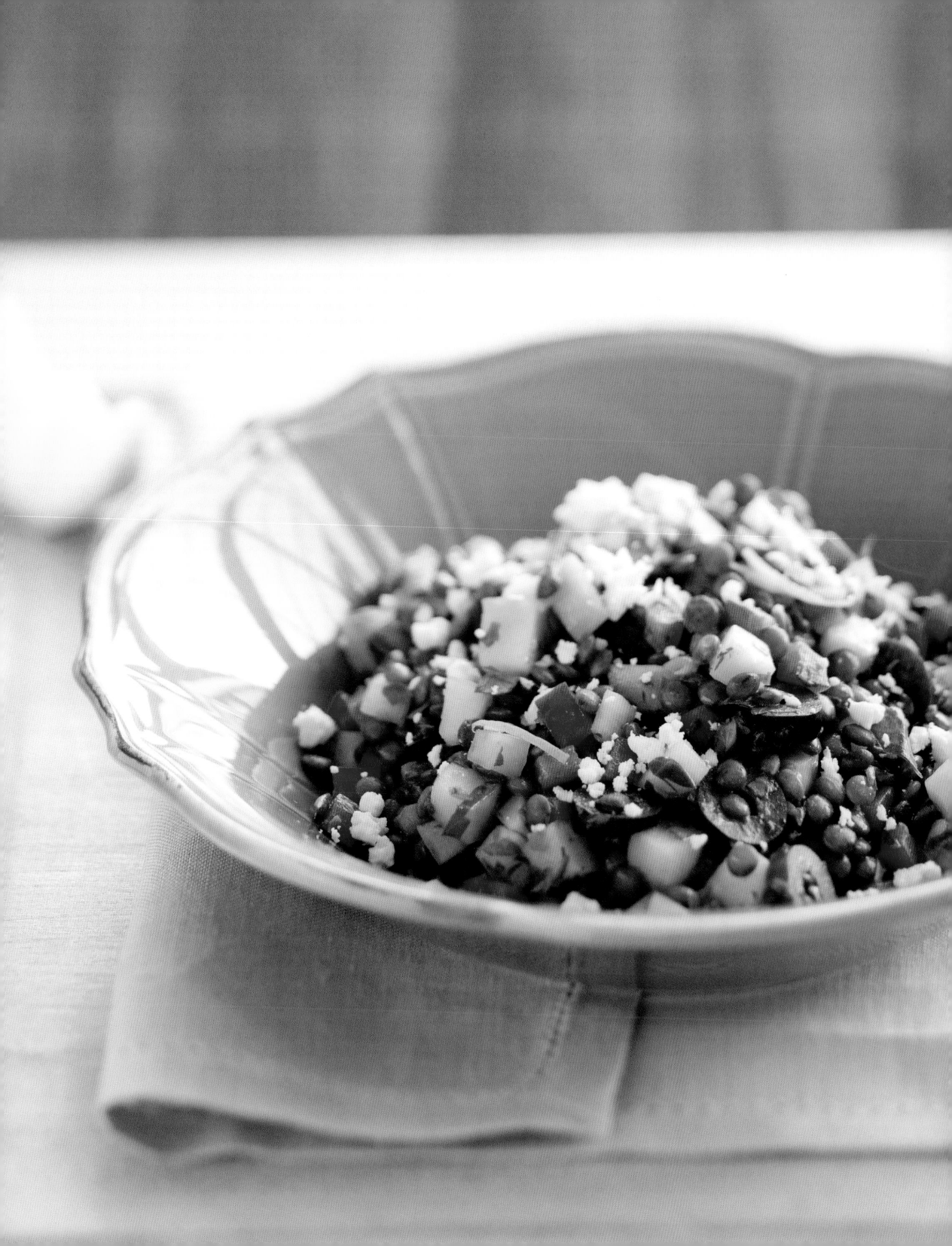

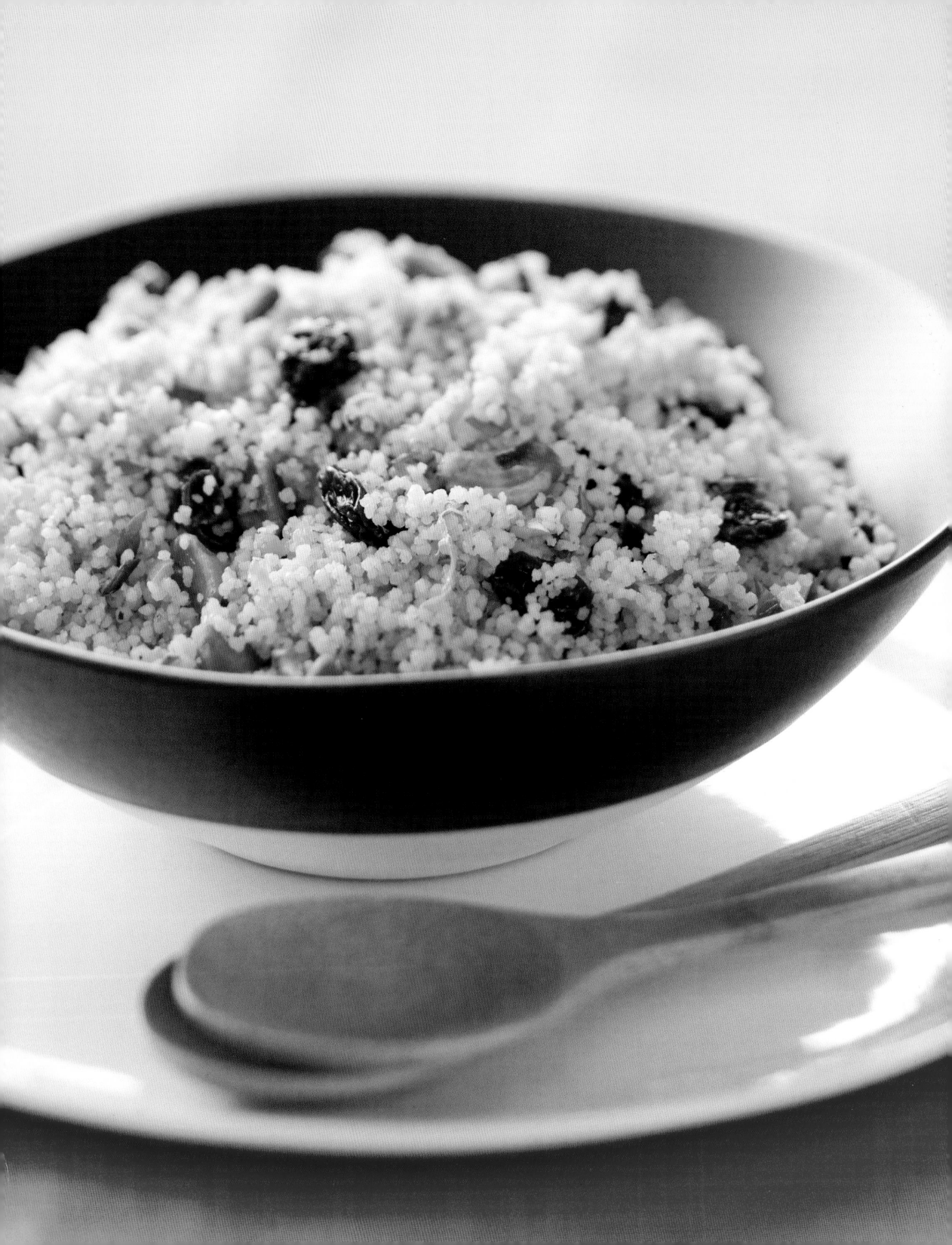

Orange Pistachio Couscous

Surprisingly, this couscous recipe has its origins in Italy. I was in Sicily, deep in the land of linguini, when out came couscous as part of our meal. "Couscous?" I thought. "That's Moroccan, not Italian." Well, it turns out that every invading army passing through Sicily left a bit of its cuisine behind. And couscous, despite the exotic name, is actually a tiny, beadlike pasta. I love it because it's easy to prepare—no huge pots of boiling water necessary, just a little steam or hot broth and, in 10 minutes, voila! It's also so soft and delicious in the mouth, like a gentle massage. Pistachios are my secret ingredient here. Most people think of them as something you only see at a ballgame or in ice cream, but their buttery texture, great vitamin content, and wonderful pale green coloring make them a great choice anytime. I love to put a dollop of Sweet and Savory Yogurt (page 189) on top of this dish. This recipe works beautifully with a drizzle of Moroccan Pesto (page 186). SERVES 6

- 1/4 cup shelled pistachios
- 1 1/2 cups whole wheat couscous, rinsed in cold water
- 1 1/2 cups boiling Magic Mineral Broth (page 54) or water
- 1 teaspoon ground cumin
- 1/2 teaspoon ground coriander
- 1 teaspoon sea salt
- 1/8 teaspoon freshly ground pepper
- 1/2 cup chopped fresh mint
- 2 scallions, white and green parts, finely chopped
- 2 tablespoons freshly squeezed lemon juice
- 2 tablespoons freshly squeezed orange juice
- 1 tablespoon orange zest
- 2 tablespoons extra-virgin olive oil
- 1/2 cup raisins

Preheat the oven to 325°F.

Spread the pistachios in an even layer on a sheet pan and bake for 7 to 10 minutes, until aromatic and slightly browned. Let cool.

Meanwhile, combine the couscous and boiling broth in a bowl, cover tightly with plastic wrap, and let sit for about 5 minutes, until the liquid is absorbed. Add the cumin, coriander, salt, and pepper and stir and fluff with a fork. Spread the couscous on a sheet pan, rake with a fork, and let cool to room temperature.

Combine the couscous, mint, scallions, lemon juice, orange juice, orange zest, olive oil, raisins, and pistachios and mix well, then do a FASS check. You may need to add a pinch or two of salt, a squeeze of lemon, or a dash of olive oil to balance the flavors.

Variation: Make this a meal in a bowl by adding 1 cup of cooked chickpeas when you stir everything together.

PREP TIME: 15 minutes · COOK TIME: 10 minutes

STORAGE: Store in an airtight container in the refrigerator for 4 days.

PER SERVING: Calories: 265; Total Fat: 10.3 g (1.3 g saturated, 5.9 g monounsaturated); Carbohydrates: 40 g; Protein: 7 g; Fiber: 6 g; Sodium: 435 mg

REBECCA'S NOTES This dish benefits from being made ahead of time. The flavor deepens as it sits.

Roasted Asparagus Pasta with White Beans and Thyme

This may come as a shock, but in Italy, pasta isn't a main dish. In fact, the average Italian meal consists of small portions of several dishes, pasta among them. In addition, pasta is usually served with sauce only, never with veggies, which are served on their own, usually later in the meal, so this combination is more what I'd call Cal-Italian. The roasted asparagus is soft and sweet and blends deliciously with the creamy cannellini beans and a healthy but not overwhelming amount of pasta. Peeling the asparagus gets rid of the stringy, sometimes tough outer layer to expose the sweet flesh underneath. Buon appetito! SERVES 6

- 1 bunch asparagus, peeled and cut diagonally into 1-inch pieces
- 2 tablespoons extra-virgin olive oil
- Sea salt
- 12 ounces penne or bowtie pasta
- 1/2 cup diced red onion
- 1 1/2 tablespoons finely chopped garlic
- Pinch of red pepper flakes
- 1 cup cooked cannellini or navy beans (see page 110)
- 1 1/2 tablespoons freshly squeezed lemon juice
- 1 tablespoon lemon zest
- 1 teaspoon fresh thyme, or 1/2 teaspoon dried
- 1/4 cup Basil Lemon Drizzle (page 177; optional)
- 1/4 cup grated organic Parmesan cheese (optional)

Preheat the oven to 400°F.

Spread the asparagus on a sheet pan, drizzle with 1 tablespoon of the olive oil, and sprinkle on 1/4 teaspoon of salt. Roast for 8 minutes (less if the asparagus is thin), shaking the sheet pan to turn the asparagus once during roasting.

Bring 4 quarts of water to a boil, then add 1/2 teaspoon of salt and the pasta and cook until al dente, checking it after 6 minutes. Drain, reserving 1/2 cup of the pasta water.

Meanwhile, heat the remaining 1 tablespoon olive oil in a large sauté pan over medium heat, then add the onion and a pinch of salt and sauté until translucent, about 4 minutes. Add the garlic and red pepper flakes, sauté for 30 seconds, then pour in 1/4 cup of the reserved pasta water to deglaze the pan.

Stir in the pasta and the remaining 1/4 cup pasta water, then add the asparagus, beans, lemon juice, lemon zest, and thyme and stir until well coated. Stir in the Basil Lemon Drizzle, the cheese, a pinch of salt, and a spritz of lemon juice and serve immediately.

Variations: For a little extra protein, add about 1 cup of diced cooked chicken. My Family's Favorite Chicken (page 111) would be a great choice.

To sneak in a serving of dark leafy greens, stir in 2 cups of chopped arugula or spinach at the very end.

"What got me through treatment was changing to a plant-based diet with a focus on fresh fruit, bean salads, and pastas."
—Laila O., ovarian cancer survivor

PREP TIME: 10 minutes · COOK TIME: 22 minutes

STORAGE: Store in an airtight container in the refrigerator for 4 days.

PER SERVING: Calories: 330; Total Fat: 5.8 g (0.7 g saturated, 3.3 g monounsaturated); Carbohydrates: 57 g; Protein: 13 g; Fiber: 6 g; Sodium: 315 mg

REBECCA'S NOTES If you're sensitive to gluten, or even if you aren't, try Tinkyada brand brown rice penne. It cooks in 12 minutes and remains al dente, which is *vero Italiano*. If you use other brands of brown rice pasta, be careful not to overcook them or they will turn mushy and fall apart. Also, unlike regular pasta, all brands of brown rice pasta need to be rinsed after cooking.

You can certainly substitute canned beans in this recipe. Use about half of a 15-ounce can and, as usual, drain and rinse, then refresh the beans with a spritz of lemon juice and a pinch of sea salt.

Forbidden Rice Salad

This recipe is like one of those beautiful American heritage quilts where every colorful swatch—or in this case ingredient—has a wonderful backstory. Forbidden rice, also called emperor's rice, got its name not because of any aristocratic connections, but rather because its deep purple hue is reminiscent of a royal cloak. As with many grains and vegetables, the rich color of forbidden rice signifies a high level of antioxidants and phytochemicals. Star anise also has anticancer properties, along with a delightful name and a light licorice flavor that's immensely appealing. This recipe calls for soaking the rice overnight, so plan ahead. SERVES 4

- 2 cups hot water
- 2 1/2-inch slices rinsed and unpeeled fresh ginger, plus 1 teaspoon minced fresh ginger
- 2 pods star anise
- Sea salt
- 1 cup forbidden rice, soaked overnight in water
- 1 tablespoon freshly squeezed lime juice
- 1 tablespoon brown rice vinegar
- 1 teaspoon mirin
- 2 tablespoons finely chopped fresh cilantro, basil, or mint
- 2 tablespoons finely diced red bell pepper

Bring the hot water, sliced ginger, star anise, and 1/4 teaspoon of salt to a boil, then stir in the rice. Cover, lower the heat, and simmer for 30 minutes, then check to see if the rice is tender.

Whisk the lime juice, rice vinegar, mirin, minced ginger, and a pinch of salt together in a mixing bowl. Add the rice and toss to combine, then stir in the cilantro and bell pepper. Serve immediately.

PREP TIME: 5 minutes (after soaking the rice overnight)

COOK TIME: 35 minutes

STORAGE: Store in an airtight container in the refrigerator for 5 to 7 days.

PER SERVING: Calories: 185; Total Fat: 1.9 g (0.5 g saturated, 0.6 g monounsaturated); Carbohydrates: 40 g; Protein: 5 g; Fiber: 4 g; Sodium: 150 mg

Simple Tuscan Farro

If you believe the ancients had something on us, you'll like farro; it's been found in archaeological digs dating back nearly twenty thousand years and was the staple that kept the Roman legions on the move. What I like about farro is that it's a whole grain, which makes it nutritionally superior to its distant relatives the refined white wheat set. Some people who are sensitive to wheat can tolerate farro because it is lower in gluten. SERVES 6

- 2 cups farro
- 6 cups water
- Juice of 1 lemon
- 6 cups Magic Mineral Broth (page 54) or water
- Sea salt
- 2 teaspoons extra-virgin olive oil
- 1 tablespoon freshly squeezed lemon juice

Place the farro in a pan or bowl with the water and juice of 1 lemon and let soak overnight, or for at least 8 hours.

Drain and rinse the farro. Bring the broth and a pinch of salt to a boil in a large saucepan, add the farro, and return to a boil. Lower the heat, cover, and simmer for 20 to 30 minutes, until tender. If there's any excess liquid, drain it off, then stir in the olive oil and 1 tablespoon of lemon juice.

PREP TIME: 5 minutes (after soaking the farro overnight)

COOK TIME: 30 minutes

STORAGE: Store in a covered container in the refrigerator for 2 days or in the freezer for 2 months.

PER SERVING: Calories: 275; Total Fat: 1.7 g (0.3 g saturated, 1.1 g monounsaturated); Carbohydrates: 56 g; Protein: 11 g; Fiber: 6 g; Sodium: 230 mg

REBECCA'S NOTES Farro is a drainable grain, so don't sweat the amount of liquid used to cook it. The texture of cooked farro is like barley, so when you taste for doneness know that you can always drain out extra water if it is finished cooking.

This is an excellent grain to freeze. Save any leftover farro in an airtight container in the freezer and use it as a creative addition to the next soup you make.

Quinoa Pilaf

Quinoa (pronounced "KEEN-wa") is its own little ecosystem, containing all of the essential amino acids that we must obtain through the diet. Put another way, quinoa brings some good nutrients to the table that the body needs to begin repairing itself. Its mild taste makes it a perfect starting point for building a pilaf, which is a Middle Eastern food fest. Pilafs are by definition seasoned dishes, and in this case all of the aromatics have great anticancer properties. About the only thing missing from this exotic, exciting dish is a belly dancer. If only I hadn't misplaced those tiny finger cymbals . . . SERVES 4

- 1 tablespoon extra-virgin olive oil
- 2 tablespoons finely diced shallot
- 1 fennel bulb, diced small
- 1 carrot, peeled and diced small
- Sea salt
- 1 cup quinoa, rinsed
- 1/2 teaspoon turmeric
- 1/4 teaspoon ground cinnamon
- 1/4 teaspoon ground cumin
- 1/4 teaspoon ground ginger
- 1/8 teaspoon ground cardamom
- 1 3/4 cups Magic Mineral Broth (page 54)
- 1/4 cup chopped fresh parsley or mint

Heat the olive oil in a saucepan over medium heat, then add the shallot, fennel, carrot, and a pinch of salt and sauté for about 3 minutes, until the vegetables start to sweat. Stir in the quinoa, turmeric, cinnamon, cumin, ginger, and cardamom, then stir in the broth and 1/2 teaspoon of salt and bring to a boil. Lower the heat, cover, and simmer for about 20 minutes, until the liquid has been absorbed and the quinoa is tender.

Remove from the heat and fluff with a fork, then add the parsley and fluff again. Do a FASS check and add a spritz of lemon juice to amp up the flavor if needed.

PREP TIME: 10 minutes · COOK TIME: 25 minutes

STORAGE: Store in an airtight container in the refrigerator for 3 days.

PER SERVING: Calories: 270; Total Fat: 9.9 g (1.3 g saturated, 5.7 g monounsaturated); Carbohydrates: 39 g; Protein: 8 g; Fiber: 6 g; Sodium: 180 mg

REBECCA'S NOTES Rinse, rinse, and rinse again! Quinoa is naturally coated with a bitter-tasting resin. To get rid of the resin, put the grain in a bowl of cool water, swish it around with your hand, then drain it in a fine-mesh sieve.

Quinoa is gluten free, which makes sense when you consider that botanically, it isn't a grain at all; it's more closely related to beets. It makes a great replacement for couscous in Orange Pistachio Couscous (page 145). It's also a great hot cereal; try it in place of oats in Best Oatmeal Ever (page 128).

WHO KNEW? Chemo and Carbs and Diabetes Risk By now, most of us know that chemo can cause muscle loss. But it can also lead to diabetes if you're not careful. Less muscle mass is a double whammy: You burn less sugar than with normal muscle levels, and you also store less sugar, in the form of glycogen, in those muscles, meaning all that unused consumed sugar stays in your body (usually in the liver, blood, and kidneys), elevating overall blood sugar levels and forcing you to use more insulin.

Dr. Jeanne Wallace says that on top of that, "when you're given chemo, you're often given a steroid that really increases the glycemic response," creating the type of blood sugar spikes and insulin surges that can predispose people to diabetes. Wallace's suggestion? While you're in treatment, forget the USDA food pyramid. It suggests 6 to 11 servings of carbs per day. You want to eat fewer carbs, so shoot for half of that if not less. When you do eat carbs, avoid refined white flour and sugar and stick with whole grains, as their higher fiber content slows the release of their sugars into the body. This may have direct anticancer benefits too, as some studies have shown that lowering blood sugar levels in animals suppressed tumor growth.

Rice Paper Moo-Shu Rolls

One of my favorite ways of getting people to enjoy eating veggies is to wrap them in rice paper rolls. If you've ever supped on Vietnamese spring rolls, you're probably familiar with these delightful translucent silky casings that hug veggies tight as a drum. They can be found in any Asian market or the Asian section of most grocery stores. The trick to working with rice paper is all in the water. In the package they look delicate, like round sheets of frosted glass, but slip them into warm water for about twenty seconds and they become soft and pliable. Put them back on the counter, add the ingredients, and wrap them just as you would a small burrito. It may take two or three tries, but I promise you'll get the knack (I've even taught the technique to kids). The result will be veggie heaven, as the rolls are easy to swallow and digest. SERVES 6

- 6 8-inch rice paper rounds
- 2 tablespoons Edamame Avocado Dip with Wasabi (page 131)
- 1 1/2 cups Warm Napa Cabbage Slaw (page 92)
- 1 1/2 cups roasted organic chicken, shredded
- 12 fresh mint leaves

REBECCA'S NOTES When you take these to go, leave them whole and wrap tightly in wax paper. Eat right away or cut when you are ready to eat!

Fill a large, shallow bowl with warm water. Soak 1 rice paper round at a time in the water until pliable, generally 30 to 60 seconds, depending on water temperature and the rice paper. Place the softened rice paper on a work surface and carefully spread 1 teaspoon of the edamame dip on the bottom third of the rice paper, leaving 2 1/2 inches between the dip and the edges of the paper. Place 1/4 cup of the slaw on top of the dip and 1/4 cup of the shredded chicken on top of the slaw, then lay 2 mint leaves over the filling. Fold the right and left sides of the paper in—over the filling, compressing the filling slightly. Fold the bottom edge up and over the filling, then tightly roll the entire thing away from your body, pressing gently to make a compact roll.

Moisten your finger with warm water and run it along the inside edge of the flap that remains at the top of the roll, then press the moistened edge against the roll to seal. Repeat with the remaining ingredients. Cut the rolls in half on the diagonal with a sharp knife before serving.

PREP TIME: 10 minutes · COOK TIME: Not applicable

STORAGE: Store in a covered container in the refrigerator for 3 days.

PER SERVING: Calories: 140; Total Fat: 4.7 g (1 g saturated, 1.8 g monounsaturated); Carbohydrates: 11 g; Protein: 12 g; Fiber: 1 g; Sodium: 250 mg

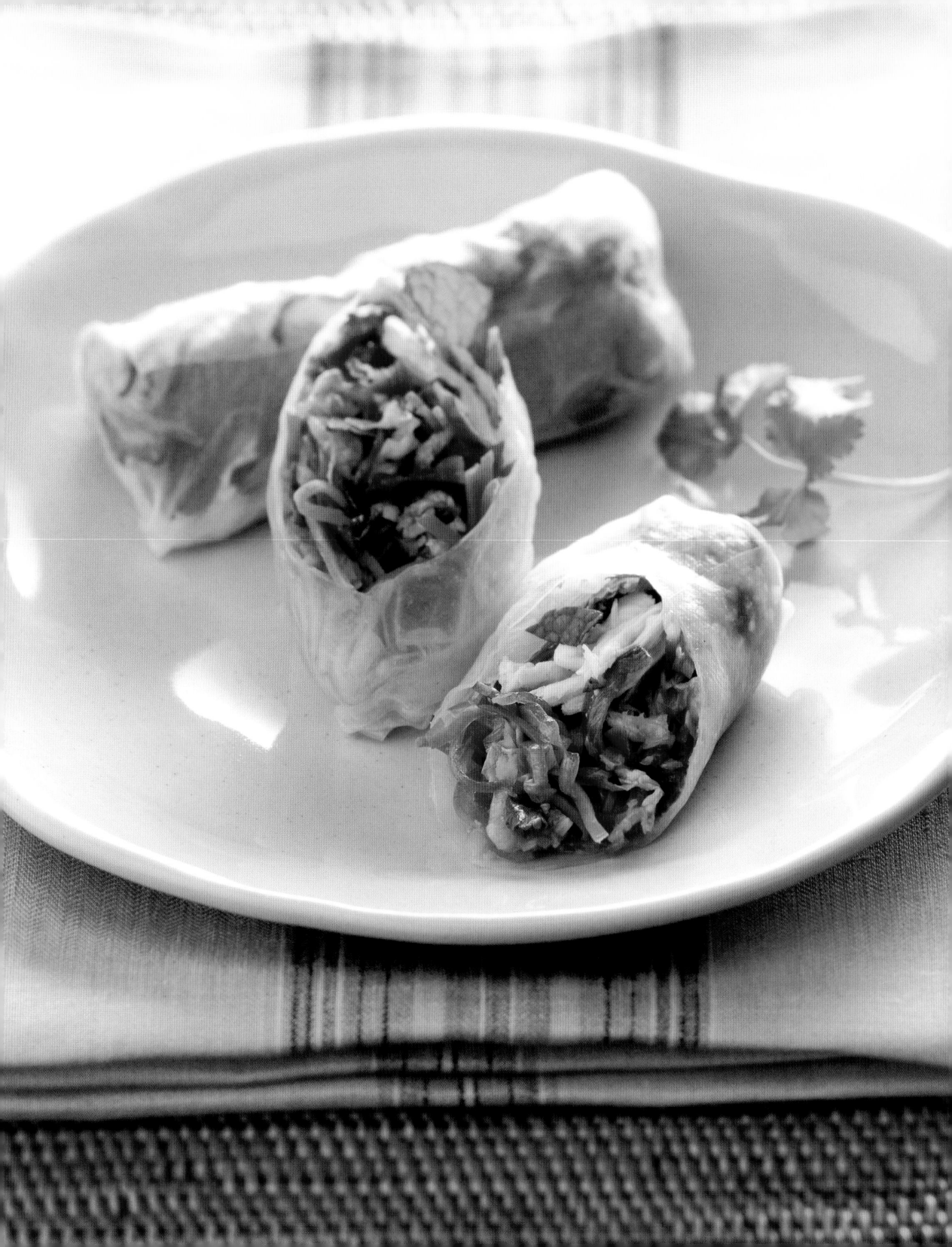

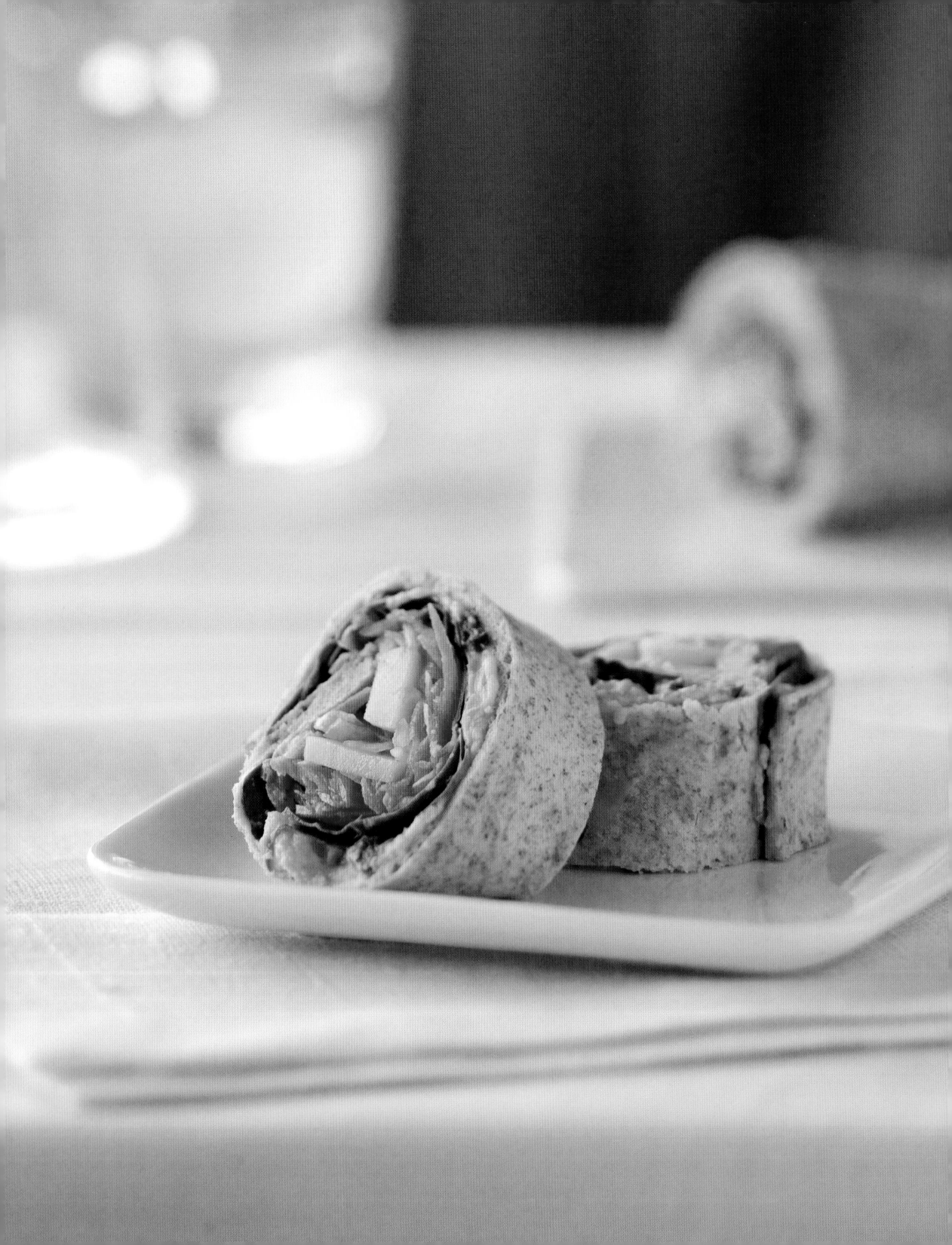

Curried Hummus and Vegetable Pinwheels

These wraps are a quick, healthy pick-me-up. When people ask me "Why curried hummus?" I always answer "Why not?" Curry is one of my favorite spices to use, and doubly so if I'm working with folks dealing with cancer. Turmeric and its subcomponent, curcumin, are common curry ingredients that have tumor-inhibiting and appetite-stimulating properties. Here I'm using hummus to transport the curry because it's a great canvas that blends well with spices and veggies. The pinwheel turns this into a simple finger food, easy to prep, grab, and go. And if you're wondering why I added mango, just take a bite. And another. And another . . . SERVES 4

- 4 8-inch spelt or whole wheat tortillas
- 1 cup Curried Hummus (page 133)
- 2 cups baby spinach, washed and dried
- 3/4 cup peeled and shredded carrot
- 3/4 cup peeled, seeded, and grated cucumber
- 1/2 cup thinly sliced mango (optional)

Place a tortilla on a flat work surface. Spread 1/4 cup of the hummus over the tortilla, leaving a 3/4-inch border all the way around. Lay one-fourth of the spinach, carrot, cucumber, and mango over the hummus, then roll up into a tube, sushi style. Glue down the top edge with a smear of hummus. Trim the ends, then slice the roll in half on the diagonal or, alternatively, cut crosswise into 1-inch pinwheels. Repeat with the remaining ingredients.

PREP TIME: 10 minutes · COOK TIME: Not applicable

STORAGE: Store in a covered container in the refrigerator for 3 days.

PER SERVING: Calories: 340; Total Fat: 8.8 g (0.8 g saturated, 2.6 g monounsaturated); Carbohydrates: 53 g; Protein: 12 g; Fiber: 10 g; Sodium: 835 mg

CHAPTER 7

Tonics and Elixirs

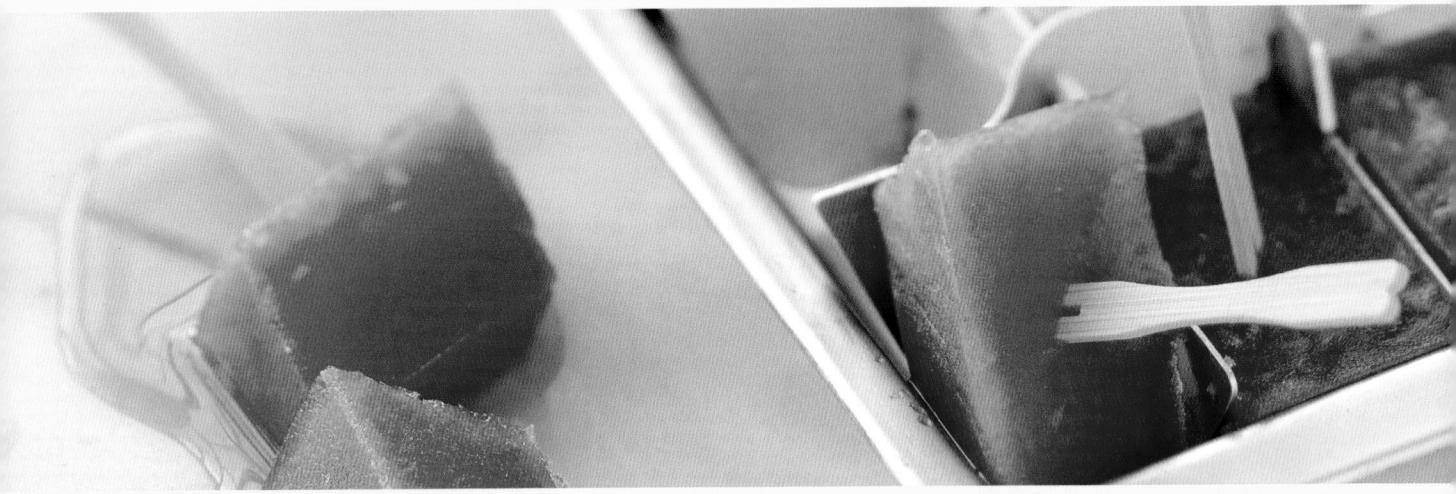

156 *Annemarie's Calming Kudzu Elixir*

157 *Commonweal's Most Nourishing and Healing Tea*

158 *Cantaloupe Granita with Mint*

161 *Mouthwatering Watermelon Granita*

162 *Ginger Peppermint Green Tea*

162 *Green Tea Ginger Lemonade*

163 *Cinnamon Ginger Tea*

163 *Ginger Tea Spritzer*

164 *Ginger Ale with Frozen Grapes*

166 *Chocolate Banana Smoothie*

167 *Mango Coconut Smoothie*

169 *Peach Ginger Smoothie*

169 *Triple Berry Smoothie*

170 *Pineapple Ginger Smoothie*

171 *Papaya Pineapple Smoothie*

There's something about reaching for a cold one that just works, yes? Whether you're playing softball, sitting on a sun-drenched porch, or coming in from working in the garden, a tall, ice-filled glass of a favorite beverage is guaranteed to slake your thirst and put a smile on your face. And, of course, the same goes for a mug of steaming liquid love on a frosty day. Pop a cinnamon stick in that tea, cider, or hot chocolate and you're halfway to a happy nap.

A choice libation is always emotionally satisfying, but it can be a real lifeline for people dealing with the head, neck, and mouth issues particular to certain cancers and treatments. I saw this firsthand with my father, as he battled and beat throat cancer. The radiation treatments left his throat so sore that he really couldn't eat. The only way for him to get nutrition was through the various smoothies that soothed his pain while delivering vital nutrients to his body.

The smoothie recipes in this chapter are great for getting delicious nourishment where it needs to go. Their coolness and creaminess make them fantastic for anyone dealing with mouth sores or swallowing issues due to radiation or surgery. They're all nutrient dense, so anyone having a tough time with tummy problems or weight loss can get a lot of benefit from just a few sips. And they all taste wonderful, which isn't always easy to accomplish when you're including ground flaxseeds or whey powder, as many nutritionists recommend. And if your doctor has suggested that you avoid cold drinks, fret not; all of these recipes can also be enjoyed at room temperature. For those suffering from mouth sores, I'd suggest the Peach Ginger Smoothie (page 169; omit the ginger) and Chocolate Banana Smoothie (page 166), as they have little or no acid to cause irritation.

While people with swallowing issues can greatly benefit from the smoothies, everyone in treatment will benefit from drinking more beverages, and with all of the different recipes in this chapter, you should find something you like. Getting enough to drink is important for several reasons. Dehydration is a common but often hard-to-detect side effect of treatment. By the time you feel symptoms of serious dehydration—dizziness, nausea, cramps, impaired thinking—you could be heading for a trip to the hospital. Most folks think drinking water is enough to stay hydrated. Not necessarily. Water without added electrolytes and minerals can pass right through the body, in the process taking much-needed nutrients right out of the bloodstream. Also, anyone who is dealing with a metallic taste in their mouth is likely to find tap water extremely unpalatable. If you've ever tasted distilled water, you'll know what I mean.

Staying hydrated with the tonics and elixirs in this chapter can also lessen nausea, replenish nutrients lost because of diarrhea, and counteract the constipating effects of pain medications, especially opiates. Of course, they're also refreshing in the extreme and contain many anticancer spices, herbs, and fruits.

Now that's worthy of a toast!

Annemarie's Calming Kudzu Elixir

My mentor, Annemarie Colbin, is both a pioneer in the field of nutrition and healing and an extremely generous woman. The founder of the cooking school I attended, the Natural Gourmet Institute for Health and Culinary Arts, Annemarie has a PhD in nutrition and is the author of Food and Healing, *considered a bible among chefs who believe in using food to support health. She's graciously allowed me to use this recipe from that book; it's a stress-relieving elixir that's a calmative in a cup. The only thing I've done is add a little ginger and cinnamon. For those days when you need a hug pronto and there's no one around to soothe your nerves, this kudzu concoction will do the trick.* MAKES 1 CUP

- 1 1/2 tablespoons kudzu root powder
- 1 cup cold, unfiltered apple juice
- 1/8 teaspoon grated fresh ginger (optional)
- 1 teaspoon vanilla extract
- 1/4 teaspoon ground cinnamon

WHO KNEW? Kudzu for an Upset Tummy While there are many good medications available to control nausea and stomach problems, folks always are asking me about nutritional options. I threw the question to Dr. Keith Block, and he suggested kudzu. In fact, Keith said, "I find kudzu better than most antidiarrheal medications in terms of binding a patient's bowels when they have loose stools." Hey, anything that keeps you from wearing out the carpet between the bed and the bathroom is worth a try.

In a small pot, mix the kudzu into the cold apple juice, stirring until dissolved. Stir in the ginger, vanilla, and cinnamon and bring to a boil over medium-low heat, stirring constantly until the liquid thickens and becomes translucent. Serve hot or cold.

Variations: For a cozy and soothing pudding, follow Annemarie's original recipe, leaving out the ginger and cinnamon, and increase the amount of kudzu to 2 tablespoons.

For a more nutrient-dense pudding, swirl 1 tablespoon of tahini into the mixture as soon as it thickens.

PREP TIME: 3 minutes · COOK TIME: 5 minutes

STORAGE: Drink immediately!

PER SERVING: Calories: 170; Total Fat: 0 g (0 g saturated, 0 g monounsaturated); Carbohydrates: 39 g; Protein: 0 g; Fiber: 0 g; Sodium: 30 mg

CULINARY RX Regarding kudzu, Annemarie says, "I was looking for ways to make puddings that didn't require milk or eggs. I turned to kudzu, which was being used in macrobiotic circles as a remedy for digestive disorders. It thickens the same way as cornstarch does—by being dissolved in a cold liquid and then heated while stirring. I loved my hot peanut apple kudzu breakfast pudding. After a few days of eating it, I began to realize I was feeling exceedingly mellow. My desire to argue seemed to vanish. I slept really deeply. Soon enough, I thought, 'This is a great stress-reducer!' Eventually I put it in my book *Food and Healing*, and in my classes on kitchen pharmacy. Everybody who had it in class got very relaxed. It's also great for calming down kids. So I will take credit for discovering this wonderful natural remedy that tastes like dessert, and hope many people learn to enjoy it!"

Commonweal's Most Nourishing and Healing Tea

You may have heard the slogan "You've tried the rest; now try the best." That's the way I feel about this tea recipe. It was developed ages ago by the fantastic folk at the Commonweal Cancer Help Program, a renowned retreat for patients and caregivers, and they've been very kind in allowing me to share their recipe with you. When I am cooking at commonweal, I often make about six quarts a day so I'll have some on hand for anyone who comes through the door, and still, it's never enough. The blend of ginger, cloves, cinnamon, and cardamom is like a backrub in a cup. It turns me into absolute mush, it's so good.

MAKES 8 CUPS

- 1/3 cup sliced peeled fresh ginger, cut 1/4 inch thick
- 10 cups water
- 3 tablespoons coriander seeds
- 1 1/2 tablespoons cardamom pods
- 4 cinnamon sticks
- 5 whole cloves
- 1 1/2 cups rice milk or almond milk
- 1 to 3 tablespoons maple syrup
- 1 teaspoon vanilla extract

Combine the ginger and water in a saucepan, and bring to a boil. Lower the heat, cover, and simmer for 30 minutes.

Add the coriander, cardamom, cinnamon, and cloves and continue to simmer for an additional 20 minutes.

Strain the tea through a fine-mesh sieve into a clean saucepan. (I recommend that you save the spices; see Rebecca's Notes.) Add the rice milk and maple syrup and gently reheat without boiling for 2 to 3 minutes, until warm. Stir in the vanilla, then taste. Add more milk or sweetener if you like. Serve hot or cold.

PREP TIME: 5 minutes · COOK TIME: 55 minutes

STORAGE: Store in an airtight container in the refrigerator for 1 week.

PER SERVING: Calories: 40; Total Fat: 0.9 g (0 g saturated, 0.6 g monounsaturated); Carbohydrates: 8 g; Protein: 0 g; Fiber: 1 g; Sodium: 15 mg g

REBECCA'S NOTES The tea will keep in the refrigerator for up to 2 weeks without the milk and sweetener, so you may want to set some aside prior to adding the milk and sweetener.

Recycle the spices that are strained out of the tea and use them to make another, smaller batch of tea. They'll keep in the refrigerator for 4 to 5 days. To make more tea, combine the spices and 6 cups of water and bring to a boil. Add 2 tablespoons of peeled fresh ginger slices. Simmer for 30 minutes, then strain the tea and discard the spices. Add sweetener and milk to taste and reheat without boiling for 2 to 3 minutes. Remove from the heat and stir in the vanilla before serving.

Cantaloupe Granita with Mint

When treatment side effects dry out the body—and believe me, that's a fairly common occurrence—granitas come to the rescue. Granitas are similar to Italian ices in consistency, which makes them great for people with mouth sores, and melons are full of water, so they're great for rehydration. In fact, melons in any form are a wonderful source of fluids and nutrients. Eaten on an empty stomach (and that's the best way to consume them, as they can cause an awful lot of tummy rumbling when combined with other food), melons require little stomach action and go right into the small intestine, allowing quick absorption of their nutrients. And here's a fun fact: Cantaloupes are named after the Italian town Cantalupo, which means "howl of the wolf." No telling if there's a run on cantaloupes there whenever the moon is full . . .

SERVES 6

- 1/4 cup boiling water
- 1 cup fresh mint leaves, loosely packed, plus 10 fresh mint leaves, finely chopped
- 6 cups chopped cantaloupe
- 1/4 cup agave nectar
- 2 tablespoons freshly squeezed lime juice

REBECCA'S NOTES To make frozen fruit pops, see the Variation on page 161.

Use caution when opening the freezer door while the granita is freezing. You want to end up with this frozen delight in your belly and not on the bottom of the freezer!

Pour the boiling water over the 1 cup of mint leaves, cover, and steep for 30 minutes. Strain the liquid and discard the mint leaves.

Put the cantaloupe in a food processor or blender and process on high speed until smooth.

Add the agave nectar, lime juice, mint infusion, and the 10 chopped mint leaves to the food processor or blender and pulse to combine. Transfer to a freezer-safe 8 by 10-inch pan with sides at least 2 inches high and freeze for 1 hour.

Use a fork to rake the mixture, breaking up the frozen parts into smaller bits and pushing them toward the center, like a pile of leaves. Return the granita to the freezer and repeat the raking process twice more at 30 minute intervals until entirely frozen.

PREP TIME: 30 minutes · COOK TIME: 2 hours in the freezer

STORAGE: Store in an airtight container in the freezer for 3 weeks.

PER SERVING: Calories: 95; Total Fat: 0.3 g (0.1 g saturated, 0 g monounsaturated); Carbohydrates: 24 g; Protein: 1 g; Fiber: 2 g; Sodium: 25 mg

"For my mouth sores, I found that sorbets in different flavors provided an anesthetic relief and, of course, everyone loves them!"
—Suzanne W., cancer survivor

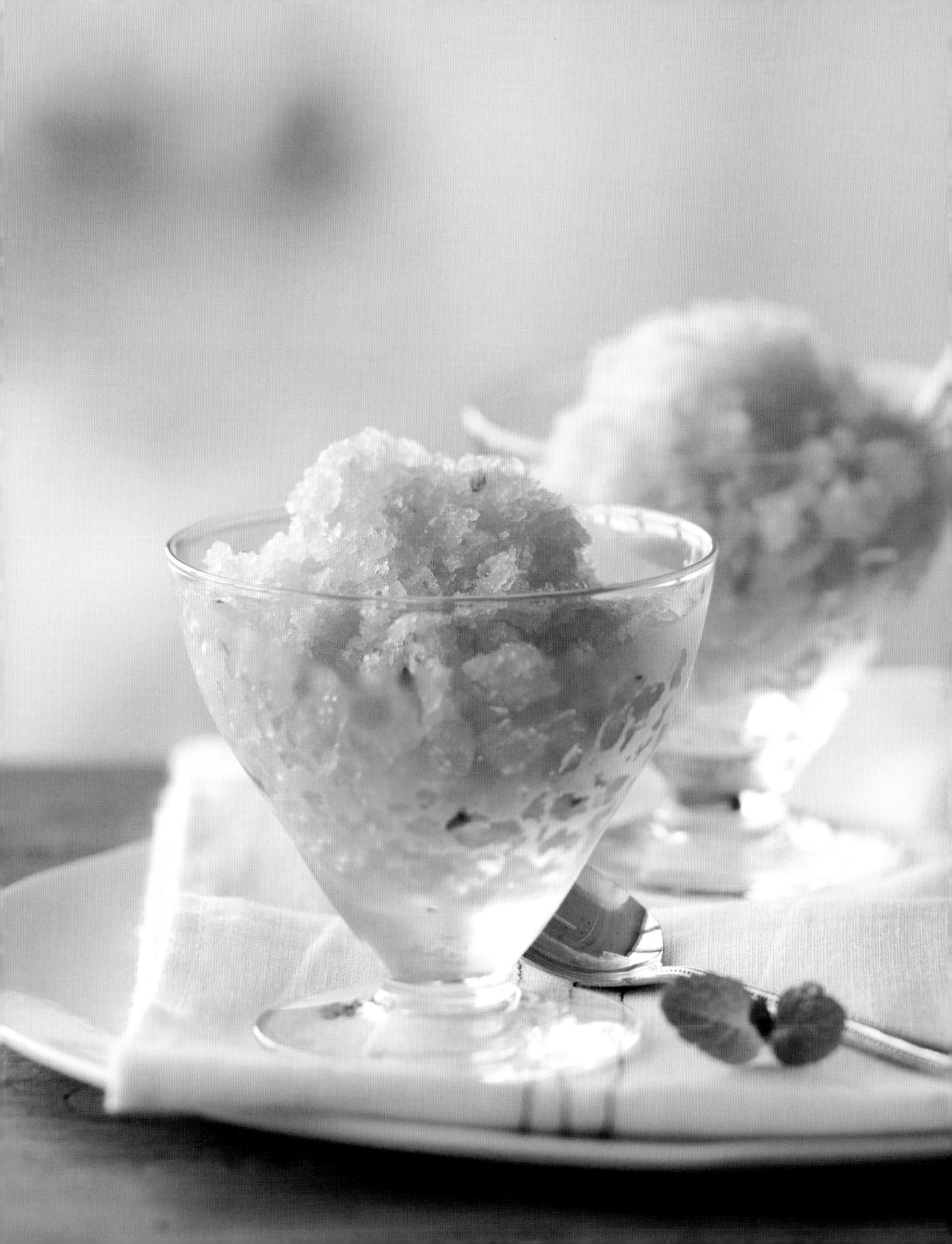

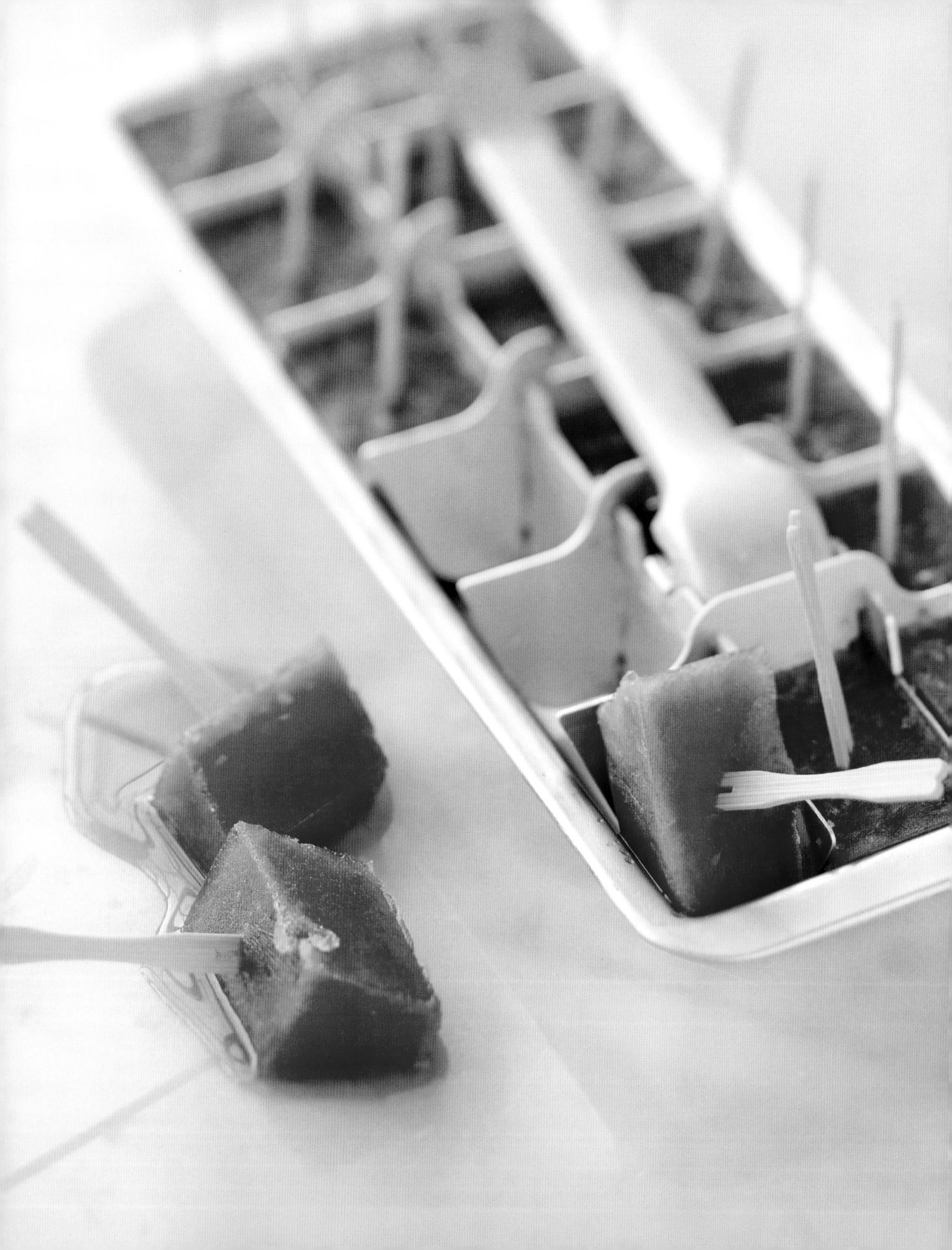

Mouthwatering Watermelon Granita

My freezer ended up with warning notes all over it after I made this granita. I put the liquid into a shallow pan in the freezer, and only a few minutes later I completely forgot it was in there. I opened the slide-out freezer drawer and was hit with a tidal wave of red. It wasn't quite like the elevator door opening in The Shining, *but it was pretty bad. I figured, "Okay, fool me once, shame on you." I swabbed out the whole freezer, put the food back in, made another batch, put that in the freezer, and left the kitchen. A few minutes later my husband, Gregg, wandered into the kitchen. Pause. "Beccaaa!!" Okay, fool me twice, shame on me. Once I cleaned off Gregg and the freezer (in that order), I made a third batch, and up went the warning notes. Success!* SERVES 6

2 cups chopped watermelon
2 1/2 tablespoons freshly squeezed lime juice
2 teaspoons agave nectar

Put the watermelon in a food processor or blender and process on high speed until smooth.

Add the lime juice and agave nectar to the food processor or blender and pulse to combine. Transfer to a freezer-safe 8 by 10-inch pan with sides at least 2 inches high and freeze for 1 hour.

Use a fork to rake the mixture, breaking up the frozen parts into smaller chunks and pushing them toward the center like a pile of leaves. Return the granita to the freezer and repeat the raking process twice more at 30 minute intervals until entirely frozen.

Variation: A fun variation on any granita is fruit drops, which I think of as a frozen version of Tootsie Pops, especially the part where you get to the sweet middle. Pour the liquid mixture into an ice cube tray, then stick a few blueberries into each of the compartments. They'll end up suspended in the middle after the liquid freezes. Put a toothpick or popsicle stick into each while they freeze and you can enjoy the fruit drops straight up, or skip the sticks and use them in beverages. Either way, these fruit drops are a treat for the eyes, and great for people with mouth sores or anyone who wants to stay hydrated.

PREP TIME: 8 minutes · COOK TIME: 2 hours in the freezer

STORAGE: Store in an airtight container in the freezer for 3 weeks.

PER SERVING: Calories: 20; Total Fat: 0 g (0 g saturated, 0 g monounsaturated); Carbohydrates: 7 g; Protein: 0 g; Fiber: 0 g; Sodium: 0 mg

Ginger Peppermint Green Tea

This tea is a little like a mother's gentle belly rub for a sick child, as both peppermint and ginger have qualities that relax the smooth muscles that surround the intestine. MAKES 4 CUPS

- 4 cups water
- 4 1/2-inch slices peeled fresh ginger
- 1 green tea bag
- 1 peppermint tea bag
- 1 tablespoon freshly squeezed lemon juice
- 1 teaspoon agave nectar or honey

Bring the water and ginger to a boil in a saucepan, then lower the heat, cover, and simmer for 10 minutes. Remove from the heat, add the green and peppermint tea bags, and steep for 10 minutes.

Remove the tea bags and ginger, then stir in the lemon juice and agave nectar. Serve hot, or chill for at least 1 hour before serving over ice.

PREP TIME: 3 minutes · COOK TIME: 25 minutes

STORAGE: Store, covered, in the refrigerator for 5 days.

PER SERVING: Calories: 10; Total Fat: 0 g (0 g saturated, 0 g monounsaturated); Carbohydrates: 2 g; Protein: 0 g; Fiber: 0 g; Sodium: 0 mg

Green Tea Ginger Lemonade

Green tea is great for you—and many of its compounds are being studied for their anticancer benefits, but it can be astringent and bitter. Here I've added ginger and lemon with either honey or agave to really knock out the bitterness. The result is a refreshing lemonade that's far healthier than the average store-bought blend. If you really want to amp up the sweetness, squeeze in a few oranges as well. MAKES 4 CUPS

- 4 cups water
- 4 1/2-inch slices peeled fresh ginger
- 2 green tea bags
- 1 tablespoon freshly squeezed lemon juice
- 2 teaspoons agave nectar or honey

Bring the water and ginger to a boil in a saucepan, then lower the heat, cover, and simmer for 10 minutes. Remove from the heat, add the tea bags, and steep for 10 minutes.

Remove the tea bags and ginger, stir in the lemon juice and agave nectar, and chill for at least 1 hour before serving over ice.

PREP TIME: 3 minutes · COOK TIME: 25 minutes, plus 1 hour for chilling

STORAGE: Store, covered, in the refrigerator for 5 to 7 days.

PER SERVING: Calories: 15; Total Fat: 0 g (0 g saturated, 0 g monounsaturated); Carbohydrates: 3 g; Protein: 0 g; Fiber: 0 g; Sodium: 0 mg

CULINARY RX Green tea has lots of wonderful antioxidants known as catechins. (Don't you love these names?) Studies have shown that catechins inhibit cancer cell growth and blood flow to tumors, but there's a catch: Green tea's catechins are absorbed far better if the contents of the intestine are slightly acidic. Enter the lemon! One study showed that adding a little citric acid to green tea boosted absorption of catechins by a whopping 500 percent. That's a mighty powerful pucker!

Cinnamon Ginger Tea

I've been playing with ginger in its various forms for years. From an Ayurvedic (traditional eastern Indian medicine) perspective, ginger "fires" the body's digestive hearth, to make the stomach and colon more efficient in metabolizing food. Here I've combined ginger with cinnamon's round, sweet flavor to create a modified Chai tea with some great health benefits. Cinnamon regulates blood sugar, while both ginger and cinnamon contain tumor inhibitors. This tea is a great way to wake up both your taste buds and your tummy. MAKES 4 CUPS

4 cups water
4 1/2-inch slices peeled fresh ginger
1 cinnamon stick
2 teaspoons honey

Bring the water, ginger, and cinnamon stick to a boil in a saucepan, then lower the heat, cover, and simmer for 10 minutes.

Remove and discard the ginger and cinnamon stick, stir in the honey, and serve immediately.

PREP TIME: 3 minutes · COOK TIME: 15 minutes
STORAGE: Store, covered, in the refrigerator for 5 days.
PER SERVING: Calories: 13; Total Fat: 0 g (0 g saturated, 0 g monounsaturated); Carbohydrates: 3 g; Protein: 0 g; Fiber: 0 g; Sodium: 0 mg

Ginger Tea Spritzer

This cool, refreshing drink tastes wonderful, and can also help combat nausea. MAKES 1 CUP OF SYRUP

3 ginger tea bags
2 cups boiling water
1/4 teaspoon honey
1/4 teaspoon freshly squeezed lemon juice
Sparkling water

Put the tea bags in a small saucepan, pour the boiling water over them, and steep for 15 minutes.

Put the saucepan over medium heat and cook until the tea is reduced by half. Stir in the honey and lemon juice, then let cool to room temperature. To serve, put 2 tablespoons of the ginger syrup in a glass and add sparkling water.

REBECCA'S NOTES For a change, try making this recipe with both chamomile and ginger tea bags, or a chamomile ginger blend, if you can find that.

PREP TIME: 3 minutes · COOK TIME: 20 minutes
STORAGE: Store the syrup, covered, in the refrigerator for 5 days.
PER SERVING: Calories: 0; Total Fat: 0 g (0 g saturated, 0 g monounsaturated); Carbohydrates: 0 g; Protein: 0 g; Fiber: 0 g; Sodium: 0 mg

CULINARY RX A staple of folk medicine in countries around the world, ginger also has some solid science behind it. It's long been studied for its antinausea properties. A study in the *British Journal of Anaesthesia* suggested that ginger is helpful in controlling nausea in a variety of situations, including stomach distress induced by chemotherapy. The American Cancer Society notes that, in addition to helping with nausea and motion sickness, ginger might slow tumor growth.

Ginger Ale with Frozen Grapes

Ginger is one of your best friends during chemo, both for its flavor, which can spark even the most jaded taste buds, and for its tummy-soothing properties. A lot of people think store-bought ginger ale will do the trick, but the actual ginger content in most commerical varieties is minimal. Plus, you often get a whole host of other garbage (can you say high fructose corn syrup?) that you'd be better off without. Enter this recipe, which uses straight-up ginger syrup so you can control the amount of zing in your tonic. The frozen grapes serve the same purpose as your basic ice cubes, but also sneak a bunch of healthy minerals and phytochemicals into the brew. MAKES ABOUT 2 CUPS SYRUP

- 4 cups water
- 2 cups sliced unpeeled fresh ginger
- 2 tablespoons freshly squeezed lemon juice
- 2 tablespoons honey
- Frozen seedless grapes
- Sparkling water
- Mint sprigs, for garnish

Bring the water and ginger to a boil in a saucepan, then lower the heat, cover, and simmer for 1 hour. Uncover and continue to simmer for 30 minutes.

Strain the infusion through cheesecloth and discard the ginger. Stir in the lemon juice and honey and let cool to room temperature.

For each serving, add 1/4 cup of the ginger syrup to a glass with frozen grapes, then fill the glass with sparkling water and garnish with a sprig of mint.

REBECCA'S NOTES You can also use this ginger syrup to make a hot beverage. Just stir 3 tablespoons of the syrup into 1 cup of hot water, then add more honey or lemon if you like.

PREP TIME: 5 minutes · COOK TIME: 1 hour 30 minutes

STORAGE: Store the ginger syrup in an airtight container in the refrigerator for 7 days. Store the grapes in a resealable plastic bag in the freezer for 3 months.

PER SERVING: Calories: 50; Total Fat: 0.2 g (0.1 g saturated, 0 g monounsaturated); Carbohydrates: 12 g; Protein: 0 g; Fiber: 1 g; Sodium: 5 mg

"Be kind to yourself. Remember that you and your body need to heal and recover. The downtime you need is more important than the 'up time' you want to get back to."
—Ty H., cancer survivor

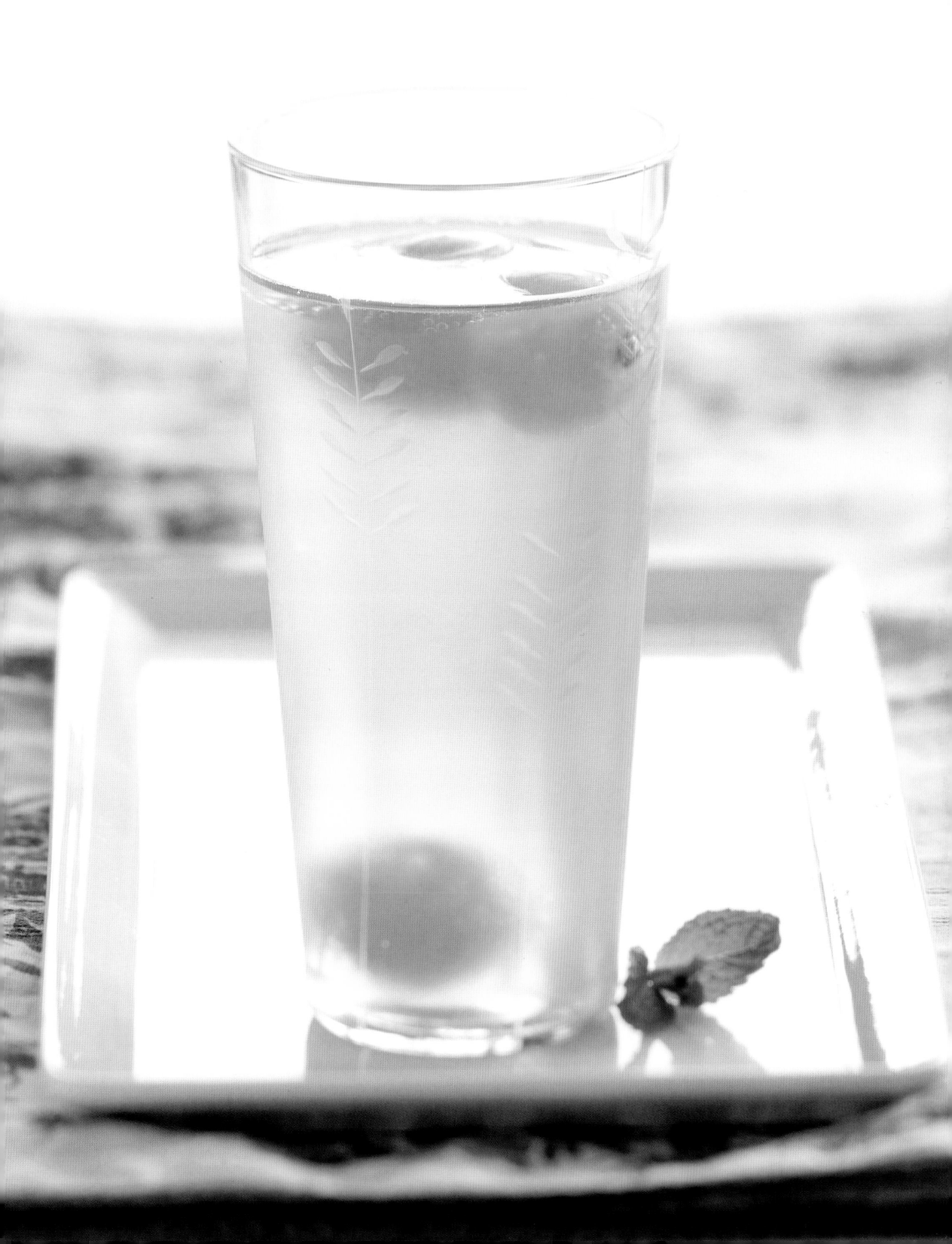

Chocolate Banana Smoothie

There's this old restaurant called Field's near where I used to live in Baltimore. Every town has a place like this—or at least used to—with a soda counter, red plastic stools, and sweet-and-sour elderly waitresses in pink candy striper outfits. Going to Field's was like making a pilgrimage, except instead of seeking wisdom we desired to attain the perfect milkshake. I think this smoothie gives Field's a run for its money—without creating the world's largest sugar spike. A little almond butter is the secret ingredient, creating a creamy goodness that will make you want to twirl around in your seat. MAKES 3 1/2 CUPS

- 3 cups unsweetened almond milk (or substitute rice or soy milk)
- 2 frozen bananas
- 2 tablespoons unsweetened cocoa powder
- 1 1/2 tablespoons almond butter
- 1 tablespoon finely ground flaxseeds
- 1/2 teaspoon maple syrup
- 1/4 teaspoon vanilla extract
- Pinch of sea salt
- 4 ice cubes (optional; see Rebecca's Notes)

Put all of the ingredients in a blender and process until smooth. Do a FASS check and add a couple drops of lemon juice to perk up the flavor if needed. Serve immediately.

Variations: For a more chocolaty flavor, add 2 1/2 tablespoons cocoa powder. Chocolate goodness!

Add 1 tablespoon of unrefined virgin coconut oil for additional healthy fat and calories.

For more protein, add a scoop of whey protein powder.

PREP TIME: 5 minutes · COOK TIME: Not applicable

STORAGE: Store in an airtight glass container in the refrigerator for 2 days. Shake well or blend again before serving.

PER SERVING: Calories: 165; Total Fat: 8 g (0.5 g saturated, 2.8 g monounsaturated); Carbohydrates: 22 g; Protein: 4 g; Fiber: 4 g; Sodium: 270 mg

REBECCA'S NOTES The ice cubes in this shake will make a big difference in thickening up the smoothie. If this is the consistency you prefer, add the optional ice cubes along with the frozen bananas.

It's much easier to peel bananas before they're frozen. Once they're peeled, store them in a resealable plastic bag and pop them in the freezer. They're a delicious snack on their own, and great to have on hand for smoothies and frozen drinks. If you don't have frozen bananas on hand and want to make this shake right away, use room-temperature bananas and be sure to include the ice cubes.

Mango Coconut Smoothie

Coconut and mango in one drink? Yum! Coconut is one of those foods that tastes so amazing, you can't possibly believe it's also good for you. It's kind of like waking up to find out that chocolate is guaranteed to grow back your hair and help you run a seven-minute mile. Coconut milk and coconut oil, which is a variation in this recipe, both contain lauric acid. Guess what else contains lauric acid? Mother's milk. And like that most elemental of foods, the lauric acid in coconut milk and oil has antiviral and antibacterial properties. And as for fat, although coconut contains saturated fat, it's assimilated better by the body because it's vegetable based, not animal based (like butter). But forget all the science for a moment. You want to do the happy dance? Drink this. MAKES 3 CUPS

- 1 1/2 cups chopped mango
- 1 cup water
- 1/2 cup freshly squeezed orange juice
- 1/4 cup coconut milk
- 1 tablespoon freshly squeezed lime juice
- 1 tablespoon finely ground flaxseeds or flax oil
- 4 ice cubes
- 1 teaspoon agave nectar

Combine all of the ingredients in a blender and process until smooth. Serve immediately.

Variations: Add 1 tablespoon of unrefined virgin coconut oil for additional healthy fat and calories.

For more protein, add a scoop of whey protein powder.

PREP TIME: 5 minutes · COOK TIME: Not applicable

STORAGE: Store in an airtight glass container in the refrigerator for 2 days. Shake well before serving.

PER SERVING: Calories: 130; Total Fat: 5.5 g (3.7 g saturated, 0.5 g monounsaturated); Carbohydrates: 22 g; Protein: 2 g; Fiber: 3 g; Sodium: 5 mg

WHO KNEW? Whey to Go! According to Keith Block, MD, whey has benefits beyond just helping to keep weight on. It can also help carry glutathione into your cells. Why should that make you deliriously happy? Because studies show that glutathione protects healthy cells from adverse effects, while also making cancer cells more susceptible to chemotherapy. Neat.

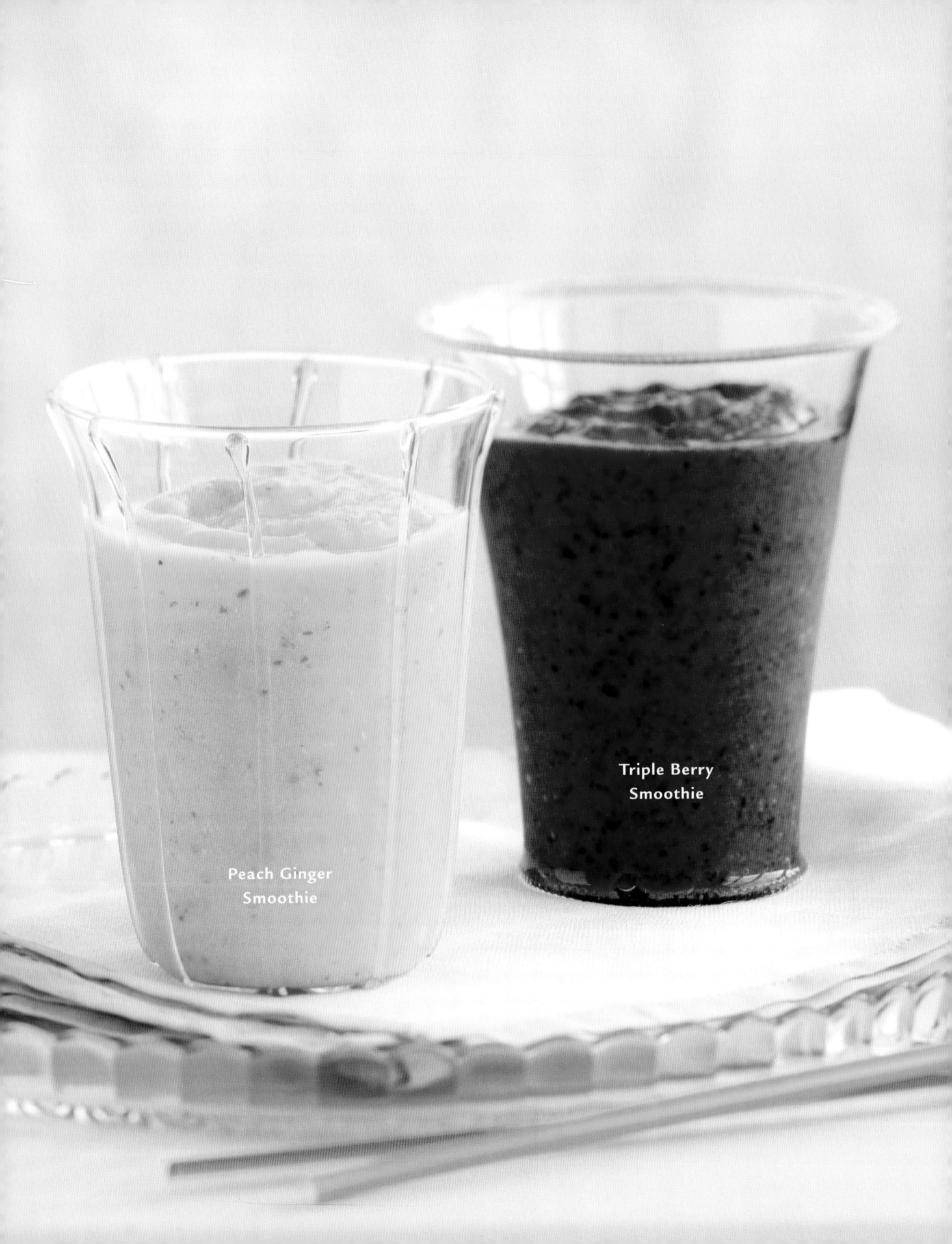
Triple Berry
Smoothie
Peach Ginger
Smoothie

Peach Ginger Smoothie

When I was a kid, nothing could compare to hearing the jingling bells of the ice cream man; it meant I got a Creamsicle. Looking for that taste again and to create something kids would adore, I came up with this recipe. One note: If you have a sensitive mouth or throat issues, omit the ginger to avoid irritation.

MAKES 4 1/2 CUPS

- 1 1/4 cups peach nectar
- 3/4 cup organic plain yogurt
- 1 teaspoon minced fresh ginger
- 3 cups frozen peaches, or 3 cups fresh peaches, pitted and chopped
- 1 tablespoon finely ground flaxseeds
- 1 1/2 teaspoons maple syrup
- 1/2 teaspoon vanilla extract
- 1/2 teaspoon freshly squeezed lime juice

Combine the peach nectar, yogurt, ginger, and half of the peaches in a blender and process until smooth. Add the remaining peaches, the flaxseeds, maple syrup, vanilla, and lime juice and blend until smooth and creamy. Serve immediately.

Variations: Add 1 tablespoon of unrefined virgin coconut oil for additional healthy fat and calories.

For more protein, add a scoop of whey protein powder.

PREP TIME: 5 minutes · COOK TIME: Not applicable

STORAGE: Store in an airtight glass container in the refrigerator for 2 days. Shake well again before serving.

PER SERVING: Calories: 135; Total Fat: 2.4 g (1 g saturated, 0.6 g monounsaturated); Carbohydrates: 25 g; Protein: 3 g; Fiber: 1 g; Sodium: 27 mg

Triple Berry Smoothie

A lot of people wonder why adding healthy items like flaxseeds to a decent-tasting smoothie destroys the taste. The answer is that the smoothie recipe didn't take into account the items you'd want to add. The normal fix is to add a ton of sweetener, but I don't agree with that approach, especially in recipes for cancer patients. But the berry blast of this smoothie plays well with the vital flax and whey. The abundant antioxidants make this smoothie one for the books. MAKES 3 3/4 CUPS

- 1 cup organic plain yogurt
- 1 cup water
- 1/4 cup freshly squeezed orange juice
- 1 cup frozen strawberries
- 1 1/2 cups frozen blueberries
- 1/2 cup frozen raspberries
- 1 tablespoon ground flaxseeds
- 1 teaspoon agave nectar, honey, or maple syrup

Combine the yogurt, water, and orange juice in a blender and process for a few seconds. Add the strawberries and process until well blended, then add the blueberries, raspberries, flaxseeds, and agave nectar and blend until smooth. Serve immediately.

Variations: Add 1 tablespoon of unrefined virgin coconut oil for additional healthy fat and calories.

For more protein, add a scoop of whey protein powder.

PREP TIME: 5 minutes · COOK TIME: Not applicable

STORAGE: Store in an airtight glass container in the refrigerator for 2 days. Shake well again before serving.

PER SERVING: Calories: 145; Total Fat: 4.6 g (1.8 g saturated, 1 g monounsaturated); Carbohydrates: 24 g; Protein: 4 g; Fiber: 5 g; Sodium: 40 mg

Pineapple Ginger Smoothie

Move over, Hoover. The finest vacuum we know, capable of getting a whole load of nasty stuff out of your system in a jiffy, is none other than pineapple. It contains a host of enzymes, including bromelain, which helps dissolve the mucus buildup that's so common with lung issues. It even aids in flushing fat from the body. (Liposuction in a glass. Who knew?) As for the taste, it pops like fireworks—or like the grand finale in this smoothie, due to the addition of ginger and mint. This great, refreshing smoothie is good for anyone, with just one caveat: If you have a sensitive mouth or throat issues, omit the ginger to avoid irritation. If you have a sensitive stomach, cut the amount of pineapple to two cups and add an additional banana. MAKES 3 CUPS

- 3 cups chopped fresh pineapple
- 1 frozen banana
- 1/2 cup water
- 1 teaspoon minced fresh ginger
- 1 tablespoon finely ground flaxseeds
- 2 fresh mint leaves

Combine the pineapple, banana, water, ginger, and flaxseeds in a blender and process until smooth. Add the mint leaves and blend briefly, only until the mint leaves are just incorporated. Serve immediately.

Variations: Add 1 tablespoon of unrefined virgin coconut oil for additional healthy fat and calories.

For more protein, add a scoop of whey protein powder.

PREP TIME: 5 minutes · COOK TIME: Not applicable

STORAGE: Store in an airtight glass container in the refrigerator for 2 days. Shake well again before serving.

PER SERVING: Calories: 100; Total Fat: 1.1 g (0.1 g saturated, 0.2 g monounsaturated); Carbohydrates: 24 g; Protein: 1 g; Fiber: 3 g; Sodium: 0 mg

Papaya Pineapple Smoothie

Both papaya and pineapple have a lot of enzymes that aid digestion. If you're having digestive difficulty, drinking some of this smoothie before a meal will help lessen bloating and indigestion. MAKES 3 1/4 CUPS

- 1/4 cup chopped papaya
- 2 cups chopped fresh pineapple
- 8 ice cubes
- 1 cup rice milk or almond milk
- 1/2 cup freshly squeezed orange juice
- 1/4 cup coconut milk
- 1 tablespoon finely ground flaxseeds
- 1/2 teaspoon freshly squeezed lime juice
- 1/2 teaspoon maple syrup

Combine all of the ingredients in a blender and process until smooth. Serve immediately.

Variations: Add 1 tablespoon of unrefined virgin coconut oil for additional healthy fat and calories.

For more protein, add a scoop of whey protein powder.

If you use frozen fruit, leave out the ice cubes as the smoothie will be thick enough without them.

PREP TIME: 5 minutes · COOK TIME: Not applicable

STORAGE: Store in an airtight glass container in the refrigerator for 2 days. Shake well again before serving.

PER SERVING: Calories: 125; Total Fat: 4.7 g (2.8 g saturated, 0.7 g monounsaturated); Carbohydrates: 21 g; Protein: 2 g; Fiber: 2 g; Sodium: 20 mg

CULINARY RX Papayas have vitamin C, which is an antioxidant and may also reduce absorption of cancer-causing nitrosamines. They also contain folic acid, which has been shown to minimize cervical dysplasia and certain cancers.

CHAPTER 8

Dollops of Yum!

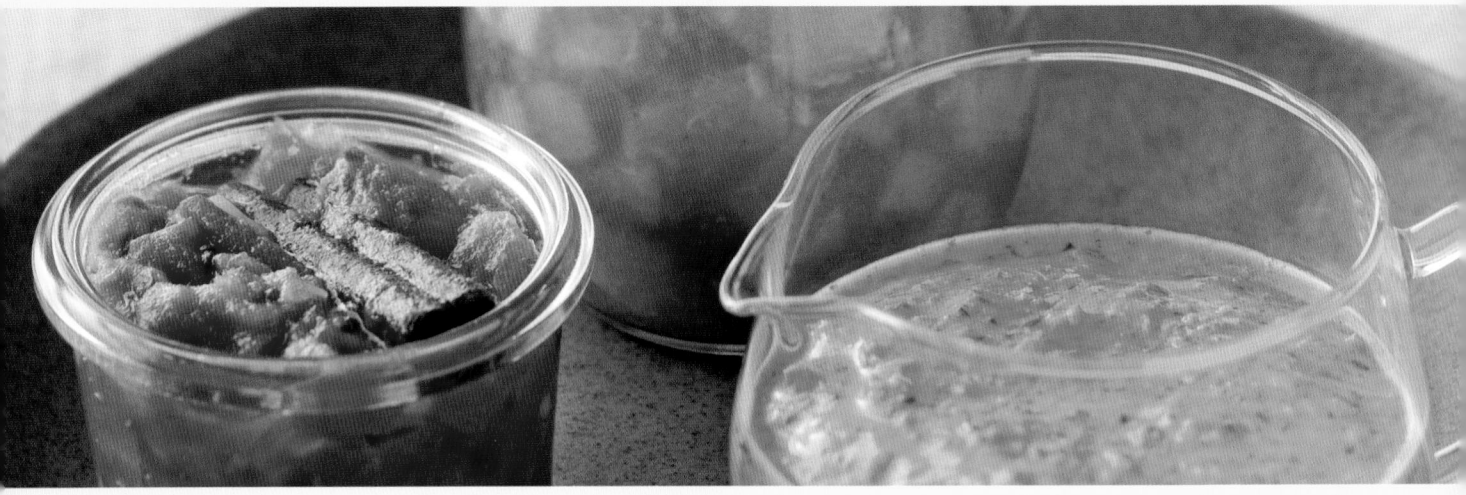

175 *Apricot Pear Chutney*
176 *Tomato Mint Chutney*
177 *Basil Lemon Drizzle*
178 *Avocado Dressing*
178 *Avocado Cream*
180 *Cashew Cream*
181 *Pistachio Cream*
181 *Cilantro Lime Vinaigrette*
182 *Zesty Lemon Fennel Vinaigrette*
183 *Dried Fruit Compote*
184 *Seasonal Stewed Fruit*
185 *Blueberry Compote*
185 *Mango and Avocado Salsa*
186 *Olive and Caper Relish*
186 *Moroccan Pesto*
187 *Parsley Basil Drizzle*
188 *Signora's Tomato Sauce*
189 *Sweet and Savory Yogurt*

Accessories? I can see why people might look at the dollops that follow and think of them as the culinary equivalent of a jaunty chapeau peacock feather or a fabulous consignment store bling ring. Pistachio Cream? Basil Lemon Drizzle?! Tomato Mint Chutney?!? At first glance, they may seem like add-ons, albeit tasty ones. However, there's a whole lot more to these dollops of yum. In their own way, they're like Allen to Burns, Kermie to Miss Piggy, or a bee to a buttercup—a complement that makes the whole shebang fly. And that's the way I'd like you to look at these dollops: not as afterthoughts, but as the cherry that makes the sundae truly irresistible.

In some cases, these recipes play an integral role in creating the taste and texture of a dish. Take vinaigrettes: They play an obvious role with salads, but I also like them as marinades for fish and meat. There's nothing like a dish that's marinated until the meat is so tender that it practically dissolves in your mouth.

Remember, people in treatment often need this kind of additional palate pleasure, especially if they have impaired taste buds or a constant metallic tang in the mouth. The drizzles are useful here. I tell my clients that they're an example of working from the outside in, ensuring that the first thing that hits the tongue has an explosive burst of flavor. Without this coaxing, some people may not feel like working their way through the more subtle flavors of the rest of the food—and the accompanying nutrients.

The dollops here not only enhance the dishes they adorn, in many cases they also help carry the flavor of the dish. They're designed to move taste around the mouth, seeking those islands of taste buds that are in the best shape to transmit maximum flavor. When I recommend that dollop X—say Tomato Mint Chutney—goes with dish Y—for example, Middle Eastern Chickpea Burgers—you can take it to the bank. (Okay, maybe to the table. Banks aren't so reliable these days.)

These dollops serve another purpose: They provide more delicious, nutrient-dense calories, which is so important for people who are trying to keep weight on, so use them whenever you can. I've designed many of these dollops to go with multiple dishes. Apricot Pear Chutney complements five of the recipes in this book, and Olive and Caper Relish also plays nicely off five. The Basil Lemon Drizzle is great over almost any fish dish or salad you can imagine. My advice? Always keep plenty of dollops on hand (I've also designed them to store nicely), because you'd hate to have a dish go out half-dressed. What would the neighbors say?

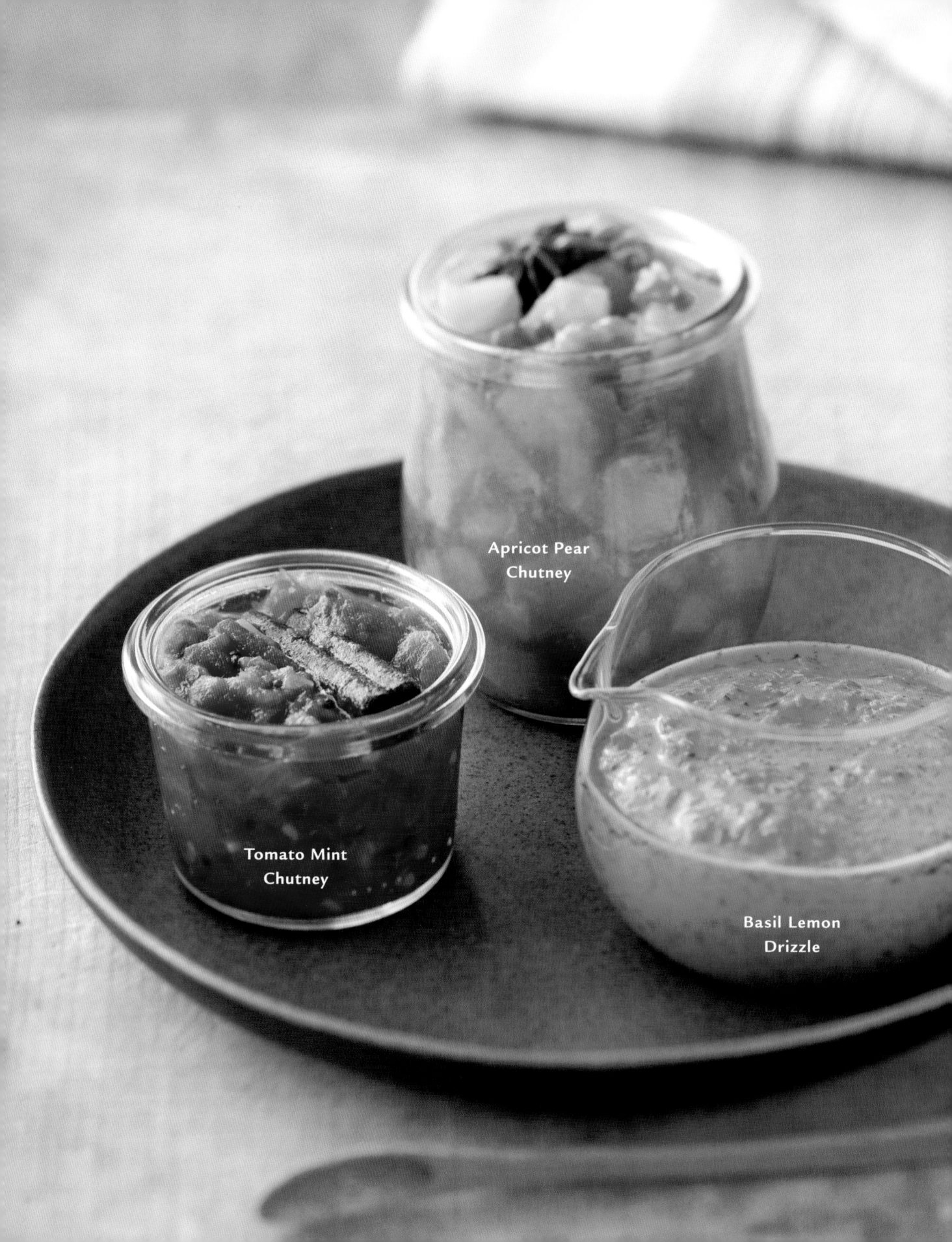
Apricot Pear
Chutney
Tomato Mint
Chutney
Basil Lemon
Drizzle

Apricot Pear Chutney

Chutney is a relish, but believe me, it doesn't taste anything like the relish you're probably used to. Here the mellow sweetness of the pears plays perfectly against the tartness of the apricots. The sour-sweet combo leaves those taste buds wanting more, kind of like delirious rock fans screaming for an encore, and they'll stay at the table until their demands are satisfied! This chutney is also a nutritious alternative to jam or jelly. Any pear will work for this recipe; some of my favorites are Bosc, brown Asian, or Anjou.

MAKES 4 CUPS

- 2 pounds pears, peeled, cored, and diced
- 1 1/4 cups chopped unsulfured dried apricots
- 1/2 teaspoon lemon zest
- 1/2 cup brown rice vinegar
- 1/4 cup freshly squeezed lemon juice
- 1/4 cup maple syrup
- 1/2 teaspoon minced garlic
- 1/2 teaspoon grated fresh ginger
- 1/2 teaspoon sea salt
- 1/2 teaspoon ground cinnamon
- 1/4 teaspoon ground allspice
- 1/4 teaspoon ground cardamom
- 1/4 teaspoon red pepper flakes
- 1 pod star anise (optional)

Combine all of the ingredients in a large saucepan and bring to a boil. Lower the heat to maintain a bubbly simmer and cook, stirring occasionally, for 45 to 50 minutes with the lid partially off so that the liquid begins to evaporate. Once the pears are soft but not mushy and the liquid has reduced to a thick coating over the fruit, remove the chutney from the heat. Remove the star anise (you can save it for garnish, if you like). Serve warm or at room temperature.

Goes with Curry Cauliflower Soup (page 67), Velvety Red Lentil Dahl (page 74), Spiced Sweet Potato Soup (page 72), Orange Ginger Roasted Chicken (page 117), and Middle Eastern Chickpea Burgers (page 112).

PREP TIME: 15 minutes · COOK TIME: 50 minutes

STORAGE: Store in an airtight container in the refrigerator for 7 days or in the freezer for 2 months.

PER SERVING: Calories: 20; Total Fat: 0 g (0 g saturated, 0 g monounsaturated); Carbohydrates: 5 g; Protein: 0 g; Fiber: 1 g; Sodium: 20 mg

REBECCA'S NOTES This chutney is quite versatile. A dollop is a delicious addition to many soups, and it can also be served over roasted chicken. For a sophisticated snack, spread soft goat cheese on crackers and top with a bit of the chutney.

Tomato Mint Chutney

The flavors in this wonderful chutney make it a good choice for brightening just about any dish.

MAKES 1 CUP

- 2 tablespoons extra-virgin olive oil
- 2 shallots, diced small
- 1/4 teaspoon red pepper flakes
- 1 teaspoon cumin seeds
- 1/4 teaspoon brown mustard seeds (see Rebecca's Notes)
- 2 cinnamon sticks
- 4 cups coarsely chopped fresh tomatoes or diced canned tomatoes
- 3 tablespoons maple syrup
- 1/2 teaspoon sea salt
- 1 teaspoon grated fresh ginger
- 1/4 cup loosely packed fresh mint leaves, chopped

Heat the olive oil in a large, heavy skillet over medium-low heat, then add the shallots, red pepper flakes, cumin seeds, mustard seeds, and cinnamon sticks and sauté until the shallots are golden brown, about 4 minutes. Stir in the tomatoes, maple syrup, and salt, then lower the heat and simmer for 15 to 20 minutes, until the tomato juices have evaporated.

Stir in the ginger and mint and serve warm or at room temperature.

Goes with Middle Eastern Chickpea Burgers (page 112), Velvety Red Lentil Dahl (page 74), Triple-Citrus Ginger Black Cod (page 118), My Family's Favorite Chicken (page 111), Basil Broccoli (page 78), poached salmon (page 121), and just about any brown rice, polenta, or pasta dish.

PREP TIME: 15 minutes · COOK TIME: 25 minutes

STORAGE: Store in an airtight container in the refrigerator for 3 to 4 days or in the freezer for 2 months.

PER SERVING: Calories: 35; Total Fat: 1.9 g (0.3 g saturated, 1.3 g monounsaturated); Carbohydrates: 5 g; Protein: 0 g; Fiber: 1 g; Sodium: 75 mg

REBECCA'S NOTES The brown mustard seeds in this recipe are optional. They are found in the bulk foods section of the market and add a delicious flavor.

For a less spicy chutney, lower the amount of ginger and red pepper flakes.

Basil Lemon Drizzle

"Simple is as simple does," said Forrest Gump, and when it comes to cooking, I heartily agree. This drizzle is a perfect example of FASS in action. This is the little black dress of condiments—appropriate in almost any situation. What it really comes down to is lemon zest, basil, and lemon juice, and zingo, you have a condiment that brightens and brings out the flavor in anything you put it on top of—veggies, chicken, fish, whatever. But it isn't just packed with flavor, it's also loaded with cancer-fighting properties, including anti-inflammatory agents in the basil and antioxidants in the lemon. MAKES 1/2 CUP

- 1 cup loosely packed fresh basil leaves
- 2 tablespoons freshly squeezed lemon juice
- 1 teaspoon lemon zest
- 1/4 cup extra-virgin olive oil
- 1 teaspoon maple syrup (optional)
- 1/4 teaspoon sea salt

Put all of the ingredients in a food processor and process until well blended.

Variation: For a richer drizzle that's more like pesto, add 1/4 cup pecans or walnuts when you process the ingredients.

Goes with Cooling Cucumber Avocado Soup (page 70), Minestrone (page 64), Roasted Red Roma Tomato Soup (page 69), Creamy Broccoli and Potato Soup (page 75), Italian White Bean Soup (page 57), Lemon Mustard Salmon Salad (page 109), Nana's Egg Salad (page 114), Easy Eggs in a Cup (page 102), Basil Broccoli (page 78), Mediterranean Lentil Salad (page 142), Simple Tuscan Farro (page 148), Tuscan Farro and Bean Salad (page 107), and, as you might guess from this list, a myriad other savory dishes.

PREP TIME: 5 minutes · COOK TIME: Not applicable

STORAGE: Store in an airtight container in the refrigerator for 7 to 10 days or in the freezer for 2 months.

PER SERVING: Calories: 125; Total Fat: 14.1 g (2 g saturated, 10 g monounsaturated); Carbohydrates: 1 g; Protein: 0 g; Fiber: 0 g; Sodium: 150 mg

Avocado Dressing

This is my riff on green goddess dressing. I've omitted the buttermilk, but you won't miss it a bit, as the luscious avocado blends with the brown rice vinegar to create a mellow dressing that's ideal tossed with crunchy salads—a mix of tastes and textures that's like giving your palate an invigorating massage. MAKES 1 CUP

- 3/4 cup water
- 2 tablespoons extra-virgin olive oil
- 2 tablespoons brown rice vinegar
- 2 tablespoons freshly squeezed lime juice
- 1 teaspoon agave nectar
- 1/2 teaspoon sea salt
- 1/2 ripe avocado
- 1/4 cup loosely packed chopped fresh basil
- 1 clove garlic, chopped

Combine all of the ingredients in a blender or food processor and blend until smooth and creamy.

Goes with all of your favorite salads, or on top of fish or chicken.

PREP TIME: 5 minutes · COOK TIME: Not applicable

STORAGE: Store in an airtight container in the refrigerator for 1 to 2 days.

PER SERVING: Calories: 25; Total Fat: 2.4 g (0.3 g saturated, 1.7 g monounsaturated); Carbohydrates: 1 g; Protein: 0 g; Fiber: 0 g; Sodium: 75 mg

Avocado Cream

Putting avocado and cream in the same title is almost redundant; avocados by their very nature have one of the creamiest textures in the fruit kingdom, as any guacamole lover can attest. Avocado has fantastic proportions of healthy fats, vitamins, and minerals, especially potassium. In fact, avocados contain more potassium than bananas, making them ideal for combating the potassium loss that can occur because of dehydration. Whether on a cracker or over a dish, this creamy dollop guarantees you both fantastic taste and superb nutrition. MAKES 1 CUP

- 1 ripe avocado, pitted and peeled
- 1/4 cup loosely packed fresh cilantro (optional)
- 1 tablespoon water
- 1 tablespoon freshly squeezed lime juice
- 1/4 teaspoon sea salt

REBECCA'S NOTES Want a little heat? Add a pinch of cayenne. Want a bright taste? Add a few tablespoons of chopped fresh mint.

Combine all of the ingredients in a blender or food processor and process until smooth. Do a FASS check. You may want to add some extra lime juice or a pinch of salt.

Goes with Rockin' Black Bean Soup (page 71) and Black Bean Hummus (page 132), and also makes a great sandwich spread.

PREP TIME: 5 minutes · COOK TIME: Not applicable

STORAGE: Store in an airtight container in the refrigerator for 3 days.

PER SERVING: Calories: 15; Total Fat: 1.3 g (0.2 g saturated, 0.8 g monounsaturated); Carbohydrates: 1 g; Protein: 0 g; Fiber: 1 g; Sodium: 40 mg

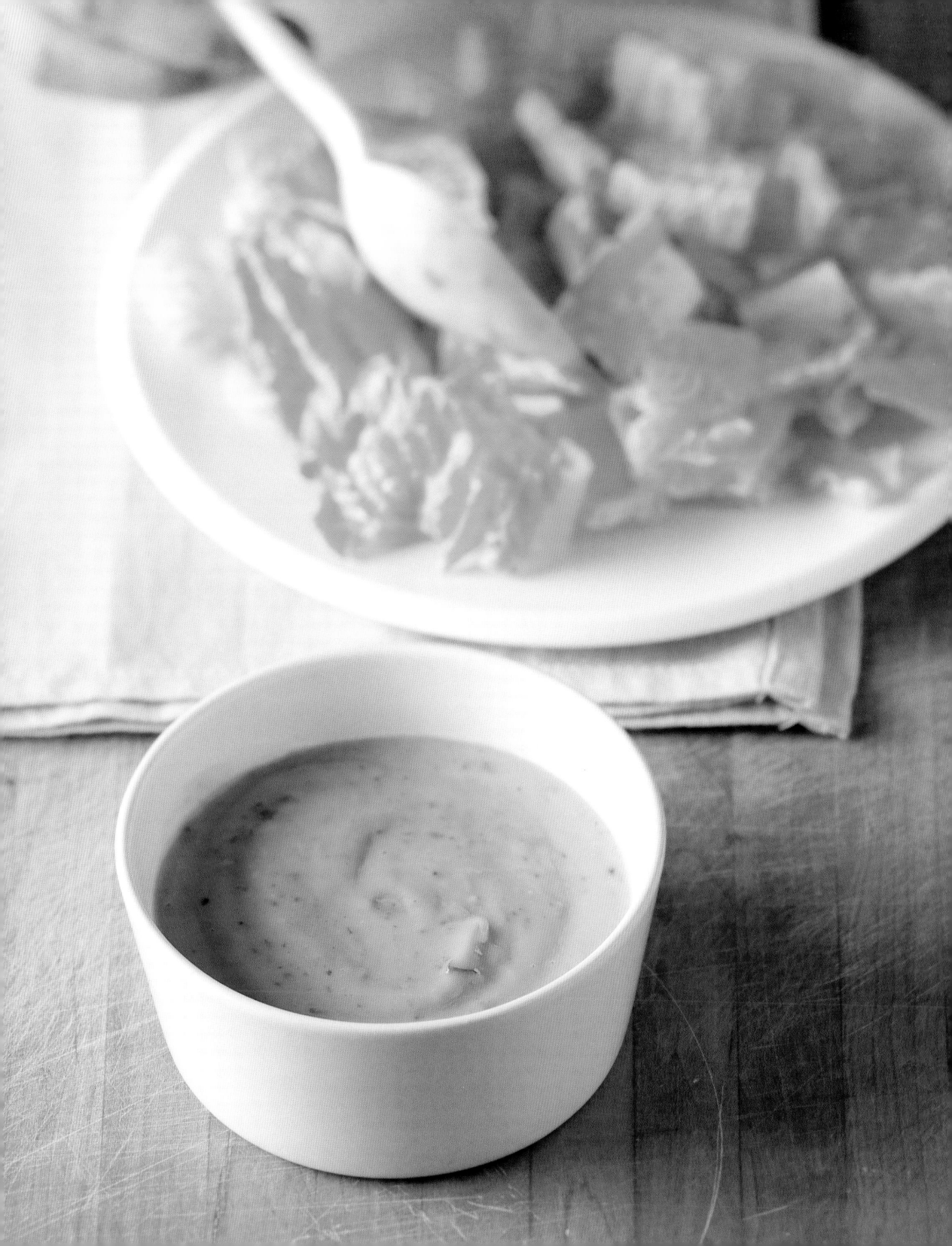

Cashew Cream

You know that old Sesame Street *song that goes, "One of these things is not like the others . . ."? Put a cashew next to butter and margarine, and you'll probably think, "Hey, I know which one of these doesn't belong." Think again. I've pleased many a client who swears by butter but wants to go dairy free by substituting nut creams, in this case pulverized cashews. Not only is the taste fulfilling and delightful, nuts are far better for you than any store-bought buttery spread made from corn oil.*

MAKES ABOUT 3 1/2 CUPS

- 2 cups raw cashews
- 2 cups water
- 2 teaspoons freshly squeezed lemon juice or orange juice
- 1/2 teaspoon sea salt
- 1/8 teaspoon freshly ground nutmeg

Grind the cashews in a mini food processor or nut grinder to give them a head start in the blender. (If you have a Vita-Mix, you can skip this step.) Put the water in a blender, then add the lemon juice, salt, nutmeg, and cashews and blend until creamy smooth. This takes several minutes, but your taste buds will reap the rewards of your patience.

Variations: Substitute other nuts, such as almonds, pecans, pistachios, or hazelnuts.

For a variation that's similar to pesto, add 1 1/2 cups fresh basil. This is great tossed with your favorite pasta or rice.

If you want more citrus flavor without an acidic taste, add 1 teaspoon lemon or orange zest.

Goes with Emerald Greens with Orange (page 84), Warm and Toasty Cumin Carrots (page 93), Creamiest Buckwheat (page 138), Creamy Millet (page 136), Simple Tuscan Farro (page 148), and Poached Pears with Saffron Broth (page 203). Cashew Cream is also a tasty and nutritious addition to any smoothie.

PREP TIME: 5 minutes · COOK TIME: Not applicable

STORAGE: Store in an airtight container in the refrigerator for 2 weeks or in the freezer for 2 months.

PER SERVING: Calories: 30; Total Fat: 2.2 g (0.4 g saturated, 1.2 g monounsaturated); Carbohydrates: 2 g; Protein: 1 g; Fiber: 0 g; Sodium: 20 mg

Pistachio Cream

When I was in high school, my idea of a great time was sitting on the floor with my best friend Jill and devouring a huge bag of pistachios while we discussed which cute boys we had crushes on. By the time we were done, we were knee-deep in shells and soul-deep in feminine solidarity. Little did I know we were also improving our health. Turns out those pistachios are their own wellness center, rich in potassium (for cell fluid balance and nerve function), magnesium (for enzymes that help catalyze the body's energy), thiamine (for appetite stimulation), and vitamin B_6 (for protein absorption). MAKES 1 1/2 CUPS

1 cup water
2 teaspoons freshly squeezed lemon juice
1/4 teaspoon sea salt
1 cup raw pistachios

Combine all of the ingredients in a blender and blend until very smooth.

Goes with Summer's Best Zucchini Soup (page 73) and Poached Pears with Saffron Broth (page 203).

PREP TIME: 5 minutes · COOK TIME: Not applicable

STORAGE: Store in an airtight container in the refrigerator for 2 weeks or in the freezer for 2 months.

PER SERVING: Calories: 30; Total Fat: 2.4 g (0.3 g saturated, 1.2 g monounsaturated); Carbohydrates: 2 g; Protein: 1 g; Fiber: 1 g; Sodium: 25 mg

Cilantro Lime Vinaigrette

Vinaigrettes, at least the way we design them, have a double purpose. They're a wonderful addition to kick up greens and put their taste over the top. But I also like them as marinades for fish and meats. There's nothing like a dish that's marinated until the meat is so tender that it practically slides off the bone and into your mouth. In Middle-Eastern cuisine, some dishes are marinated for days. Okay, so few us are that patient—and in truth it's really not necessary. Even just a little cuddle time between a dish and these vinaigrettes/marinades is enough to make any meal succulent. I like the Cilantro Lime Vinaigrette as a marinade for fish and chicken recipes. MAKES 1/2 CUP

3 1/2 tablespoons freshly squeezed lime juice
2 teaspoons brown rice vinegar
1/4 teaspoon sea salt
1/4 teaspoon ground cumin
Pinch of cayenne
3/4 teaspoon agave nectar or honey
1/4 cup extra-virgin olive oil
2 teaspoons finely chopped fresh cilantro

Combine all of the ingredients and whisk until thoroughly blended.

Goes with Mixed Greens with Edamame, Radish, and Avocado (page 91) and Cucumber, Jicama, and Mango Salad (page 83). In addition, this vinaigrette makes a great marinade for fish and chicken.

PREP TIME: 5 minutes · COOK TIME: Not applicable

STORAGE: Store in an airtight container in the refrigerator for 7 days.

PER SERVING: Calories: 65; Total Fat: 7 g (1 g saturated, 5 g monounsaturated); Carbohydrates: 1 g; Protein: 0 g; Fiber: 0 g; Sodium: 75 mg

Zesty Lemon Fennel Vinaigrette

Like the Cilantro Lime Vinaigrette, this recipe works wonderfully with salads or as a quick way to dress up fish or meat. The lemon kick makes this a great partner for My Family's Favorite Chicken (page 111).

MAKES 1/2 CUP

- 1 teaspoon fennel seeds
- 3 tablespoons freshly squeezed lemon juice
- 1 teaspoon agave nectar
- 1/2 teaspoon minced shallot
- 1/4 teaspoon sea salt
- 1/4 cup extra-virgin olive oil

REBECCA'S NOTES Although toasting the fennel seeds may seem like a time-consuming and unnecessary step, I assure you that it isn't. Toasting unleashes the natural oils of the fennel seeds, coaxing out their tremendous flavor and healing properties.

Toast the fennel seeds in a small sauté pan over medium heat, shaking a few times for even toasting, until they become aromatic and start to brown slightly. Be careful that they don't burn. Let cool slightly, then pulse a couple of times in a spice grinder or clean coffee grinder, just until the fennel is broken up a bit.

Transfer to a small bowl and stir in the lemon juice, agave nectar, shallot, and salt. Slowly pour in the olive oil, whisking all the while, and continue whisking until smooth. Transfer to a small container with a fitted lid and shake well. Do a FASS check. Depending on the type and taste of the lemons, you may want to add a teaspoon of olive oil or a pinch of salt.

Goes with My Family's Favorite Chicken (page 111), as a marinade. It also makes a good marinade for fish and is wonderful drizzled over roasted asparagus and other vegetables.

PREP TIME: 5 minutes · COOK TIME: 1 minute

STORAGE: Store in an airtight container in the refrigerator for 5 to 7 days.

PER SERVING: Calories: 65; Total Fat: 7 g (1 g saturated, 5 g monounsaturated); Carbohydrates: 1 g; Protein: 0 g; Fiber: 0 g; Sodium: 75 mg

Dried Fruit Compote

This is an absolute go-to dish for people taking pain medication. Why? Because many pain meds, especially opiates, can stop up the works, if you get my meaning. This isn't your typical fiber-laden, tasteless concoction. (Can you say bran muffin?) In addition to prunes, the traditional remedy, this compote also includes dried apricots and cherries, and we've also brought ginger and cardomom to the party. The result is a delicious compote that smells incredible while it's cooking and goes great over oatmeal or on toast. For those days when you need a kick start, this blend will nudge you in the right direction. Believe me, it works. Before cooking the compote, it's best to soak the fruit for a few hours, or preferably overnight, so plan ahead. This is great served warm or at room temperature. MAKES 4 TO 5 CUPS

- 1 cup pitted prunes
- 1 cup unsulfured dried apricots
- 1 cup dried cherries or raisins
- 3 cinnamon sticks
- 6 cardamom pods, or 1/4 teaspoon ground cardamom
- 1/2 teaspoon chopped fresh ginger, or 1/4 teaspoon ground ginger
- Pinch of sea salt
- 1/4 teaspoon freshly squeezed lemon juice

Combine the prunes, apricots, cherries, cinnamon, cardamom, ginger, and salt in a saucepan and add water to cover. Soak overnight, if possible, or for a few hours before cooking.

Bring the mixture to a boil over high heat, then lower the heat and gently simmer for about 1 hour, until the fruit is very, very soft and the liquid is syrupy. Stir in the lemon juice and remove from the heat. Remove and discard the cinnamon sticks.

Goes with Best Oatmeal Ever (page 128), Creamy Millet (page 136), and Creamiest Buckwheat (page 138).

PREP TIME: 5 minutes · COOK TIME: 1 hour

STORAGE: Store in an airtight container in the refrigerator for 7 days or in the freezer for 2 months.

PER SERVING: Calories: 303; Total Fat: 0 g (0 g saturated, 0 g monounsaturated); Carbohydrates: 70 g; Protein: 3 g; Fiber: 12 g; Sodium: 85 mg

REBECCA'S NOTES You can use dried apples, pears, figs, or any combination of dried fruit to equal 3 cups.

The compote is a versatile condiment that crosses culinary boundaries and can be used on both sweet and savory dishes. Stir it into yogurt, spoon it alongside a sweet potato, or serve it atop oatmeal. You can even use it like jam: spread a dollop on a piece of toast with almond butter.

Seasonal Stewed Fruit

A foodie friend of mine was in the hospital for leukemia treatments when his caregiver called me. Our buddy wasn't having a great day, and it didn't help that his doctors were saying he couldn't have his favorite pick-me-up food, fruit. Now this is a guy who can eat a quart of strawberries at a sitting. In a sense the docs were right; raw fruit can contain bacteria, a problem for people with low white blood cell counts, which show they're prone to infection. But I had a solution. I told his caregiver, "He can have fruit; you just have to cut it up and heat it thoroughly to kill off the germs." The docs had no objections, the caregiver came in with a beautiful medley of stewed seasonal fruit, and my friend was thrilled. So if you're concerned about raw fruits, this is the recipe for you. The heat, along with a little bit of lemon juice and a pinch of sea salt, breaks down the fruit's fiber, making it soft but not mushy. I used apricots and cherries here, but any fruit in season will do. MAKES 1 1/4 CUPS

- 4 large apricots, pitted and quartered
- 1 teaspoon freshly squeezed lemon juice
- Pinch of sea salt
- 10 cherries, stemmed and pitted
- 1 teaspoon agave nectar

REBECCA'S NOTES This fruit is warm and comforting and is the perfect topping for hot cereal, like Best Oatmeal Ever (page 128), Creamiest Buckwheat (page 138), or Creamy Millet (page 136).

Combine the apricots, lemon juice, and salt in a small saucepan over low heat and cook, stirring occasionally, until the fruit begins to soften, about 10 minutes. Stir in the cherries, cover, and cook, stirring often, until all of the fruit has softened, about 5 minutes. Remove from the heat and stir in the agave nectar. Serve hot, at room temperature, or chilled.

Variations: Make a yogurt parfait. Let cool the fruit to room temperature, then spoon 1/4 cup of plain organic yogurt into a glass, spoon in 1/4 cup of fruit, repeat with another layer of yogurt and then fruit. Serve topped with a sprinkle of Maple-Glazed Walnuts (page 144).

Substitute 2 cups of any seasonal fruit that is available at your local farmers' market or grocery store. Some of my favorite duets are: apples with pears, strawberries with rhubarb, and nectarines or peaches with blueberries. Cook firmer fruits first, and adjust the cooking time as needed.

PREP TIME: 10 minutes · COOK TIME: 15 minutes

STORAGE: Store in an airtight container in the refrigerator for 3 to 5 days.

PER SERVING: Calories: 30; Total Fat: 0.2 g (0 g saturated, 0 g monounsaturated); Carbohydrates: 7 g; Protein: 1 g; Fiber: 1 g; Sodium: 75 mg

Blueberry Compote

Blueberries contain lots of pectin, which helps soothe the stomach, and one of their active compounds can help prevent cancer cells from getting nourishment. MAKES 1 1/4 CUPS

- 1 1/2 cups frozen blueberries
- 1 teaspoon freshly squeezed orange or lemon juice
- 1 teaspoon orange or lemon zest
- 1 teaspoon maple syrup
- 1/4 teaspoon ground ginger

Combine all of the ingredients in a small saucepan over medium heat. Cook, stirring occasionally, for 3 to 4 minutes, until the mixture bubbles, pulls away from the sides of the pan, and becomes syrupy.

Variation: If you have fresh blueberries, all the better. Just add 2 tablespoons of water to the recipe.

Goes with Best Oatmeal Ever (page 128), Creamy Millet (page 136), and Creamiest Buckwheat (page 138).

PREP TIME: 5 minutes · COOK TIME: 10 minutes

STORAGE: Store in an airtight container in the refrigerator for 7 days or in the freezer for 2 months.

PER SERVING: Calories: 30; Total Fat: 0.4 g (0 g saturated, 0 g monounsaturated); Carbohydrates: 8 g; Protein: 0 g; Fiber: 2 g; Sodium: 0 mg

Mango and Avocado Salsa

Avocado sure knows how to tango with mango. As a taste and texture combo, it's one of the most refreshing two-steps I've come across. Mangoes are sweet, but not overly so. Avocados are creamy, but with some heft. Together, they make for a fantastic salsa that's especially great for people dealing with a metallic taste in the mouth due to treatment. With the added perkiness of the red bell pepper, cilantro, and lime, this salsa whirls around the dance floor of your palate. MAKES 2 CUPS

- 1 cup diced mango
- 1 cup diced avocado
- 3 tablespoons finely diced red bell pepper
- 3 tablespoons finely chopped fresh cilantro
- 2 tablespoons freshly squeezed lime juice
- 1 tablespoon extra-virgin olive oil
- 1/4 teaspoon sea salt
- Pinch of cayenne

Mix all of the ingredients together then do a FASS check. For optimal flavor, let the salsa sit for 30 minutes.

Variations: Substitute tomatoes or papaya for the mango.

For a beautiful fall salsa, and the ultimate antioxidant rush, substitute 1/2 cup of pomegranate seeds for the mango.

Goes with My Family's Favorite Chicken (page 111), as well as fish, grilled chicken, and salads.

PREP TIME: 20 minutes · COOK TIME: Not applicable

STORAGE: Store in an airtight container in the refrigerator for 4 days.

PER SERVING: Calories: 30; Total Fat: 2.3 g (0.3 g saturated, 1.6 g monounsaturated); Carbohydrates: 3 g; Protein: 0 g; Fiber: 1 g; Sodium: 40 mg

Olive and Caper Relish

In baseball, the utility man is the one who can do everything. He keeps four different gloves on hand in case he's called on to play catcher, first base, the infield, or the outfield. I suppose he also does the team's laundry between games of a doubleheader. I think of capers as my utility guys, capable of blending into many dishes from eggs to polenta. Capers, which are actually flower buds, are usually pickled. They may be tiny, but they pack a flavorful punch. Here, they're blended with chopped olives and lemon zest to create a mouth-popping relish. MAKES 1/2 CUP

- 1/3 cup pitted kalamata olives, rinsed and chopped
- 2 teaspoons capers, rinsed and chopped
- 1 teaspoon extra-virgin olive oil
- 1/4 teaspoon freshly squeezed lemon juice
- 1/8 teaspoon lemon zest
- 2 tablespoons chopped fresh basil

Stir all of the ingredients together.

Goes with Baked Citrus Halibut with Tomato Sauce (page 123), My Family's Favorite Chicken (page 111), Nana's Egg Salad (page 114), Lemon Mustard Salmon Salad (page 109), and Creamy Polenta (page 134). This relish is also great on a variety of fish, chicken, pasta, and rice dishes, or use it as a sandwich spread or a topping for crostini.

PREP TIME: 5 minutes · COOK TIME: Not applicable

STORAGE: Store in an airtight container in the refrigerator for 7 days.

PER SERVING: Calories: 20; Total Fat: 2 g (0.3 g saturated, 1.5 g monounsaturated); Carbohydrates: 1 g; Protein: 0 g; Fiber: 0 g; Sodium: 110 mg

Moroccan Pesto

This dazzling emerald green sauce is incredibly versatile. MAKES 1 CUP

- 1 cup tightly packed fresh parsley
- 1/2 cup tightly packed fresh cilantro or basil leaves
- 6 fresh mint leaves
- 1/2 teaspoon ground cumin
- 1/2 teaspoon paprika
- 1 clove garlic, chopped
- 1/4 cup extra-virgin olive oil
- 3 tablespoons freshly squeezed lemon juice
- 1/4 teaspoon salt
- 2 tablespoons water (optional)

Combine all of the ingredients in a food processor and process until well blended. Do a FASS check to see whether you need to add another squeeze or two of lemon juice, and add water to achieve the desired consistency.

Goes with poached salmon (page 121) My Family's Favorite Chicken (page 111), Triple Citrus Black Cod (page 118), and Middle Eastern Chickpea Burgers (page 112).

PREP TIME: 5 minutes · COOK TIME: Not applicable

STORAGE: Store in airtight container in the refrigerator for 7 days or in the freezer for 2 months.

PER SERVING: Calories: 35; Total Fat: 3.6 g (0.5 g saturated, 2.5 g monounsaturated); Carbohydrates: 1 g; Protein: 0 g; Fiber: 0 g; Sodium: 40 mg

Parsley Basil Drizzle

Drizzles and dollops are very helpful for people who are dealing with impaired taste buds as a result of treatment. Drizzles are a bit like Roman candles; they light up the palette. They're lighter than dollops, but don't be fooled; the parsley in this drizzle is like a whiff of pure oxygen. It's that energizing. MAKES 1/2 CUP

- 1/4 cup tightly packed fresh basil leaves
- 1/2 cup tightly packed fresh flat-leaf parsley leaves
- 2 tablespoons freshly squeezed lemon juice
- 1 tablespoon water
- 1/4 teaspoon sea salt
- 1/4 cup extra-virgin olive oil

REBECCA'S NOTES This is the base recipe for pesto. If you want a richer, thicker sauce, add 1/4 cup of pine nuts or chopped walnuts along with the herbs.

Combine the basil, parsley, lemon juice, water, and salt in a blender or food processor and process until finely chopped. With the motor running, slowly pour in the olive oil and continue to process until very smooth. Do a quick FASS check. If the drizzle tastes too sour, add another pinch of salt.

Goes with Cooling Cucumber Avocado Soup (page 70), Minestrone (page 64), Roasted Red Roma Tomato Soup (page 69), Creamy Broccoli and Potato Soup (page 75), Italian White Bean Soup (page 57), Lemon Mustard Salmon Salad (page 109), Nana's Egg Salad (page 114), My Family's Favorite Chicken (page 111), Easy Eggs in a Cup (page 102), Basil Broccoli (page 78), Mediterranean Lentil Salad (page 142), Simple Tuscan Farro (page 148), and Tuscan Farro and Bean Salad (page 107). It's also great over poached eggs (see page 115).

PREP TIME: 5 minutes · COOK TIME: Not applicable

STORAGE: Store in an airtight container in the refrigerator for 3 days. Shake well before serving.

PER SERVING: Calories: 60; Total Fat: 7 g (1 g saturated, 5 g monounsaturated); Carbohydrates: 1 g; Protein: 0 g; Fiber: 0 g; Sodium: 75 mg

Signora's Tomato Sauce

I cooked for a lot of crazy signoras when I lived in Italy, and one of them whipped me into shape by insisting that the tomatoes for tomato sauce be put through a food mill first. For the uninitiated, it's kind of like an old coffee mill, but with a more tightly geared hand crank. In would go the roasted tomatoes, and each crank by hand would squeeze them through holes in the side of the mill. I needed a tube of Bengay for my arms after the first batch, but the result is a far lighter sauce than any store-bought variety. If you're not up for the workout, just lightly pulse the tomatoes in a food processor. SERVES 6

- 4 pounds Roma tomatoes, halved
- 2 tablespoons extra-virgin olive oil
- Sea salt
- 1 onion, diced small
- 2 carrots, scrubbed and diced small
- 2 cloves garlic, chopped
- 2 cups loosely packed fresh basil leaves, chopped

CULINARY RX Tomatoes have been touted for having lycopene, a well-studied antioxidant that appears to have protective properties against many types of cancer. A few tricks can help you coax a little more lycopene out of these colorful orbs. Heat is one key. Tomatoes grown in hot weather produce more lycopene, and cooking boosts the availability of this phytochemical. Ohio State University scientists decided to do a little home cooking and found that using oil and a second round of heat (260°F for 40 minutes) created a tomato sauce that allowed participants to absorb 55 percent more lycopene. If tomatoes aren't your thing, watermelon is also high in lycopene.

Preheat the oven to 400°F.

Gently squeeze the tomatoes by hand to remove excess seeds, then put them in a bowl and toss with 1 tablespoon of the olive oil and 1/2 teaspoon of salt. Place the tomatoes, cut side down, in a single layer on sheet pans and roast for 20 to 30 minutes, until the skins are just browning and the juices are bubbly. Let cool for 5 minutes, then lift off the skins with a fork.

Meanwhile, heat the remaining 1 tablespoon olive oil in a large saucepan, then add the onion and a pinch of salt and sauté until golden, about 5 minutes. Add the carrots, garlic, and 1/4 teaspoon of salt and continue to sauté until the carrots become just tender, about 5 minutes.

Lift the tomatoes off the sheet pans and transfer to a food processor, then pour in any pan juices. Add the carrot mixture and the basil and pulse until pureed but still a little chunky.

Transfer back into the saucepan and stir in 1/4 teaspoon of salt. Do a FASS check. Tomatoes can sometimes be acidic, so you may want to add a pinch of sweetener and another pinch of salt.

Variation: If fresh tomatoes aren't available, you can substitute two 28-ounce cans of plum tomatoes.

Goes with baked halibut (page 123), Creamy Polenta (page 134), and a wide variety of pasta dishes.

PREP TIME: 20 minutes · COOK TIME: 30 minutes

STORAGE: Store in an airtight container in the refrigerator for 5 days or in the freezer for 2 months.

PER SERVING: Calories: 120; Total Fat: 5.4 g (0.8 g saturated, 3.5 g monounsaturated); Carbohydrates: 17 g; Protein: 4 g; Fiber: 5 g; Sodium: 230 mg

Sweet and Savory Yogurt

Yogurt is a wonderful international culinary staple that's been subverted by American agribusiness. Contrary to popular belief, genuine yogurt is anything but the thick, overly sweetened blend you're likely to find in the refrigerated section at your local grocery store. Designed as quickie substitutes for breakfast, too often they're laden with copious sugar for a rapid ride on the glucose express. Real yogurt—the healthier version known to the rest of the world—is generally much lighter. It's also served in a wider variety of contexts, such as Indian raitas, *served as a condiment, and Greek* tzatziki, *a combination of cucumbers and yogurt served as a dip, condiment, or spread. Yogurt (the name is Turkish) is meant to refresh, and this version is an ideal topping on cucumbers, lamb, or Middle Eastern Chickpea Burgers (page 112). When I first proposed this blend, one of my recipe testers looked at the long list of ingredients and asked, "all this for yogurt?" And then she took a taste . . .* MAKES 4 CUPS

- 20 unsulfured dried apricots
- 2/3 cup golden raisins
- 1/3 cup finely chopped and loosely packed fresh flat-leaf parsley
- 1/3 cup finely chopped and loosely packed fresh cilantro
- 1/3 cup finely chopped and loosely packed fresh mint leaves
- 1/3 cup coarsely chopped Maple-Glazed Walnuts (page 141)
- 1 tablespoon extra-virgin olive oil
- 1 1/2 teaspoons maple syrup
- 1 teaspoon freshly squeezed lemon juice
- 1/4 teaspoon sea salt
- 1/4 teaspoon ground cumin
- 1/8 teaspoon ground cinnamon
- 2 cups organic plain yogurt

Soak the apricots and raisins separately in hot water for 10 minutes, then drain well and pat dry. Set aside the raisins and chop the apricots into bite-size pieces. Stir all of the ingredients together until thoroughly combined, then do a FASS check. You may want to add a pinch of salt, a spritz of lemon juice, or a bit more sweetener.

Cover tightly and chill for 15 minutes before serving.

Variations: Add 1 1/2 to 2 teaspoons of curry powder.

In place of the parsley, cilantro, and mint, you can substitute 1/3 cup each of finely chopped and loosely packed fresh dill, basil, and thyme.

Goes with Middle Eastern Chickpea Burgers (page 112), Orange Pistachio Couscous (page 145), Quinoa Pilaf (page 149), Mediterranean Lentil Salad (page 142), and Poached Salmon with Moroccan Pesto (page 121).

PREP TIME: 20 minutes · COOK TIME: 15 minutes (plus 15 minutes to chill)

STORAGE: Store in a covered container in the refrigerator for 3 to 5 days.

PER SERVING: Calories: 350; Total Fat: 12.9 g (3.6 g saturated, 4.3 g monounsaturated); Carbohydrates: 52 g; Protein: 7 g; Fiber: 4 g; Sodium: 270 mg

CHAPTER 9

Sweet Bites

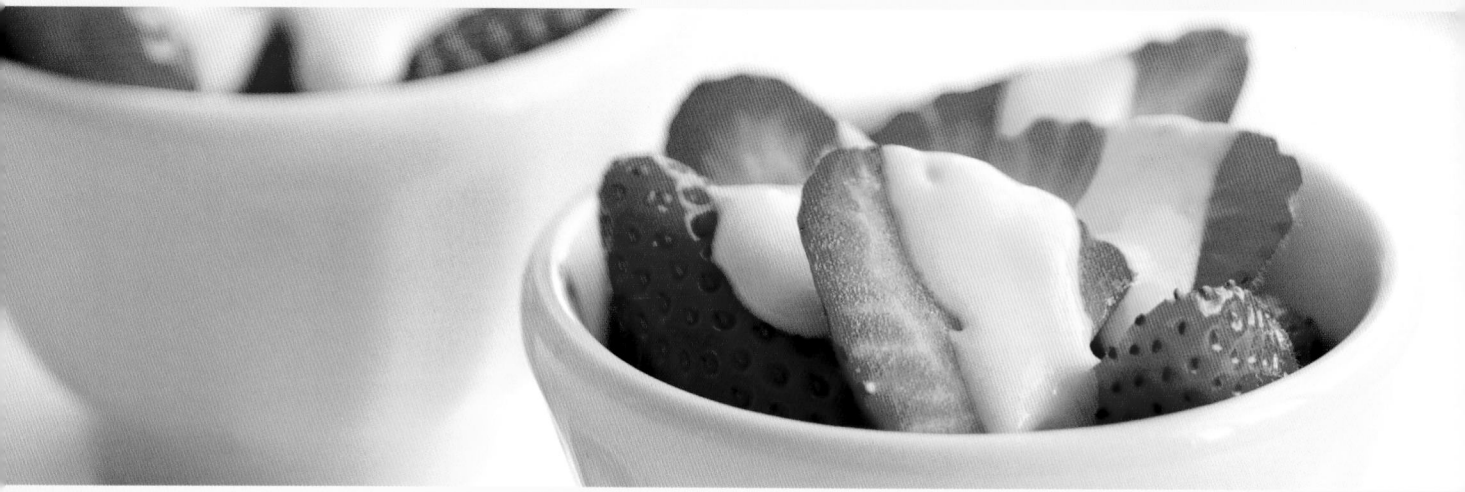

192 *Almond Muffin Mania*

194 *Baked Apples Filled with Dates and Pecans*

195 *Chocolate Tapioca Pudding*

197 *Cardamom Maple Mini Macaroons*

198 *Coconut Rice Pudding*

200 *Great Pumpkin Custard*

201 *Wendy's Date Nut Truffles*

203 *Poached Pears with Saffron Broth*

204 *Strawberries with Mango Coconut "Sabayon"*

207 *Triple Ginger Snap Cookies with Pecans*

Somewhere along the line, I discovered that I was completely and utterly missing the baking gene. At first I was horrified; I felt like a computer programmer who couldn't figure out Windows. Then I learned that most chefs can cook or bake, but not both. I guess it's kind of a left brain versus right brain thing, or like yin and yang. This is why I thank the heavens above for Wendy Remer, überbaker, master chocolatier, breast cancer survivor, dear, dear friend, and the confectionary magician who helped me come up with these recipes.

I absolutely knew I had to have Sweet Bites in this book, because I firmly believe that if someone is cut off from a food group they love, including desserts and sweets, they're at risk for disconnecting from food altogether. The challenge was coming up with desserts that weren't full of empty calories and foods the experts suggested avoiding during treatment.

So I talked to Wendy, sounding for all the world like a kid on Santa's lap with a wish list a mile long: "I'd like a coconut rice pudding and ginger cookies. And wouldn't be great if we did a cardamom macaroon? And for chocolate lovers, we must have a truffle. Oh, and by the way, no refined sugar or white flour. And the recipes should avoid gluten and dairy, if possible."

Wendy gave me a look like I had just asked her to tie a knot in a cherry stem with just her mouth. "Uh," she said, flatly, "I'll see what I can do."

What she did was incredible. Unbelievable. Yum to a factor of ten. Wendy lives nearby, and each time she cooked a new batch of something, we were like secret agents. "Meet me at the bottom of the hill," Wendy would say, and we'd both rush there like it was a pivotal moment in human history. Sometimes we didn't even make it to the parking lot for our taste test. We'd just plop down curbside, out would come, say, those cardamom macaroons, and, *munch, munch,* we'd nod and compare notes, and off Wendy would go to tweak the recipe. We knew she'd gotten it right when she called and said, "I'll bring 'em right over, if I have any left."

"Why wouldn't you have any left?" I asked.

"Well," she replied, "they kinda keep disappearing."

I have a feeing you're about to have a similar experience.

Almond Muffin Mania

A little saying around my kitchen is "If it's white, it's just not right." Many white products, espcially white sugar and white flour, have been processed to the point where they've been stripped of both color and nutrients. Nutritionists say these foods contain empty calories, meaning calories without meaningful amounts of vitamins, minerals, and other micronutrients. Empty calories aren't a good idea for anyone, and they're a definite no-no for people already dealing with diminished appetites. These muffins aren't the monsters so often seen in bakeries—they're smaller and healthier, but no less flavorful. The basic recipe, which is delicious on its own, is built on a foundation of spelt flour, agave nectar, and almonds, which are packed with nutrients. I've also provided a couple of variations below, for chocolate orange muffins and ginger lemon muffins; all three versions have one thing in common: They're little bites of powerful joy! MAKES 24 MINI MUFFINS

- 1 1/2 cups almond meal
- 1/2 cup spelt flour
- 1 tablespoon baking powder
- 1/8 teaspoon sea salt
- 1/3 cup agave nectar
- 1/2 cup mashed banana
- 1/4 cup organic milk, almond milk, rice milk, or soy milk
- 2 organic eggs
- 1/4 cup unrefined virgin coconut oil, almond oil, or a neutral-flavored extra-virgin olive oil
- 1 1/2 teaspoons almond extract
- 1/2 teaspoon vanilla extract

REBECCA'S NOTES Mini muffin tins come in a variety of sizes. I prefer using tins with a wide base, around 1 1/2 inches in diameter. Don't despair if you can find that exact size, as most anything will work.

To prevent muffins from sticking to the bottom of the pan, make sure you grease the pan really, really, really well. Then, after baking you must exercise patience and allow the muffins to cool completely before removing them from the tin.

Preheat the oven to 350°F. Prepare a mini muffin tin by generously oiling each cup.

Combine the almond meal, spelt flour, baking powder, and salt in a bowl and stir with a whisk until very well combined. Separately, combine the agave nectar, mashed banana, milk, eggs, oil, almond extract, and vanilla and whisk until smooth. Add the wet mixture to the dry and mix well with a rubber spatula.

Spoon the batter into the muffin cups, filling each about three-quarters full. Bake for 13 to 15 minutes, until a muffin springs back when touched in the center. Let cool on a wire rack for 15 minutes, then gently run a knife or small offset spatula around the sides of the muffins to loosen them before turning them out.

Variations: To make chocolate orange muffins, replace 1/4 cup of the flour with 1/4 cup unsweetened cocoa powder. Omit the extracts and instead add 1 tablespoon of orange zest or 1 teaspoons of orange oil (not orange extract) to the wet ingredients. Fold 1/3 cup chopped chocolate or mini chocolate chips into the batter once it's mixed.

For ginger lemon muffins, add 1 teaspoon of ground ginger to the dry ingredients. Omit the extracts, and instead add 3 tablespoons of finely chopped peeled fresh ginger, 2 to 3 tablespoons of lemon zest, and 1 tablespoon of freshly squeezed lemon juice to the wet ingredients.

For gluten-free muffins, replace spelt flour with brown rice flour.

PREP TIME: 7 minutes · COOK TIME: 15 minutes (plus time to cool)

STORAGE: Store in an airtight container at room temperature for 5 to 7 days or in the freezer for 2 months.

PER SERVING: Calories: 100; Total Fat: 6.4 g (2.4 g saturated, 0.4 g mono-unsaturated); Carbohydrates: 8 g; Protein: 3 g; Fiber: 1 g; Sodium: 75 mg

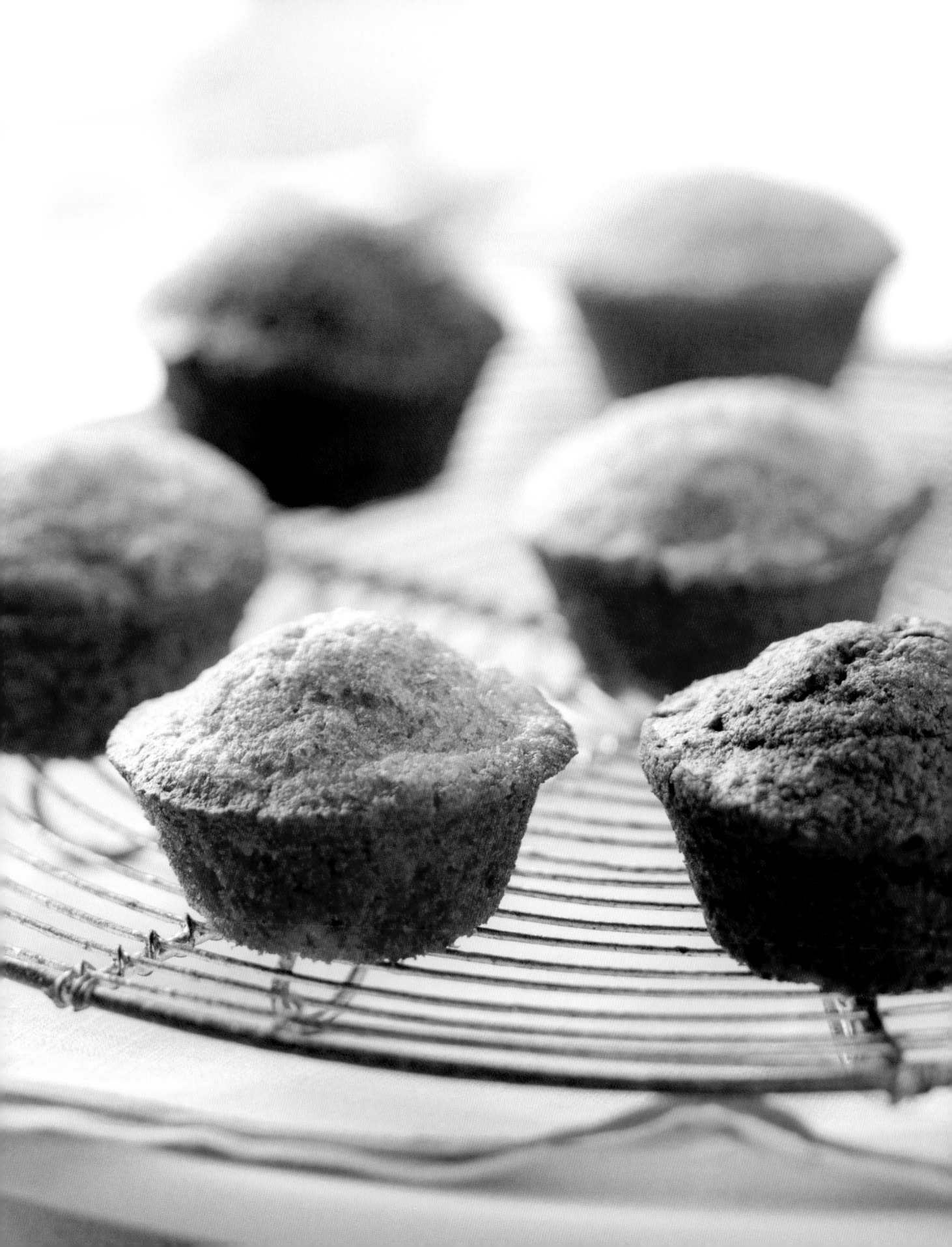

Baked Apples Filled with Dates and Pecans

When I told my friend about this baked apple dish, he said it reminded him of an old folk recipe. When he was little and had an upset tummy, his Russian grandmother would cut up an apple and leave it out on the counter for a few minutes, until it began to brown. His grandmother would then say, "Come eat, tatellah" (an affectionate way of saying, "little man" in Yiddish). Lo and behold, a few minutes later his stomach felt better. He always figured it was love at work (and, of course, it was), but years later he found out there was also some science involved: As they brown—or cook, in this case—apples release pectin, which naturally soothes the belly. Baking makes the pectin and the rest of the apple easier to digest. In this recipe, the apples are complemented by a whole host of tasty morsels and spices—toasted pecans, dates, orange zest, and cinnamon—and as they bake, they smell heavenly. SERVES 4

- 1/4 cup finely chopped toasted pecans (see page 97)
- 1/4 cup pitted and finely diced Medjool dates
- Zest and juice of 1 orange
- 1/4 teaspoon ground cinnamon
- 1/4 teaspoon sea salt
- 4 baking apples, such as Pink Lady, Pippin, or McIntosh
- 1 tablespoon organic butter (optional)
- Unfiltered apple juice, for baking

REBECCA'S NOTES If you don't have dates or pecans, be creative! You can substitute currants or raisins and walnuts or almonds, and if nuts are a problem, you can simply omit them. You can use clarified butter if you like, or for a dairy-free version use coconut oil.

Use a melon baller to scoop out the apple core; it's important to keep the base intact.

Preheat the oven to 350°F.

Combine the pecans, dates, orange zest and juice, cinnamon, and salt in a small bowl and stir to combine.

Core the apples, leaving half an inch at the bottom, and peel the top edges. Stuff the apples with the pecan filling, then dot the butter on top or melt the butter and brush it on the apple tops.

Put the apples in a baking pan, pour in about 1 inch of apple juice, and cover tightly with foil. Bake for 40 to 60 minutes, until the apples are tender but not mushy. Test for doneness by poking a fork into the apples; they should be tender and yield easily to pressure.

Serve warm, drizzled with the warm apple juice from the baking pan.

PREP TIME: 20 minutes · COOK TIME: 60 minutes

STORAGE: Store in an airtight container in the refrigerator for 3 days.

PER SERVING: Calories: 205; Total Fat: 5.8 g (0.5 g saturated, 3.1 g monounsaturated); Carbohydrates: 41 g; Protein: 2 g; Fiber: 7 g; Sodium: 150 mg

Chocolate Tapioca Pudding

One of the reasons comfort foods are such a big part of this book is that in times of stress, it's natural to seek out foods that have never let you down. So it is with tapioca pudding, a staple throughout the world. The cassava root, which is made into tapioca pearls, is rich in carbohydrates and gluten free, making this dessert a good treat for people who want to maintain weight without taxing the digestive system. A little chocolate sweetens the package, making this an ideal dessert to eat by the fireplace. Be sure to use very high-quality chocolate to enhance the yum factor. You can make tapioca without presoaking, but plan on an extra 10 to 20 minutes of cooking time. SERVES 8

- 1/2 cup small pearl tapioca
- 2 cups water, for soaking
- 3 cups organic milk, almond milk, rice milk, or soy milk
- 1/8 teaspoon sea salt
- 2 organic eggs
- 1/3 cup maple syrup
- 1/3 cup finely chopped bittersweet or semisweet chocolate
- 2 teaspoons vanilla extract

WHO KNEW? The Moo Blues
If you like milk and dairy products, here's a reason to think about which products you allow in your house. Commercially raised dairy cows are generally little milk factories. That's good for the breeder, but it means the cows also tend to have a lot of insulin-like growth factors (IGFs) in their milk. One such factor, IGF-1, has been linked to tumor progression. The commercial corn feed these cows are given may also be problematic, as it's high in undesirable omega-6 fatty acids. Experts suggest that if you're going to consume dairy products, seek out organic versions from grass-fed cows for a better nutritional mix.

Soak the tapioca in the water overnight.

Drain the tapioca and discard the liquid. Combine the milk and salt in a heavy bottomed saucepan and bring almost to a simmer; tiny bubbles will form around the edges of the pan. Stir in the tapioca and bring to a boil, stirring constantly, then turn down the heat as low as possible and cook, stirring frequently, for 10 to 15 minutes, until tapioca pearls have swollen and are translucent and tender. (If the tapioca is not presoaked, the extra cooking time will come in here.)

Whisk the eggs and maple syrup together in small bowl, then gradually add 1 cup of the tapioca mixture to the eggs while whisking constantly. Whisk the egg mixture back into the saucepan with the tapioca and continue to cook over very low heat, stirring constantly, until the pudding is bubbling gently. Cook for about 5 minutes, until somewhat thickened. The pudding will do most of its thickening while it cools, so don't overcook it at this point or the texture will be rubbery texture.

Remove from the heat and stir in the chopped chocolate. Let stand for 1 minute, then stir until the chocolate has melted and is thoroughly mixed into the pudding. Stir in the vanilla.

Transfer to a heatproof bowl or serving dish and serve warm or chilled. If you're serving it chilled and want to prevent a skin from forming, place a piece of parchment paper directly on the surface of the pudding and refrigerate for at least 2 hours.

PREP TIME: 5 minutes (after soaking the tapioca overnight)
COOK TIME: 25 minutes
STORAGE: Store in an airtight container in the refrigerator for 3 to 5 days.
PER SERVING: Calories: 180; Total Fat: 6.1 g (3.2 g saturated, 1.2 g monounsaturated); Carbohydrates: 26 g; Protein: 6 g; Fiber: 0 g; Sodium: 95 mg

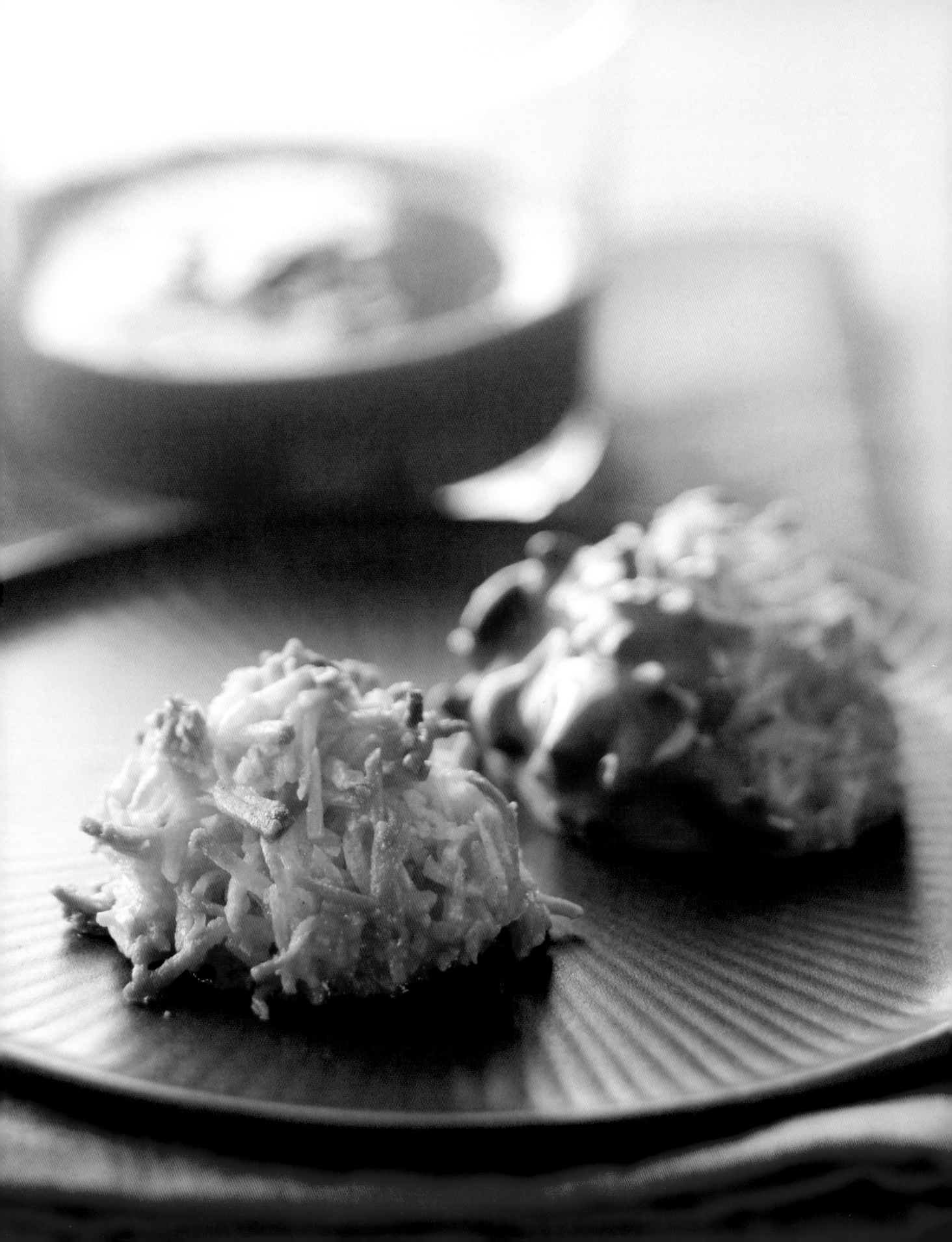

Cardamom Maple Mini Macaroons

I knew I wanted to do a cardamom macaroon recipe for this book because my grandmother, Doris, got me hooked on them when I was knee-high. My baker for this book, Wendy Remer, also has macaroon fever. These bite-size morsels are made using organic maple syrup with either a tad of brown rice syrup or honey for just the right amount of sweet. Meanwhile, cardamom adds a warm, spicy touch, while also aiding digestion and possibly slowing tumor growth. MAKES 24 MACAROONS

2 organic egg whites

1/2 cup maple syrup

1 tablespoon brown rice syrup or honey

Pinch of sea salt

1 1/2 cups unsweetened shredded coconut

2 tablespoons all-purpose unbleached white flour

1/2 teaspoon vanilla extract

1/4 teaspoon ground cardamom

REBECCA'S NOTES If you want a sweeter macaroon, bake these with honey. For a more mellow sweet taste that isn't over the top, use the brown rice syrup.

Preheat the oven to 325°F and line a baking sheet with parchment paper.

Combine the egg whites, maple syrup, brown rice syrup, and salt in a saucepan over medium heat and cook, stirring constantly, until just warm, about 1 minute. Add the coconut, flour, vanilla, and cardamom and continue to cook, stirring constantly, until the mixture just begins to sizzle and is slightly dry, about 2 minutes. Remove from the heat and let cool for a few minutes.

Using a teaspoon and your fingers, form the dough into 24 small mounds on the prepared pan. Bake for 20 to 25 minutes, until golden brown. Let cool completely before serving.

Variation: For a more decadent dessert, dip the macaroons in chocolate. Chop your favorite dark chocolate and place it in a dry metal or glass bowl and set it over a pan of gently simmering hot water (or use a double boiler if you have one). Stir the chocolate constantly until just melted, then remove it from the heat. Now for the fun part: Dip the macaroons into the melted chocolate, then place them on a pan or plate lined with wax or parchment paper. Chill in the refrigerator until the chocolate hardens, then enjoy!

PREP TIME: 10 minutes · COOK TIME: 20 minutes

STORAGE: Store in an airtight container at room temperature for 5 to 7 days.

PER SERVING: Calories: 55; Total Fat: 3 g (2.7 g saturated, 0.1 g monounsaturated); Carbohydrates: 7 g; Protein: 1 g; Fiber: 1 g; Sodium: 20 mg

Coconut Rice Pudding

Rice pudding is a soothing must-have for many people. The challenge here was figuring out how to create a delicious, healthier version that still had all of that creamy goodness without too much dairy. After a lot of tinkering together with my dessert maven, Wendy, we found that combining coconut milk—which has great nutritional qualities—and regular milk gave us the taste and consistency we were looking for, with a kick of flavor coming from the cardamom and orange. If you want to go completely dairy free, see the variation below. SERVES 6

- 1/4 cup Arborio rice
- 2 cups water
- 2 1/2 cups organic milk
- 3/4 cup coconut milk
- 2 tablespoons maple syrup
- 1/4 teaspoon ground cardamom
- Pinch of sea salt
- 1/2 teaspoon orange zest
- 2 teaspoons vanilla extract
- 1/4 cup raisins or currants (optional)
- Dried Fruit Compote (page 183), Blueberry Compote (page 185), or Seasonal Stewed Fruit (page 184), for serving

Combine the rice and water in a heavy bottomed saucepan and bring to a boil. Lower the heat and simmer gently, uncovered, for 10 minutes.

Drain the rice, rinse the saucepan, then put the milk, coconut milk, maple syrup, cardamom, and salt in the saucepan and bring to a boil. Stir in the rice, turn down the heat to medium-low, and simmer gently, stirring occasionally for about 30 minutes; during the last 10 minutes of cooking, stir more frequently to prevent sticking or scorching. The pudding is done when the rice is tender and starts to stick to the bottom of the pan and the pudding has the consistency of loose oatmeal. It will thicken as it cools.

Remove from the heat and stir in the orange zest, vanilla, and raisins. Transfer to a heatproof bowl or serving dish and serve warm or chilled. If you're serving it chilled and want to prevent a skin from forming, place a piece of parchment paper directly on the surface of the pudding and chill for at least 2 hours. Top with compote just before serving.

Variations: To make a dairy-free version of this recipe, use 2 1/4 cups of soy milk or rice milk in place of the regular milk and increase the amount of coconut milk to 1 cup. The dairy-free version will take about 5 minutes less to cook.

To increase the yum factor, and for a bit of crunch, sprinkle some toasted coconut or sliced almonds on top before serving.

PREP TIME: 5 minutes · COOK TIME: 40 minutes

STORAGE: Store in an airtight container in the refrigerator for 3 to 5 days.

PER SERVING: Calories: 455; Total Fat: 9.4 g (7.2 g saturated, 1.1 g monounsaturated); Carbohydrates: 84 g; Protein: 7 g; Fiber: 12 g; Sodium: 177 mg

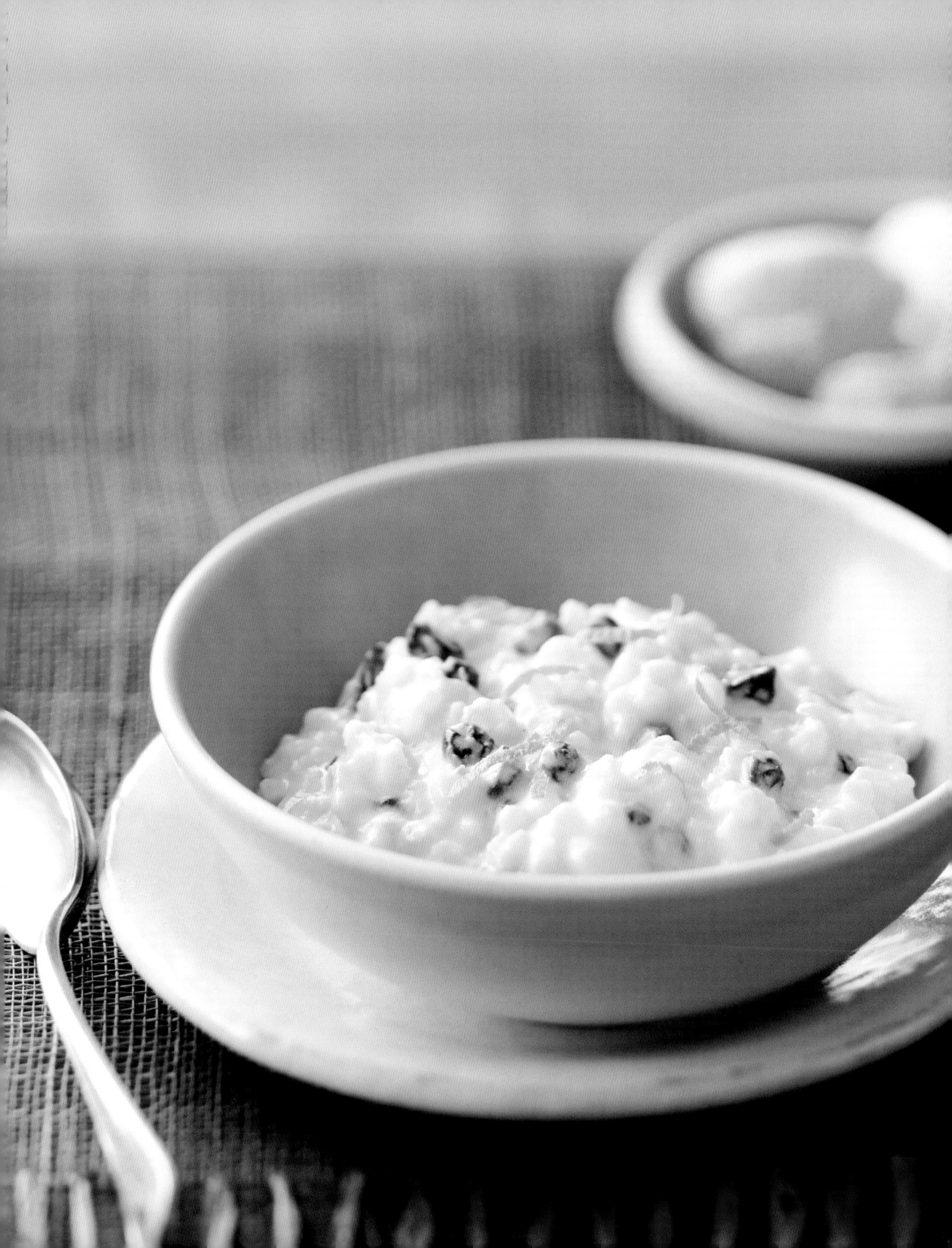

Great Pumpkin Custard

When I was in college, I always loved coming home at the holidays—in part because of my mother's pumpkin pie. I still love pumpkin, as does my husband, so this recipe is for him. I was looking for something that could deliver that awesome pumpkin taste without a fat-laden crust, and the homey familiarity of custard provided a perfect vehicle. SERVES 6

1 cup canned pumpkin puree
3/4 teaspoon ground cinnamon
1/2 teaspoon sea salt
1/2 teaspoon ground ginger
1/8 teaspoon ground cardamom
Pinch of freshly grated nutmeg
2 organic eggs
1/3 cup maple syrup
1 teaspoon vanilla extract
1 cup organic milk or soy milk

REBECCA'S NOTES Make sure that the baking pan you use to hold the ramekins has sides that are at least 3 inches high. This will ensure that the hot water you pour in doesn't slosh over when you transfer the pan to and from the oven.

Preheat the oven to 325°F.

Stir the pumpkin, cinnamon, salt, ginger, cardamom, and nutmeg together in a large bowl. In a smaller bowl, beat the eggs lightly, then whisk in the maple syrup, vanilla, and milk. Whisk the egg mixture into the pumpkin mixture until well combined.

Pour the custard into 6 1/2-cup ramekins. Place the ramekins in a baking pan and add enough hot water to the dish to come up 2 inches high around the ramekins. Carefully transfer to the oven and bake for 45 to 55 minutes, until a knife inserted into the center comes out clean. Serve warm or chilled.

PREP TIME: 5 minutes · COOK TIME: 60 minutes
STORAGE: Store in an airtight container in the refrigerator for 3 days.
PER SERVING: Calories: 110; Total Fat: 3.2 g (1.4 g saturated, 1 g monounsaturated); Carbohydrates: 18 g; Protein: 4 g; Fiber: 1 g; Sodium: 240 mg

"My tidbit for cancer survivors is that whatever you liked to eat B.C. (before cancer) may not work A.C. (after cancer). I always liked bread and crackers, but the dry mouth and swallowing issues from oral cancer made those foods difficult. Nothing tasted good at first except homemade egg custard."
—Roberta R., lymphoma survivor

Wendy's Date Nut Truffles

One day my coauthor, Mat, was reminiscing to his mom, Clair, about an ice cream store he worked at while in college. "I told her that I got so sick of ice cream that for two years after I quit I couldn't go near it." At which point Clair mentioned that as a girl she worked for years at the chocolate counter at Gimbel's, one of New York's famous retailers. Gimbel's let you eat as much chocolate as you liked on the job, so long as you didn't take any home. "I asked Mom if she ever got sick of chocolate. She just looked at me like I was nuts and said, 'Why would I?'" Which brings us to these little morsels. For chocolate aficionados, nothing provides a better fix than a truffle. My friend Wendy, an incredible chocolatier, designed these confections from a scrumptious mélange of chocolate, dates, orange zest, and ground nuts, all rolled in coconut. I could tell you that the reason to eat these is because they're high in protein and phytochemicals, but how 'bout we just call that a nice side benefit of yum! Since you're going to indulge in a chocolate dessert, be sure to make it the best by using high-quality chocolate.

MAKES 20 TRUFFLES

- 1/4 cup finely diced dried apricots
- 2 tablespoons boiling water
- 2 ounces dark chocolate with a 64 to 72 percent cacao content, finely chopped
- 1/3 cup plus 2 tablespoons almonds
- 1 cup pitted and halved Medjool dates
- 1 1/2 teaspoons orange zest, or 1/2 teaspoon orange oil (not orange extract)
- 1/8 teaspoon sea salt
- 1/2 cup unsweetened shredded coconut

REBECCA'S NOTES Cacao content is the amount of pure cocoa bean used in the chocolate; the higher the percentage, the more chocolate, which also means less sugar. Plus, the higher the cacao content, the more antioxidants in the chocolate.

Soak the diced apricots in cold water for 5 minutes.

Stir the boiling water into the chopped chocolate and let it stand for 30 seconds. Using a small whisk, stir until the chocolate is completely melted and glossy.

Coarsely grind the almonds in a food processor, then add the dates, orange zest, salt, and the chocolate mixture and process until smooth, about 1 minute. Transfer to a bowl; drain the apricots well and stir them into the chocolate mixture. Cover and chill for approximately 2 hours, until firm.

Scatter the coconut on a large plate. Scoop up approximately 1 tablespoon of the chocolate mixture and roll it into a smooth ball between your palms, then roll it in the coconut to coat. Repeat with the remaining mixture, then place the truffles in an airtight container and chill thoroughly before serving.

Variation: Substitute 1/2 cup of pecans for the almonds.

PREP TIME: 15 minutes · COOK TIME: 2 hours in the refrigerator

STORAGE: Store in an airtight container in the refrigerator for 1 week or in the freezer for 2 months.

PER SERVING: Calories: 145; Total Fat: 7.5 g (3.6 g saturated, 2.1 g monounsaturated); Carbohydrates: 19 g; Protein: 2 g; Fiber: 3 g; Sodium: 30 mg

Poached Pears with Saffron Broth

I call this "company food"—as in, what can I make for company that's easy but impressive? Poaching a pear sounds fancy, but all you're doing is simmering it in a fruity broth. The poaching softens up the pear, making it a breeze to chew and digest. The Saffron Broth turns the pears a beautiful sunset yellow color. Or if you prefer, check out the vanilla and star anise variations below. All three are light, refreshing, and nourishing; if you're looking for extra calories, top with a generous dollop of nut cream. SERVES 4

SAFFRON BROTH

4 cups pear nectar

1/4 teaspoon agave nectar

Zest of 1 lemon, in long pieces

4 inches peeled fresh ginger, cut into 1/4-inch pieces

4 teaspoons maple syrup

Generous pinch of saffron (12 to 15 threads)

2 ripe but firm pears, preferably Bosc or Comice, peeled, cut in half, seeded, and stemmed

Pistachio Cream (page 181) or Cashew Cream (page 180), for serving (optional)

REBECCA'S NOTES To seed and stem a pear beautifully, once it's cut in half, use a melon baller to scoop out the center, making sure to remove all of the seeds. Then use a sharp paring knife to make a small angled slice on each side of the core, running out from the center of the pear to the stem. This will remove a clean and even triangle-shaped piece where the stem and the core had been.

You can garnish the pears with the solids from the broth. Lemon peel, vanilla pods, star anise pods, and cloves all make beautiful garnishes.

To make the broth, stir the pear nectar, agave nectar, lemon zest, ginger, maple syrup, and saffron together in a large saucepan or 3-quart sauté pan over medium-high heat. Bring to a boil, then place the pear halves in the saucepan, flat side down. Place a piece of parchment paper over the pears and cover with a small plate to weight the pears down as they simmer. Lower the heat and simmer until the pears are tender and a knife pierces them all the way through without resistance.

Remove the pears from the saucepan. Return the liquid to the heat, bring to a lively simmer, and cook until syrupy, about 10 minutes. Taste the liquid for a quick FASS check. It may need a pinch of salt and a squeeze of lemon juice to balance the flavors.

Serve the pears drizzled with the poaching liquid and topped with a dollop of nut cream if you like.

Variations: For vanilla broth, omit the lemon zest, ginger, maple syrup, and saffron, and instead stir 2 teaspoons of agave nectar into the pear nectar. Cut a vanilla pod in half lengthwise, scrape the seeds into the saucepan, then throw in the pod. Proceed with the recipe as above.

For star anise broth, omit the lemon zest, ginger, maple syrup, and saffron, and instead stir in 4 pods of star anise, 4 whole cloves, 2 cinnamon sticks, 2 teaspoons of agave nectar, and 2 teaspoons of freshly squeezed lemon juice. Proceed with the recipe as above.

PREP TIME: 10 minutes · COOK TIME: 40 minutes

STORAGE: Store in an airtight container in the refrigerator for 3 to 5 days.

PER SERVING: Calories: 225; Total Fat: 0.2 g (0 g saturated, 0 g monounsaturated); Carbohydrates: 59 g; Protein: 1 g; Fiber: 4 g; Sodium: 15 mg

Strawberries with Mango Coconut "Sabayon"

This recipe is a little like karaoke: not exactly the original, but still a a lot of fun, and without all the production. One of my fondest kitchen memories is making the dessert or sweet topping that the French call sabayon *and the Italians call* zabaglione. *A combination of whisked egg yolks, marsala wine, and sugar, it's a high-wire act that has to go right from the heat to the plate. Get it right, and it's a froth of pure delight. Put it under the flame for a few seconds too long, and you're toast. This immensely more healthful version, which features mango and coconut, provides a similarly flavorful lightness, minus the need for perfectly timed kitchen pyrotechnics. It's great alone, or serve it drizzled over berries or rice pudding.* SERVES 4

- 1 14-ounce can coconut milk
- 1 1/2 cups chopped mango
- Pinch of sea salt
- 1/4 teaspoon agave nectar
- 1/2 teaspoon freshly squeezed lime juice
- 3 cups organic strawberries, hulled and halved
- 4 sprigs fresh mint, for garnish (optional)

Put the coconut milk in a saucepan and stir until homogenous. Stir in the mango and salt and simmer, covered, over medium-low heat until the mango is soft, 15 to 20 minutes.

Pour the mixture into a food processor, add the agave nectar and lime juice, and process until smooth. Spoon over fresh organic strawberries and serve garnished with the mint.

Variation: For a more puddinglike texture, leave out the agave nectar and lime juice and cook for an additional 10 minutes. Pour into 4 small ramekins and chill for at least 2 hours before serving.

Goes with Coconut Rice Pudding (page 198), sorbets, and fresh fruit, especially strawberries.

PREP TIME: 5 minutes · COOK TIME: 20 minutes

STORAGE: Store in an airtight container in the refrigerator for 5 days.

PER SERVING: Calories: 275; Total Fat: 21.7 g (18.8 g saturated, 1 g monounsaturated); Carbohydrates: 22 g; Protein: 3 g; Fiber: 5 g; Sodium: 90 mg

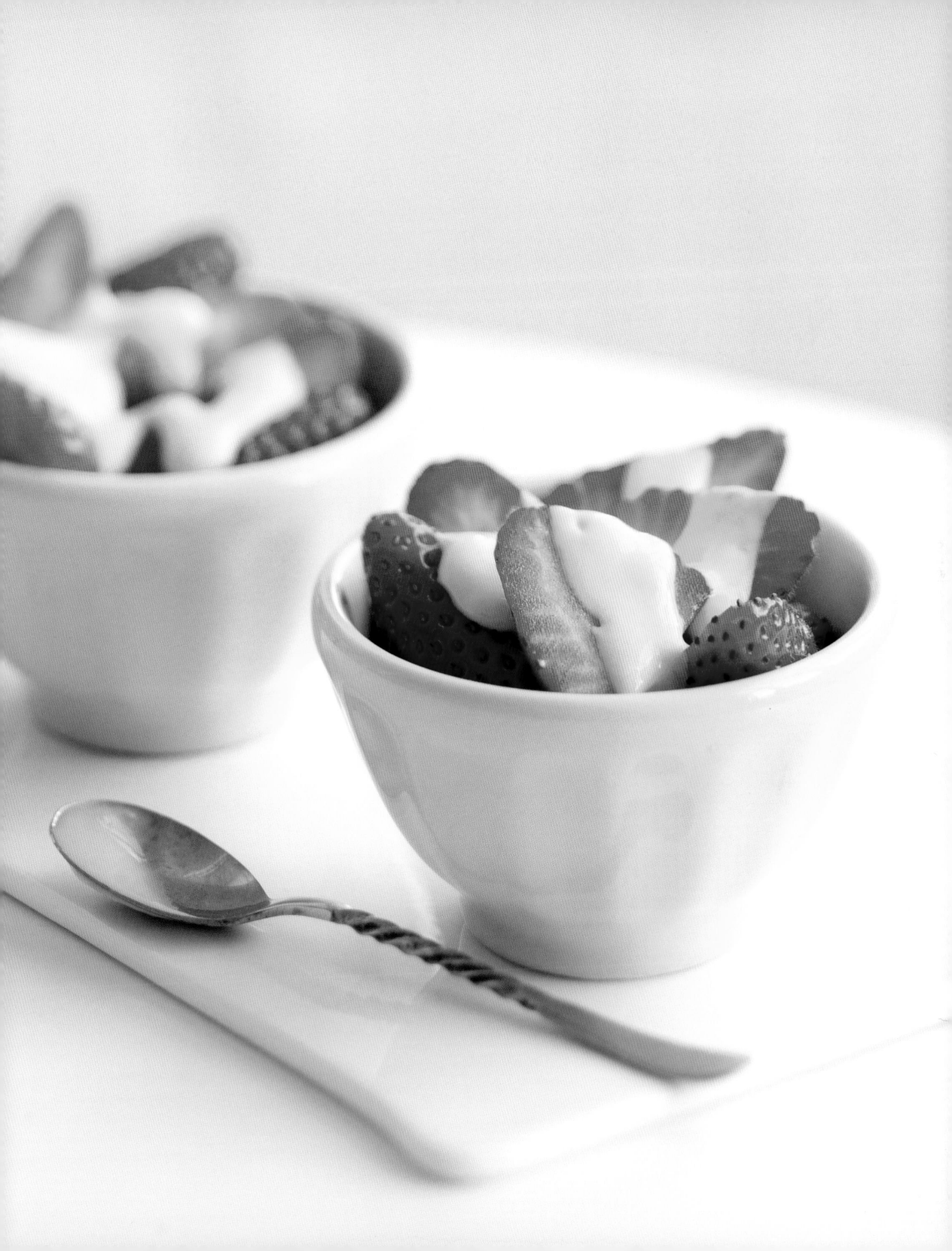

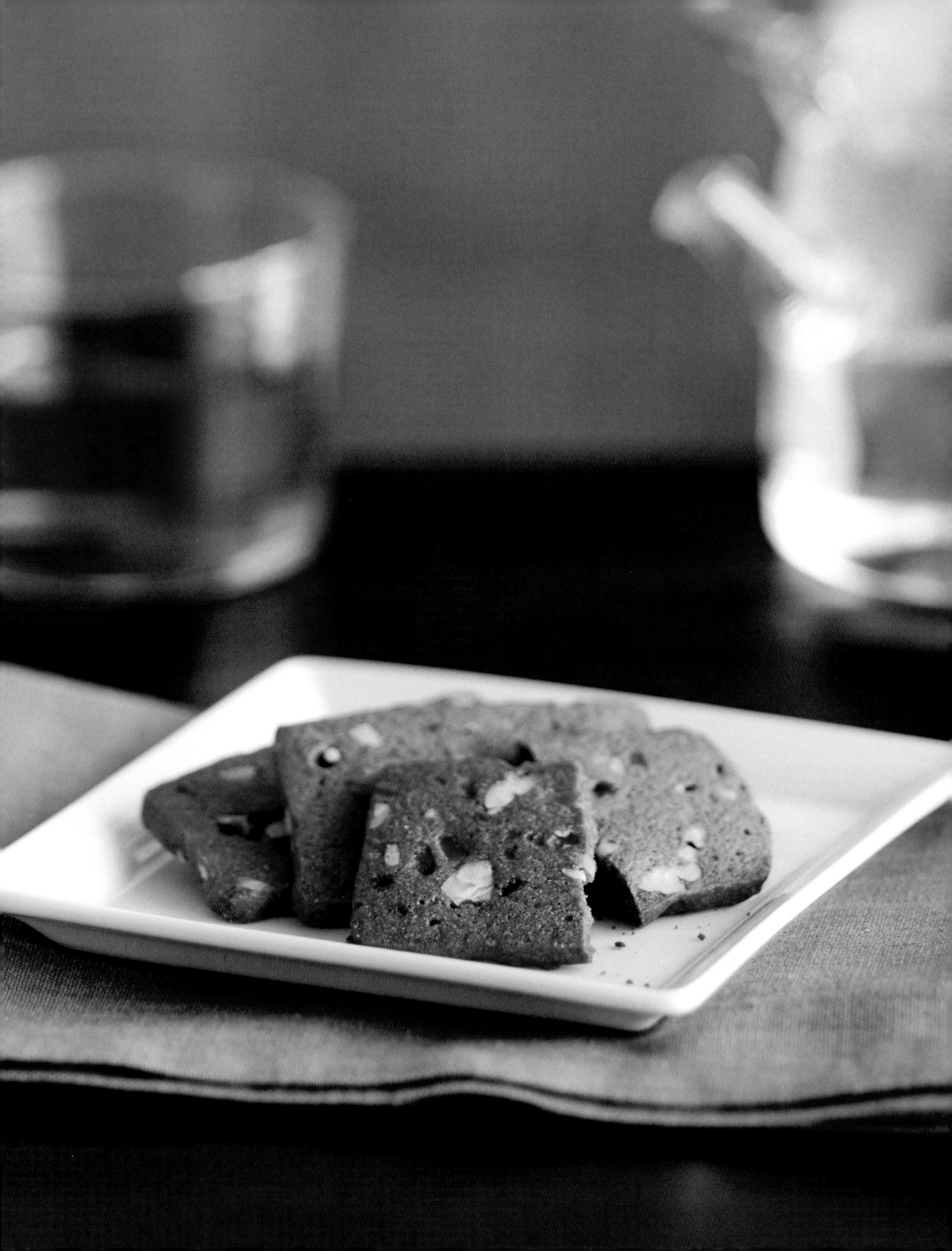

Triple Ginger Snap Cookies with Pecans

For people—and especially kids—who like crisply textured sweets, there's nothing like a ginger snap to scratch that itch. Many of my clients worry that they'll have to give up sweet treats like cookies during treatment. Nonsense. You just have to be smart about it, and this recipe shows you how: It uses quality ingredients (and no refined flour) and many cancer-fighting spices. There's just one caveat: Make the dough at least three hours before you want to bake the cookies, and preferably an entire day ahead. Once you make the dough, it can be stored in the refrigerator for up to five days. Chilling the dough makes it easier to cut the cookies and also gives the flavors a chance to come together so the cookies taste their very best. MAKES 38 COOKIES

Scant 1/2 cup unrefined virgin coconut oil, melted

2/3 cup rapadura

2 tablespoons organic butter or unrefined virgin coconut oil

1/3 cup unsulphured molasses

1 1/2 teaspoons ground cinnamon

1 tablespoon ground ginger

1/4 teaspoon ground cloves

1 1/3 cups barley flour

1 1/3 cups spelt flour

1 teaspoon baking soda

1/8 teaspoon sea salt

1 organic egg

3/4 cup chopped raw pecans

3 tablespoons chopped uncrystallized candied ginger (see Rebecca's Notes)

REBECCA'S NOTES These cookies freeze beautifully, both in dough form and baked. If freezing the dough, wrap it tightly in plastic wrap.

Rapadura is an unrefined organic sugar from the first pressing of the sugarcane with a unique caramel taste. Look for Rapunzel brand rapadura in your grocery store or find it online at www.rapunzel.com. You can also use muscovado, which is very similar.

If you can't find uncrystallized candied ginger, use the crystallized version; just rinse and pat dry before chopping.

Line a loaf pan with plastic wrap, with several inches overhanging on each side.

Combine the coconut oil, rapadura, butter, molasses, cinnamon, ginger, and cloves in a saucepan over medium heat, and cook, stirring constantly, until the mixture comes to a boil. Pour into a heatproof bowl or measuring cup and let cool to room temperature.

Combine the flours, baking soda, and salt in a large bowl and stir with a whisk. Whisk the egg into the cooled oil mixture until well combined, then pour the oil mixture into the flour mixture and mix well using a rubber spatula. Stir in the pecans and candied ginger.

Transfer the dough to the prepared loaf pan, fold the flaps of plastic wrap over the dough, and press gently into an even layer. Chill for at least 3 hours, and preferably overnight.

When you're ready to bake the cookies, preheat the oven to 400°F and line two baking sheets with parchment paper. Lift the dough from the pan, unwrap it, and cut it in half lengthwise. Rewrap one piece and return it to the fridge. Slice the other piece crosswise into very thin cookies, about the thickness of a graham cracker, and place on the prepared pans, leaving 1 inch between cookies. Bake one pan at a time for 7 to 9 minutes, until the edges begin to brown visibly. (If you have a convection oven, you can bake both pans of cookies at the same time.) Let cool on the pans for 5 minutes, then transfer to a cooling rack to cool completely.

PREP TIME: 15 minutes (plus at least 3 hours to chill the dough)

COOK TIME: 9 minutes per sheet

STORAGE: Store in an airtight container in the refrigerator for 5 to 7 days or in the freezer for 2 months.

PER SERVING: Calories: 110; Total Fat: 5.6 g (3.1 g saturated, 1.4 g monounsaturated); Carbohydrates: 14 g; Protein: 2 g; Fiber: 1 g; Sodium: 50 mg

Resources

Kitchen Equipment Suppliers

Where can you find that 16-quart stockpot or sharp chef's knife? The Internet, of course. Here's a list of reputable online retailers who ship anywhere in the United States and offer sale items on a regular basis:

Bed Bath & Beyond: www.bedbathandbeyond.com

Chef's Resource: www.chefsresource.com

Cooking.com, for everything for the household: www.cooking.com

Cooks Plus: www.cooksplus.com

Cutlery and More, for that sharp chef's knife: www.cutleryandmore.com

InstaWares Restaurant Supply, for the invaluable 16-quart stockpot: www.instawares.com

Kitchen Emporium, for airpots and insulated carafes: www.kitchenemporium.com

Metro Kitchen: www.metrokitchen.com

Sur La Table: www.surlatable.com

Vita-Mix, for the blender I use to puree everything: www.vitamix.com

Williams-Sonoma: www.williams-sonoma.com

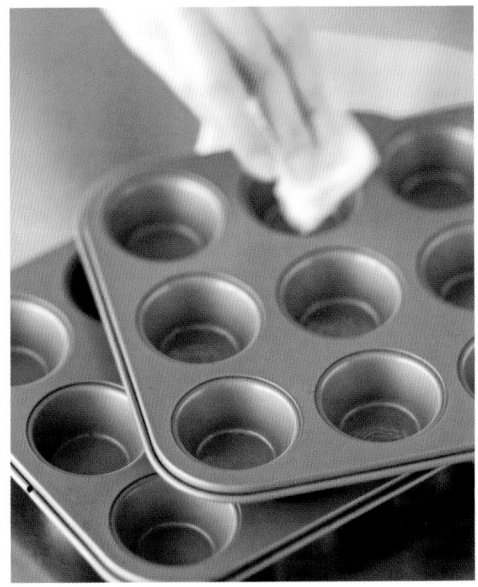

Sources for Specialty Ingredients

Arrowhead Mills, for organic and gluten-free grains and baking mixes: www.arrowheadmills.com

Bionaturae, for Italian organic fruit nectars, fruit spreads, oil, vinegars, and pastas: www.bionaturae.com

Blackwing Meats, for organic, free-range chicken: www.blackwing.com

Bob's Red Mill, for a variety of flours, including gluten-free products and almond meal: www.bobsredmill.com

Breads from Anna, for gluten-free bread and pancake mixes, pie crusts, and other goodies with outstanding taste and texture: www.breadsfromanna.com

Eden Foods, a great source for canned beans, condiments, sweeteners, soy, oils, vinegars, snack foods, and whole grains: www.edenfoods.com

Grain and Salt Society, for information on salt and sea vegetables: www.celtic-seasalt.com

Living Tree, for raw, organic, and kosher nut butters, tahini, pestos, oils, honey, and grains: www.livingtreecommunity.com

Lotus Foods, for heirloom and new rice varieties, including forbidden rice: www.lotusfoods.com

Madhava Honey, a source for agave nectar and honey: www.madhavahoney.com

Maine Coast Sea Vegetables: www.seaveg.com

Maple Valley Syrup, for organic grade B syrup: www.maplevalleysyrup.com

Pocono, for cream of buckwheat and buckwheat products: www.poconofoods.com

Purity Farms, for ghee, a clarified butter product that may be easier to digest for those who are lactose sensitive: www.purityfarms.com

Rapunzel, for organic, whole cane sugar: www.rapunzel.com

Real Salt, for natural, kosher-certified mineral sea salt: www.realsalt.com

San-J, for tamari, shoyu soy sauces, Asian cooking sauces, and Japanese salad dressings: www.san-j.com

Spectrum Naturals, for healthy cooking oils: www.spectrumorganics.com

Spicely Organics, a one-stop shop for a wide variety and comprehensive selection of spices and herbs in small packages: www.spicely.com

Tazo Teas, artisan tea blends in a variety of combinations and flavors: www.tazo.com

Traditional Medicinals, for certified organic herbal and medicinal teas: www.traditionalmedicinals.com

Vital Choice, for wild line-caught salmon and other high-quality seafood: www.vitalchoice.com

Wilderness Family Naturals, for coconut oil, milk, and more: www.wildernessnaturals.com

National Grocery and Online Shopping Markets

Diamond Organics, farm fresh, all-organic food, nationwide overnight home delivery: www.diamondorganics.com

Eat Wild, search your state to find out where you can buy local grass-fed meats, poultry, and dairy products: www.eatwild.com

Organic Kitchen, organic product resource guide for markets, farms, vineyards, and lifestyle products nationwide and locally: www.organickitchen.com

Organic Provisions, online organic grocery and supermarket: www.orgfood.com

Safeway, mainstream supermarket that carries its own line of organic food and produce products: www.safeway.com

Sun Organic Farm, organic kitchen staples, pantry items, and online ordering: www.sunorganic.com

Sunflower Farmers Markets, western U.S.-based natural- and quality-focused supermarket: www.sfmarkets.com

Trader Joe's, nationwide value grocery store with organic products: www.traderjoes.com

Whole Foods, the nation's first certified organic supermarket: www.wholefoods.com

Wild Harvest/Shaw's, the Wild Harvest branch within this East coast–based supermarket chain focuses on natural and organic products and food stuffs: www.shaws.com

Farmers' Markets

To find your local farmers' market, community supported agriculture programs, and a list of farms in your area: www.localharvest.org

The U.S. Department of Agriculture also has a nationwide farmers' market finder: www.ams.usda.gov/farmersmarkets/map.html

For more information on what is ripe in your area seasonally, and where to find organic foods grown closest to you, consult your local farmers' market or investigate the following websites:

www.eatwellguide.org
www.ams.usda.gov/farmersmarkets/map.html
www.epicurious.com/articlesguides/seasonalcooking/farmtotable/seasonalingredientmap

Nutrition Resources

My Food My Health: delicious, healthy recipes created by chefs who have been trained to cook for people with health considerations: www.myfoodmyhealth.com

USDA Nutrient Data Laboratory, for nutritional databases on every food from apples to zucchini: www.nal.usda.gov/fnic/foodcomp

The World's Healthiest Foods, for information on subjects related to nutrition and health: www.whfoods.com

Resources for Living with Cancer

The American Cancer Society: www.americanccancersociety.com

The American Institute for Cancer Research: www.aicr.org

American Society of Clinical Oncology: www.cancer.net

Association of Cancer Online Resources: www.acor.org

Cancer Advocacy, National Coalition for Cancer Survivorship: www.canceradvocacy.org

CancerCare: www.cancercare.org

Caring4Cancer: www.caring4cancer.com

Commonweal Cancer Help Program: www.commonweal.org

The National Cancer Institute: www.cancer.gov

Oncology Resources: www.cancerconsultants.com

Smith Farm Center for Healing and the Arts: www.smithfarm.com

Caregiving Resources

How to organize a group to care for someone who is seriously ill: www.sharethecare.org

Lotsa Helping Hands can help you or someone you love to easily organize family members and friends to pitch in and help: www.lotsahelpinghands.com

Resources for keeping friends and family in the loop: www.carepages.com and www.caringbridge.com

Recommended Reading

Abrams, D., and A. Weil. *Integrative Oncology.* New York: Oxford University Press, 2008.

Beliveau, R., and D. Gingras. *Foods That Fight Cancer: Preventing Cancer through Diet.* Toronto: McClelland and Stewart, 2006.

Block, K. *Life Over Cancer: The Block Center Program for Integrative Cancer Treatment.* New York: Bantam, 2009.

Capossela, C., and S. Warnock. *Share the Care: How to Organize a Group to Care for Someone Who Is Seriously Ill.* New York: Fireside Books, 2004.

Ensminger, A. H. *Food for Health: A Nutrition Encyclopedia.* Clovis, CA: Pegasus Press, 1986.

Geffen, J. *The Journey through Cancer: Healing and Transforming the Whole Person.* New York: Three Rivers Press, 2006.

Lerner, M. *Choices in Healing: Integrating the Best of Conventional and Complementary Approaches to Cancer.* Cambridge: MIT Press, 1998.

Mateljan, G. *The World's Healthiest Foods: Essential Guide for the Healthiest Way of Eating.* Seattle, WA: World's Healthiest Foods, 2006.

Murray, M. and J. Pizzorno. *The Encyclopedia of Healing Foods.* New York: Atria Books, 2005.

Onstad, D. *Whole Foods Companion: A Guide for Adventurous Cooks, Curious Shoppers, and Lovers of Natural Foods.* White River Junction, VT: Chelsea Green Publishing, 2004.

Bibliography

Aggarwal, B. B., and Shishodia, S. (2004). "Suppression of the nuclear factor-kappaB activation pathway by spice-derived phytochemicals: Reasoning for seasoning." *Annals of the New York Academy of Sciences* 1030:434–441. PMID: 15659827.

Alarcon de la Lastra, C., Barranco, M. D., Motilva, V., and Herrerias, J. M. (2001). "Mediterranean diet and health: Biological importance of olive oil." *Current Pharmaceutical Design* 7(10):933–950. PMID: 11472248.

American Cancer Society. (2007). "Lycopene." July 12. www.cancer.org/docroot/ETO/content/ETO_5_3X_Lycopene.asp

American Cancer Society. (2000). "Prevention Colorectal Cancer." March 7. www.cancer.org/docroot/NWS/content/NWS_1_1x_Eat_Right_to_Prevent_Colorectal_Cancer.asp

American Cancer Society. (2007). "Quercetin." June 19. www.cancer.org/docroot/ETO/content/ETO_5_3x_Quercetin.asp

American Cancer Society. (2007). "Shiitake mushroom." July 12. www.cancer.org/docroot/ETO/content/ETO_5_3x_Shiitake_Mushroom.asp

American Cancer Society. (2007). "Wild Yam." June 19. www.cancer.org/docroot/ETO/content/ETO_5_3X_Wild_Yam.asp

Balendiran, G., Dabur R., and Fraser, D. (2004). "The role of glutathione in cancer." *Cell Biochemistry and Function* 22(6): 343–352.

Blomhoff, R., Carlsen, M. H., Andersen, L. F., and Jacobs, D. R., Jr. (2006). "Health benefits of nuts: Potential role of antioxidants." *British Journal of Nutrition* 96(Suppl 2):S52–S60. PMID: 17125534.

Boyles, S. (2003). "Eggs may lower breast cancer risk: vegetable oils and fiber also may be protective." March 16. http://women.webmd.com/news/20030221/eggs-may-lower-breast-cancer-risk

Caldwell, E. (2008). "Turning up the heat on tomatoes boosts absorption of lycopene." August 21. http://extension.osu.edu/~news/story.php?id=4789

Canene-Adams, K., Lindshield, B. L., Wang, S., Jeffery, E. H., Clinton, S. K., and Erdman, J. W., Jr. (2007). "Combinations of tomato and broccoli enhance antitumor activity in Dunning R3327-H prostate adenocarcinomas." *Cancer Research* 67(2):836–843. PMID: 17213256.

Cao, Y., and Cao, R. (1999). "Angiogenesis inhibited by drinking tea." *Nature* 398(6726):381.

Chen, C. Y., and Blumberg, J. B. (2008). "Phytochemical composition of nuts." *Asia Pacific Journal of Clinical Nutrition* 17(Suppl 1):329–332.

Chen, D., Daniel, K. G., Kuhn, D. J., et al. (2004). "Green tea and tea polyphenols in cancer prevention." *Frontiers in Bioscience* 9:2618–2631. PMID: 15358585.

Cheng, A., Has, C. H., Lin, J. K., et al. (2001). "Phase I clinical trial of curcumin, a chemopreventative agent, in patients with high-risk or pre-malignant lesions." *Anticancer Research* 21(4B):2895–2900.

Cotterchio, M., Boucher, B., Kreiger, N., et al. (2007). "Dietary phytoestrogen intake—lignans and isoflavones—and breast cancer risk." *Cancer Causes and Control* (19)3: 259–272.

Crowell, P., (1999). "Prevention and therapy of cancer by dietary monoterpenes." *Journal of Nutrition* 129:775–778.

Cumashi, A., Ushakova, N. A., Preobrazhenskaya, M. E., et al. (2007). "A comparative study of the anti-inflammatory, anticoagulant, antiangiogenic, and antiadhesive activities of nine different fucoidans from brown seaweeds." *Glycobiology* 17(5):541–552.

Dietrich, M., Traber, M.G., Jacques, P., Cross, C.E., Hu, Y., Block, G. (2006). "Does gamma-tocopherol play a role in the primary prevention of heart disease and cancer?" *Journal of the American College of Nutrition* 25(4):292–299.

Edris, A. E., and Farrag, E. S. (2003). "Antifungal activity of peppermint and sweet basil essential oils and their major aroma constituents on some plant pathogenic fungi from the vapor phase." *Die Nahrung* 47(2):117–121.

Elgayyar, M., Draughon, F. A., Golden, D. A., and Mount, J. R. (2001). "Antimicrobial activity of essential oils from plants against selected pathogenic and saprophytic microorganisms." *Journal of Food Protection* 64(7):1019–1024. PMID: 11456186.

Erhardt, J. G., Meisner, C., Bode, J. C., and Bode, C. (2003). "Lycopene, beta-carotene, and colorectal adenomas." *American Journal of Clinical Nutrition* 78(6):1219–1224.

Fowke, J. H., Chung, F. L., Jin, F., et al. (2003). "Urinary isothiocyanate levels, brassica, and human breast cancer." *Cancer Research* 63(14):3980–3986. PMID: 12873994.

Galeone, C., Pelucchi, C., Levi, F., et al. (2006). "Onion and garlic use and human cancer." *American Journal of Clinical Nutrition* 84(5):1027–1032.

George, S. L., Polascik, T. J., Albala, M., et al. (2007). "Impact of flaxseed supplementation and dietary fat restriction on prostate cancer proliferation and other biomarkers: Results of a phase II randomized controlled trial (RCT) using a presurgical model." *Journal of Clinical Oncology, 2007 ASCO Annual Meeting Proceedings Part I,* 25(Suppl 18):1510.

George Mateljan Foundation. (2008). "The world's healthiest foods: Kale." www.whfoods.com/genpage.php?tname=foodspice&dbid=38

"Ginger 'could halt bowel cancer'" (2003). http://news.bbc.co.uk/2/hi/health/3221547.stm 29

Golden E., Lam P., Kardosh A., Gaffney K. (2009). "Green tea polyphenols block the anticancer effects of bortezomib and other boronic acid-based proteasome inhibitors." *Journal of the American Society of Hematology* http://blood-journal.hematologylibrary.org/cgi/content/abstract/blood-2008-07-171389v1

Honan, W. (2004). "Researchers rewrite first chapter for the history of medicine." http://www.nytimes.com/2004/03/02/science/02MEDI.html?ex=1393563600&en=c3177ebac2572d43&ei=5007&partner=USERLAND

Hou, D., Kai, K., Li, J., et al. (2003). "Anthocyanidins inhibit activator protein 1 activity and cell transformation: structure-activity relationship and molecular mechanisms." *Carcinogenesis* http://carcin.oxfordjournals.org/cgi/content/abstract/bgg184v1

Iberg, A.J., Chen, J.C., Zhao, H., Hoffman, S.C., Comstock, G.W., and Helzlsouer, K.J. (2000). "Household exposure to passive cigarette smoking and serum micronutrient concentrations." *American Journal of Clinical Nutrition* 72(6):1576–82.

Jankun, J., Selman, S. H., Swiercz, R., et al. (1997). "Why drinking green tea could prevent cancer." *Nature* 387(6633):561.

Karadeniz, F., Durst, R. W., and Wrolstad, R. E. (2000). "Polyphenolic composition of raisins." *Journal of Agricultural and Food Chemistry* 48(11):5343–5350. PMID: 11087484.

Kato K., Takahashi, S., Cui, L., et al. (2000). "Suppressive effects of dietary genistin and daidzin on rat prostate carcinogenesis." *Japan Journal of Cancer* 91(8):786–791.

Kawa, J. M., Taylor, C. G., and Przybylski, R. (1996). "Buckwheat concentrate reduces serum glucose in streptozotocin-diabetic rats." *Journal of Agricultural and Food Chemistry* 51(25):7287–7291. PMID: 14640572.

Kim, Y. (2004). "Will mandatory folic acid fortification prevent or promote cancer?" *American Journal of Clinical Nutrition* 80(5):1123–1128.

Linus Pauling Institute. (2007). "Molybdenum." http://lpi.oregonstate.edu/infocenter/minerals/molybdenum

Linus Pauling Institute. (2005). "Ligans: hormone-associated cancers." http://lpi.oregonstate.edu/infocenter/phytochemicals/lignans

Li, T., Molteni, A., Latkovich, P., Castellani, W., and Baybutt, R. C. (2003). "Vitamin A depletion induced by cigarette smoke is associated with the development of emphysema in rats." *Journal of Nutrition* 133(8):2629–34. PMID: 12888649.

Lui R. (2002). "Long-cooked corn higher in antioxidant." www.psa-rising.com/eatingwell/corn/cooked-phenolics-0802.htm

Marimuthu, S., Adluri, S., Venugopal, M., (2007). "Ferulic acid: therapeutic potential through its antioxidant property." *Journal of Clinical Biochemical Nutrition* 40(2): 92–100. PMCID: PMC2127228.

Minakshi De, Amit Krishna De, Sen, P., and Banerjee, A. (2000). "Antimicrobial properties of star anise." *Phytotherapy Research*16(1): 94–95.

Miyazawa, K., Kasuga, I., Minemura, K., et al. (2003). "Apoptosis induction of vitamin K2 in lung carcinoma cell lines: the possibility of vitamin K2 therapy for lung cancer." *International Journal of Oncology* 23(3):627–32. PMID: 12888897.

Mujumdar, A. M., Dhuley, J. N., Deshmukh, V. K., et al. (1990). "Anti-inflammatory activity of piperine." *Japanese Journal of Medical Science and Biology* 43(3):95–100. PMID: 2283727.

National Cancer Institute, "Glycosaminoglycan." http://www.cancer.gov/templates/db_alpha.aspx?CdrID=44206

National Cancer Institute, "Piperine extract." www.cancer.gov/Templates/drugdictionary.aspx?CdrID=440023

National Cancer Institute, "Psoralen." http://www.cancer.gov/templates/db_alpha.aspx?CdrID=44900

National Cancer Institute, "Salvia." http://www.cancer.gov/templates/drugdictionary.aspx?CdrID=574480

Nevin, K. G., and Rajamohan, T. (2004). "Beneficial effects of virgin coconut oil on lipid parameters and in vitro LDL oxidation." *Clinical Biochemistry* 37(9):830–835. PMID: 15329324.

Nimptsch R., Rohrmann S., Linseisen, J. (2008). "Dietary intake of vitamin K and risk of prostate cancer in the Heidelberg cohort of the European Prospecetive Investigation into Cancer and Nutrition (EPIC-Heidelberg)." *American Journal of Clinical Nutrition* 87(4):985–992.

Nutrition Data. (2008). "Beans, kidney, all types, mature seeds, cooked, boiled, without salt." www.nutritiondata.com/facts/legumes-and-legume-products/4297/2

Nutrition Data. (2008). "Lentils, raw." www.nutritiondata.com/facts/legumes-and-legume-products/4337/2

Ogbolu, D. O., Oni, A. A., Daini, O. A., and Oloko, A. P. (2007). "In vitro antimicrobial properties of coconut oil on *Candida* species in Ibadan, Nigeria." *Journal of Medicinal Food* 10(2):384–387. PMID: 17651080.

Ouellet, V., Marois, J., Weisnagel, S.J., Jacques, H. (2007). "Dietary cod protein improves insulin sensitivity in insulin-resistant men and women." *Diabetes Care* (11):2816–21. PMID: 17682120.

Prakash P., Krinsky, N. I., Russell, R. M. (2000). "Retinoids, carotenoids, and human breast cancer cell cultures: a review of differential effects." *Nutrition Reviews* 58(6):170–176.

Queensland Institute of Medical Research (2008). "Bromelain: new cancer fighting properties uncovered." www.thehealthierlife.co.uk/natural-health-articles/cancer/bromelain-cancer-fighting-properties-00075.html

Sartippour, M. R., Seeram, N. P., Rao, J. Y., and Moro, A. (2008). "Ellagitannin-rich pomegranate extract inhibits angiogenesis in prostate cancer in vitro and in vivo." *International Journal of Oncology* 2(2):475–80. PMID: 18202771.

Schmandke, H. (2005) "Betalains in beetroot and prickly pear fruit." www.cababstractsplus.org/abstracts/Abstract.aspx?AcNo=20053038235

Sengupta, A., Ghosh, S., and Bhattacharjee, S. (2005). "Dietary cardamom inhibits the formation of azoxymethane-induced aberrant crypt foci in mice and reduces COX-2 and iNOS expression in the colon." *Asian Pacific Journal of Cancer Prevention* 6(2):118–22. PMID: 16101317.

Sereiti, M. R., Abu-Amer, K. M., and Sen, P. (1999). "Pharmacology of rosemary (*Rosmarinus officinalis* Linn.) and its therapeutic potentials." *Indian Journal of Experimental Biology* 37(2):124–30. PMID: 10641130.

Stoner, G. (2001). "Black raspberries show multiple defenses in thwarting cancer." http://researchnews.osu.edu/archive/canberry.htm

Wood, R. (1988). *The Whole Foods Encyclopedia.* New York: Prentice-Hall Press.

Yuan, J. M., Stram, D. O., Arakawa, K., Lee, H. P., and Yu, M. C. (2003). "Dietary cryptoxanthin and reduced risk of lung cancer: The Singapore Chinese Health Study." *Cancer Epidemiology, Biomarkers and Prevention* 12(9):890–898.

Yuan, Y. V., and Walsh, N. A. (2006). "Antioxidant and antiproliferative activities of extracts from a variety of edible seaweeds." *Food and Chemical Toxicology* 44(7):1144–1150.

Index

A

Abrams, Donald, 3, 97, 136
agave nectar, anti-inflammatory uses of, 29
allspice/allspice berries, as aid to digestion, 29
Almond Muffin Mania, 192, 193
almonds, anti-inflammatory uses of, 29–30
anemia, foods for, 11
angiogenesis, copper and, 135
anise/aniseed, uses of, 29
Annemarie's Calming Kudzu Elixir, 156
antioxidants, about, 98
Anytime Bars, 126–127
anytime foods for
    anemia side effects, 11
    constipation, 12
    fatigue side effects, 12–13
    neutropenia side effects, 13
    radiation side effects, 17
    sore mouth and difficulty swallowing, 14
    weight loss, 14
appetite
    loss of, 20–22
    during treatment, 18–19, 125
apples, anti-inflammatory uses of, 30
Apricot Pear Chutney, 174, 175
apricots, anti-inflammatory uses of, 30
asparagus, anti-inflammatory uses of, 30
Avocado Cream, 178
avocados, anti-flammatory uses of, 30
Avocado Dressing, 178, 179

B

Baby Bok Choy with Yam and Ginger, 80
Baked Apples Filled with Dates and Pecans, 194
Baked Citrus Halibut with Tomato Sauce, 123
bananas
    electrolytes and, 30
    freezing, 166
barley, anti-inflammatory uses of, 30
basil, anti-inflammatory uses of, 30–31, 177
Basil Broccoli, 78, 79
Basil Lemon Drizzle, 174
bay leaf, abdominal cramps/gas and, 31
beans and lentils, anti-inflammatory uses of, 31
beets, anti-inflammatory uses of, 31
bell peppers, anti-inflammatory uses of, 31
Bella's Carrot, Orange, and Fennel Soup, 65
Best and Worst Fish Choices, 122
Best Oatmeal Ever, 128
beta-cryptoxanthin, lung cancer and, 33
Beyond Just Good Cornbread, 129
Black Bean Hummus, 132
black pepper, as digestion aid, 31
Block, Keith
    on benefits of whey, 167
    on taking care of oneself during treatment, 87
blueberries, anti-inflammatory uses of, 31
Blueberry Compote, 185
Brazil nuts, anti-inflammatory uses of, 31
broccoli, anti-inflammatory uses of, 31–32
Broffman, Michael, 114, 142
buckwheat, anti-inflammatory uses of, 32

C

cabbage, anti-inflammatory uses of, 32
cacao, about, 201
cancer diagnosis, impact of, 2
cancer-fighting ingredients, 28
cancer treatment, overview, 43
Cannellini Bean Dip with Katamata Olives, 132
cantaloupe, about, 158
cantaloupe, anti-inflammatory uses of, 32
Cantaloupe Granita with Mint, 158, 159
caraway, as appetite stimulant, 32
cardamom, as digestion aid, 32
Cardamom Maple Mini Macaroons, 196, 197
carrots, anti-inflammatory uses of, 32
Cashew Cream, 180
cashews, anticancer uses of, 32
catechins, about, 162
Catherine's Magic Green Tea Rice, 135
cauliflower, anti-inflammatory uses of, 32–33
Center for Mind-Body Medicine, 2–3
chemo resistance, about, 109
chemotherapy
    diabetes and, 149
    high fat foods and, 14
    lack of appetite during, 125
chicken
    benefits of eating, 101
    how to pound, 111
    using leftovers, 117
Chicken and Broccoli Stir-Fry with Cashews, 105
Chicken Magic Mineral Broth Broth, 55
Chicken Vegetable Soup with Ginger Meatballs, 58, 59
Chinese spices, 27, 28
Chocolate Banana Smoothie, 166
Chocolate Tapioca Pudding, 195
chutney, variations for, 175
Cilantro Lime Vinaigrette, 181
Cinnamon Ginger Tea, 163
cloves, as digestion aid, 33
coconut, benefits of, 167
coconut milk/coconut oil, anti-inflammatory uses of, 33
Coconut Rice Pudding, 198, 199
Commonweal's Most Nourishing and Healing Tea, 157
complete proteins, about, 101
compotes, about, 183
constipation, general recommendations for, 11
cooking and reheating tips, 50
Cooling Cucumber Avocado Soup, 70
corn, antioxidants and, 33
corticosteroids, immune function and, 44
Cozy Comfy Chicken and Rice, 106
cranberries, anti-inflammatory uses of, 34
Creamiest Buckwheat, 138
Creamy Broccoli and Potato Soup, 75
Creamy Millet, 136, 137
Creamy Polenta, 134
Cucumber, Jicama, and Mango Salad, 82, 83
culinary pharmacy
    overview, 28
    see also specific ingredients
culinary preferences, discovering, 26–28
cumin, anti-inflammatory uses of, 34
Curried Chicken Salad, 104
Curried Hummus, 133
Curried Hummus and Vegetable Pinwheels, 152, 153
curry, anti-inflammatory properties of, 104
Curry Cauliflower Soup, 66, 67

D

dates, 34, 201
dehydration
    about, 102
    foods for, 12
diabetes onset, chemo therapy and, 149
diarrhea, foods for, 12
dieticians, advantages of working with, 49
Dixon, Suzanne, 44, 46, 49, 98
dollops of Yum! for
    constipation, 12
    impaired taste buds, 173
    neutropenia side effects, 13
    nutrient density of, 173
Dried Fruit Compote, 183

E

Easy Eggs in a Cup, 102, 103
eating, scheduling before cancer treatments, 14
Edamame Avocado Dip with Wasabi, 130, 131
edamame (soybeans), anti-inflammatory uses of, 34–35
eggs
  anti-inflammatory uses of, 35
  benefits of eating, 101
Emerald Greens with Orange, 84, 85
empty calories, about, 192
eugenol oil, anti-inflamatory uses of, 33
exercise, importance of during treatment, 47–48

F

faro, freezing, 148
FASS, for loss of appetite, 20–21
fat, about, 20–21, 22
fatigue
  foods for, 12–13
  and radiation treatments, 14
fennel
  as a digestion aid, 35
  toasting, 182
ferulic acid, 33
fish
  benefits of eating, 101
  best and worst choices, 122
  fresh versus farmed, 123
  how to choose, 118
  how to store until use, 121
flax oils, oxidization of, 127
flaxseeds
  anti-inflammatory uses of, 35
  benefits of, 127
food storage tips, 50
foods
  culinary preferences, 26–27
  multiple cancer-fighting properties of, 3
Forbidden Rice Salad, 147

G

garlic, anti-inflammatory uses of, 35
German spices, 27
ginger
  medicinal properties of, 163
  nausea reducer, 35
Ginger Ale with Frozen Grapes, 164, 165
Ginger Peppermint Green Tea, 162
ginger syrup, 164
Ginger Tea Spritzer, 163
"good bites" to spur appetite, 46
Gordon, Jim, 2–3
Great Pumpkin Custard, 200
Green Beans with Brazil Nuts and Basil, 81
green tea
  anti-inflammatory uses of, 35
  antioxidants in, 162
Green Tea Ginger Lemonade, 162
Gregg's Stuffed Acorn Squash with Quinoa, Cranberries, and Swiss Chard, 86–87
guilt, negative aspects of, 44

H

halibut, anti-inflammatory uses of, 35
hard-boiled eggs, about, 114
honey, propolis in, 35
hospitals, bringing food into during treatments, 46–47
Hungarian Roasted Root Vegetable Potpie, 94, 95–96
Hungarian spices, 27

I

immune function, impairment of, 44
immune system, cancer treatments and, 10
Indian spices, 27, 28
insulin-like growth factors (IGFs), about, 195
Italian White Bean Soup, 57

K

kaempferol intake, and ovarian cancer risk, 33, 89
kale
  anti-inflammatory uses of, 35–36
  phytochemicals in, 89

Kale with Carrots, 88
Kale with Sweet Potatoes and Pecans, 89
kidney beans, benefits of eating, 64
Koetters, Theresa, 88
kombu
    chlorophyllins in, 36
    radiation and, 14
kudzu
    about, 156
    medicinal properties of, 36

L

laetrile, the bowel and, 36
lauric acid, about, 33, 167
leeks, anti-inflammatory uses of, 36
Lefer, Lenore, 44–45, 47
Lemon Mustard Salmon Salad, 108, 109
lemongrass, anti-inflammatory uses of, 36
lemons
    about, 20–21, 22
    anti-inflammatory uses of, 36
Lemony Greek Chicken Soup, 60
lentils. *See* beans and lentils
limes, anti-inflammatory uses of, 36

M

Magic Mineral Broth, 54
Mango and Avocado Salsa, 185
Mango Coconut Smoothie, 167
mangoes, gallbladder cancer reduction and, 36
Maple-Glazed Walnuts, 140, 141
maple syrup, levels of zinc in, 36
maple syrup, grade B, prostate cancer and, 36
Ma's Mushroom Barley Soup, 61
Mashed Cinnamon Butternut Squash, 90
Master Recipe for Cooking Beans, 110, 110 (table)
McConkie, Catherine, 135
Mediterranean diet, 123
Mediterranean Lentil Salad, 142, 143
metallic taste. *See* FASS
Mexican spices, 27, 28
Middle Eastern Chickpea Burgers, 112, 113
Middle Eastern spices, 27
millet, anti-inflammatory uses of, 36
Minestrone, 64
mint, as digestion aid, 37
miso, radiation and, 14
Mixed Greens with Edamame, Radish, and Avocado, 91
monolaurin, about, 33
Moroccan Pesto, 186
Mouthwatering Granita, 160, 161
muffin tins, about, 192
Mullin, Gerry, on hospital foods, 46
mushrooms, anti-inflammatory uses of, 37
mustard seed, as appetite stimulant, 37
mustard seeds, about, 176
My Family's Favorite Chicken, 111
myristicin, 37

N

Nana's Egg Salad, 114
nausea and vomiting, foods for, 13
Navy Bean and Sun-Dried Tomato Dip, 131
nerve roots, damage to, 22
neutropenia, soups for, 13
nori, radiation and, 14
North African (Moroccan) spices, 27
nutmeg, myristicin in, 37
nutrition
    as factor of development of cancer, 3
    optinizing by grazing, 45–47
nuts, benefits of eating, 81

O

oats, presoaking before using, 128
Olive and Caper Relish, 186
olives, types of, 106
olives/olive oil, anti-inflammatory uses of, 37
onions, anti-inflammatory uses of, 37
Orange Ginger Roasted Chicken, 117
Orange Pistachio Couscous, 144, 145
oranges, benefits of eating, 37
oregano, anti-inflammatory uses of, 37
organic foods, benefits of eating, 75 (sidebar), 101
organics, shopping for, 87
Osher Center for Integrative Medicine, 3

P

Papaya Pineapple Smoothie, 171
papayas
    antioxidants in, 171
    uses of, 38
parsley, antitumor properties of, 38
Parsley Basil Drizzle, 187
parsnips, benefits of eating, 38
Pasture Beef Bone Broth, 56
Peach Ginger Smoothie, 168, 169
pears, how to seed and stem, 102
pectin
    cancer cells and, 185
    digestability and, 194
peppermint, multi-uses for, 38
pineapple, anti-inflammatory uses of, 36, 38, 170
Pineapple Ginger Smoothie, 170
Pistachio Cream, 181
Poached Eggs with Basil Lemon Drizzle, 115
Poached Pears with Saffron Broth, 202, 203
Poached Salmon with Moroccan Pesto, 100, 120, 121
potatoes, 38
protein-building foods for
    fatigue side effects, 12
    neutropenia side effects, 13
    radiation side effects, 17
proteins, about, 101
Purple Peruvian Smashed Potatoes, 93

Q

quercetin, anti-inflammatory uses of, 30, 32
quinoa
    anti-inflammatory uses of, 38
    preparing, 149
Quinoa Pilaf, 149

R

radiation treatments
    fatigue after, 14
    sea vegetables and, 14
radishes, anti-inflammatory uses of, 38
raisins, phenolic activity in, 38
ramekins, about, 200
rapadura, where to find, 207
raspberries, anti-inflammatory uses of, 39
Remer, Wendy, 191, 197
rice, anti-inflammatory uses of, 39
Rice Paper Moo-Shu Rolls, 150, 151
Roasted Asparagus Pasta with White Beans and Thyme, 146–147
Roasted Red Roma Tomato Soup, 68, 69–70
Rockin' Black Bean Soup, 70
rosemary, anti-inflammatory uses of, 39
Russian spices, 27

S

saffron, anti-inflammatory uses of, 39
sage, therapeutic benefits of, 39
salmon
    anti-inflammatory uses of, 39
    how to poach, 121
    how to store, 121
sea salt
    about, 20–21
    as appetite stimulant, 39
sea vegetables, radiation and, 14
Seasonal Stewed Fruit, 184
seeds or nuts, how to toast, 97
sesame seeds, anti-inflamatory uses of, 39
Shredded Carrot and Beet Salad, 98, 99
side effects, about, 10-11. *See also* specific side effects
Signora's Tomato Sauce, 188
Simple Tuscan Farro, 148
smoothies
    about, 155
    how to thicken, 166
sore mouth and difficulty swallowing, 14
soups, overview, 53
soups for
    anemia side effects, 11
    constipation side effects, 11
    dehydration, 12
    fatigue side effects, 12
    nausea/vomiting side effects, 12
    neutropenia side effects, 13
    sore mouth and difficulty swallowing, 14

spelt
about, 129
anti-inflammatory uses of, 39
Spiced Sweet Potato Soup, 72
Spiced Toasted Almonds, 139, 140
spinach, carotenoids in, 39
squash, colonic benefits of, 39, 40
star anise
antimicrobial properties of, 40
uses of, 39
Stir-Fried Baby Bok Choy with Shittake Mushrooms, 97
strawberries, anti-inflammatory uses of, 39, 40
Strawberries with Mango Coconut "Sabayon," 204, 205
stress, negative aspects of, 44
Summer's Best Zucchini Soup, 73
support team, creating, 43–44, 48–49
Sweet and Savory Yogurt, 189
sweet bites for
constipation, 12
neutropenia side effects, 13
radiation side effects, 17
sweet potatoes, anti-inflammatory uses of, 39
sweet potatoes and yams, beta-carotene in, 40
Swiss chard, anti-inflammatory uses of, 39, 40

T

taste buds, effect of chemotherapy on, 20
Thai It Up Chicken Soup, 62, 63
Thai spices, 27, 28
"the power of yum," 1–2, 10
thyme, soothing nature of, 39, 40
Tinkyada brown rice penne, preparing, 147
Tomato Mint Chutney, 174, 176
tomatoes, lycopene and, 40, 188
tonics and elixirs for
constipation, 12
dehydration, 12
diarrhea, 12
fatigue, 12–13
nausea and vomiting side effects, 12
neutropenia side effects, 13
radiation side effects, 17
sore mouth and difficulty swallowing, 14
weight loss, 14
"transient taste change," 20
Tripathy, Debu, on nutrition, 115
Triple Berry Smoothie, 168, 169
Triple-Citrus Ginger Black Cod, 118, 119
Triple Ginger Snap Cookies with Pecans, 206, 207
tumors, how they function, 3
turmeric, appetite stimulant properties, 40
Tuscan Farro and Bean Salad, 107

V

vegetable sources of protein, 101
vegetables, about, 77
vegetables for
anemia side effects, 11, 12
fatigue side effects, 12
neutropenia side effects, 13
radiation side effects, 17
Velvety Red Lentil Dahl, 74

W

Wallace, Jeanne, 2–3, 47–49, 127, 135, 149
walnuts, anti-inflammatory uses of, 40
Warm and Toasty Cumin Carrots, 93
Warm Napa Cabbage Slaw, 92
weight loss, 14
Wendy's Date Nut Truffles, 201
whey, about, 167
whole foods approach, 4
working during cancer treatment, 46

Y

yams, anti-inflammatory uses of, 39
yogurt
about, 189
benefits of, 40

Z

Zesty Lemon Fennel Vinaigrette, 182

Date Due

BRODART, CO. Cat. No. 23-233 Printed in U.S.A.